Design, Development, and Integration of Reliable Electronic Healthcare Platforms

Anastasius Moumtzoglou
P&A Kyriakou Children's Hospital, Greece

A volume in the Advances in Healthcare Information Systems and Administration (AHISA) Book Series

IGI GLOBAL
DISSEMINATOR OF KNOWLEDGE

www.igi-global.com

Published in the United States of America by
IGI Global
Medical Information Science Reference (an imprint of IGI Global)
701 E. Chocolate Avenue
Hershey PA, USA 17033
Tel: 717-533-8845
Fax: 717-533-8661
E-mail: cust@igi-global.com
Web site: http://www.igi-global.com

Library of Congress Cataloging-in-Publication Data

Library of Congress Cataloging-in-Publication Data

Names: Moumtzoglou, Anastasius, 1959- editor.
Title: Design, development, and integration of reliable electronic healthcare platforms / Anastasius Moumtzoglou, editor.
Other titles: Advances in healthcare information systems and administration (AHISA) book series. 2328-1243
Description: Hershey PA : Medical Information Science Reference, [2017] | Series: Advances in healthcare information systems and administration | Includes bibliographical references and index.
Identifiers: LCCN 2016041752| ISBN 9781522517245 (hardcover) | ISBN 9781522517252 (ebook)
Subjects: | MESH: Medical Informatics | Technology Assessment, Biomedical | Telemedicine | Biomedical Technology
Classification: LCC R855.3 | NLM W 26.5 | DDC 610.285--dc23 LC record available at https://lccn.loc.gov/2016041752

This book is published in the IGI Global book series Advances in Healthcare Information Systems and Administration (AHISA) (ISSN: 2328-1243; eISSN: 2328-126X)

British Cataloguing in Publication Data
A Cataloguing in Publication record for this book is available from the British Library.

For electronic access to this publication, please contact: eresources@igi-global.com.

Advances in Healthcare Information Systems and Administration (AHISA) Book Series

Anastasius Moumtzoglou
Hellenic Society for Quality & Safety in Healthcare and P. & A. Kyriakou Children's Hospital, Greece

ISSN: 2328-1243
EISSN: 2328-126X

Mission

The **Advances in Healthcare Information Systems and Administration (AHISA) Book Series** aims to provide a channel for international researchers to progress the field of study on technology and its implications on healthcare and health information systems. With the growing focus on healthcare and the importance of enhancing this industry to tend to the expanding population, the book series seeks to accelerate the awareness of technological advancements of health information systems and expand awareness and implementation.

Driven by advancing technologies and their clinical applications, the emerging field of health information systems and informatics is still searching for coherent directing frameworks to advance health care and clinical practices and research. Conducting research in these areas is both promising and challenging due to a host of factors, including rapidly evolving technologies and their application complexity. At the same time, organizational issues, including technology adoption, diffusion and acceptance as well as cost benefits and cost effectiveness of advancing health information systems and informatics applications as innovative forms of investment in healthcare are gaining attention as well. **AHISA** addresses these concepts and critical issues.

Coverage

- IT Applications in Physical Therapeutic Treatments
- E-Health and M-Health
- Nursing Expert Systems
- Telemedicine
- Clinical Decision Support Design, Development and Implementation
- Role of Informatics Specialists
- Decision Support Systems
- Rehabilitative Technologies
- Medical Informatics
- Management of Emerging Health Care Technologies

IGI Global is currently accepting manuscripts for publication within this series. To submit a proposal for a volume in this series, please contact our Acquisition Editors at Acquisitions@igi-global.com or visit: http://www.igi-global.com/publish/.

The Advances in Healthcare Information Systems and Administration (AHISA) Book Series (ISSN 2328-1243) is published by IGI Global, 701 E. Chocolate Avenue, Hershey, PA 17033-1240, USA, www.igi-global.com. This series is composed of titles available for purchase individually; each title is edited to be contextually exclusive from any other title within the series. For pricing and ordering information please visit http://www.igi-global.com/book-series/advances-healthcare-information-systems-administration/37156. Postmaster: Send all address changes to above address.

Titles in this Series

For a list of additional titles in this series, please visit: www.igi-global.com

Cloud Computing Systems and Applications in Healthcare
Chintan M. Bhatt (Charotar University of Science & Technology, India) and S. K. Peddoju (Indian Institute of Technology Roorkee, India)
Medical Information Science Reference • copyright 2017 • 282pp • H/C (ISBN: 9781522510024) • US $205.00 (our price)

Handbook of Research on Healthcare Administration and Management
Nilmini Wickramasinghe (Epworth HealthCare, Australia & Deakin University, Australia)
Medical Information Science Reference • copyright 2017 • 825pp • H/C (ISBN: 9781522509202) • US $345.00 (our price)

Reshaping Medical Practice and Care with Health Information Systems
Ashish Dwivedi (University of Hull, UK)
Medical Information Science Reference • copyright 2016 • 399pp • H/C (ISBN: 9781466698703) • US $150.00 (our price)

M-Health Innovations for Patient-Centered Care
Anastasius Moumtzoglou (P&A Kyriakou Children's Hospital, Greece)
Medical Information Science Reference • copyright 2016 • 438pp • H/C (ISBN: 9781466698611) • US $235.00 (our price)

Improving Health Management through Clinical Decision Support Systems
Jane D. Moon (The University of Melbourne, Australia) and Mary P. Galea (The University of Melbourne, Australia)
Medical Information Science Reference • copyright 2016 • 425pp • H/C (ISBN: 9781466694323) • US $225.00 (our price)

Maximizing Healthcare Delivery and Management through Technology Integration
Tiko Iyamu (Cape Peninsula University of Technology, South Africa) and Arthur Tatnall (Victoria University, Australia)
Medical Information Science Reference • copyright 2016 • 378pp • H/C (ISBN: 9781466694460) • US $235.00 (our price)

Flipping Health Care through Retail Clinics and Convenient Care Models
Amer Kaissi (Trinity University, USA)
Medical Information Science Reference • copyright 2015 • 306pp • H/C (ISBN: 9781466663558) • US $245.00 (our price)

This book is dedicated to my mother, Maria Moumtzoglou & my daughter Maria-Georgia Moumtzoglou

Table of Contents

Detailed Table of Contents

Population Health Management (PHM) aims to provide better health outcomes for preventing diseases, closing care gaps and providing more personalized care. Since the inception of the Pap test, cervical cancer (CxCa) decreased in countries applying screening programs, involving both prevention and treatment. In this chapter, we map a PHM roadmap to CxCa screening programs, examine the effect of supporting information technology systems, and propose a suitable architecture for implementation. Notwithstanding screening programs have a tight relation to PHM; the mapping reveals numerous interventions involving additional data sources, and timeless reconfiguration. Today, the use of open source platforms allows the implementation of IT systems supporting CxCa screening, when employed in a multitier web-based architecture.

The authors present a proposal to develop intelligent assisted living environments for home based healthcare. These environments unite the chronical patient clinical history sematic representation with the ability of monitoring the living conditions and events recurring to a fully managed Semantic Web of Things (SWoT). Several levels of acquired knowledge and the case based reasoning that is possible by knowledge representation of the health-disease history and acquisition of the scientific evidence will

Healthcare robotic applications are a growing trend due to rapid demographic changes that affect healthcare systems, professionals and quality of life indicators, for the elderly, the injured and the disabled. Current technological advances in robotic systems offer an exciting field for medical research, as the interdisciplinary approach of robotics in healthcare and specifically in surgery is continuously gaining ground. This chapter features a review of current applications, from external large scale robotic devices to nanoscale swarm robots programmed to interact on a cellular level.

In this chapter, the collection and the analysis for the development of an Ob/Gyn EMR software for small Obstetrics and Gynecology organizations is analyzed. The necessary gynecological information was gathered via research concerning the needs of the practice and was organized and categorized according to its importance to the clinicians. The user interface of the developed software provides access to obstetrics, gynecological, surgical, sterilization and PAP test data, along with video and image file storage capabilities. An integrated appointment scheduling module, as well as an expected labor day prediction module, are also part of the application. The developed software is self-contained so that it can be installed on the clinician's computer or accessed within the clinic.

Alzheimer's Disease (AD) is considered one of the most debilitating illness in modern societies and the leading cause of dementia. This study is a new approach to detect early AD Electroencephalogram (EEG) temporal events in order to improve early AD diagnosis. For that, Self-Organized Maps (SOM) were used, and it was found that there are sequences of EEG energy variation, characteristic of AD, that appear with high incidence in Mild Cognitive Impairment (MCI) patients. Those AD events are related to the first cognitive changes in patients that interfered with the normal EEG signal pattern. Moreover, there are significant differences concerning the propagation time of those events between the study groups($p=0.0082<0.05$), meaning that, as AD progresses the brain dynamics are progressively affected, what is expected because AD causes brain atrophy.

An algorithm to automatically identify segments of silence or speech is presented. The algorithm was developed to measure the silence periods in spontaneous and read speech. These silence periods are one of the parameters used to know the degree of severity of stuttered speech. For this purpose the three longer disfluent events (pauses or other disfluent events) and also the percentage of silence are useful. The algorithm is based on the evaluation of the energy and the zero crossing rate of the signal compared to the threshold values previously determined in silence. One experiment with eight subjects is described using the Stuttering Severity Instrument for Children and Adults – SSI and the percentage of silence in speech. It was concluded that the percentage of silence is good enough to separate stuttered from the normal speech but alone is not capable of measuring the degree of severity of the stuttered speech.

Segmentation is a powerful procedure that could be used to extract relevant information of the images based on advanced techniques (like active contours, region growing, Markov random fields, and medical atlas analysis). For the procedures, the main task is the contour, or volume or surface representation of specific parts of the organs that could be used for the benefit of the patients under doctor evaluation. So, in real cases, the proposed process must be quick, accurate and easy to implement. The segmentation of the organ is another problem that must be considered. More complicated, more demanding the segmentation process. In our case (bronchus segmentation) a quick, effective and easy to implement procedure is proposed based on the combination of boundary tracking and region growing techniques.

When it comes to the evaluation of natural language systems, it is well acknowledged that there is a lack of common evaluation methodologies, making the fair comparison of such systems a difficult task. Many attempts to standardize this process have used a quality model based on the ISO/IEC 9126 standards. The authors have also used these standards for the definition of a weighted quality model for the evaluation of a medical speech translator, showing the relative importance of the system's features depending on the potential user (patient or doctor, developer). More recently, ISO/IEC 9126 has been replaced by a new series of standards, the 25000 or SQuaRE series, indicating that the model should be migrated to the new series in order to maintain compliance adherence to current standards. This chapter demonstrates how to migrate from ISO/IEC 9126 to ISO 25000 by using the authors' previous work as a use case.

Individualizing care must take into account the diversity of patient values and perspectives while attending to the specific needs of people must take into account the multifaceted nature of culture. Digital medicine enables digital proximity and self-care, challenges the traditional paternal model of medicine, reshapes the nature and expectations of health care delivery, emphasizes the active involvement of patients and has an enormous potential to empower patients. Moreover, the concepts of bio-objects, cultural competence, and patient-centered care could be apparently thought on a continuum with one pole representing the bio-objects and the other representing one of the health care quality dimensions, patient-centered care. All-embracing, digital medicine affects the core values of cultural competence, which are shared by patient-centered care, one of the health care quality dimensions.

Medical practice, monitoring and control guidelines enable standardization, assessment and quality improvement in healthcare. This often implies collecting and analyzing electronic medical records (EMRs) in order to calculate compliance metrics and support evidence-based decision-making. However, for these benefits to materialize a set of challenges must be overcome, including the complexity required to represent guidelines in such a way that compliance can be automatically determined with the aid of software; the combination of both structured and unstructured (narrative text) data; and cultural or political barriers. In this chapter, we present a strategy to overcome these challenges using three case studies in chronic disease for a developing country. As such, this work contributes an approach to enable the use of ICT-supported medical guideline evaluation, in order to contribute to a more reliable and context-dependent way of improving healthcare in developing countries in particular.

Informed consents, either for treatment or sensitive information use/disclosure, that protect the privacy of patient/participant information subject to law that in certain circumstances may override patient wishes, are mandatory practice in healthcare. Similarly, for protecting and respecting research participants, informed consents are also prerequisite for human subjects research. Although the healthcare industry has widely adopted Electronic Medical Record (EMR) systems, consents are still obtained and stored primarily on paper or scanned electronic documents. Integrating a consent management system for different purposes into an EMR system involves various implementation challenges. A case study, informed consent for genetic services, is used to show how genetic informed consents placed new challenges on the traditional ethical standards of informed consent, and how appropriate consents can be electronically obtained and automatically enforced using a system that combines medical workflows and hierarchically, ontologically motivated rule enforcement. Finally, this chapter describes an implementation that uses the open-source software-based addition of these components to an open-source EMR system, so that existing systems do not need to be scrapped or otherwise rendered obsolete.

For several decades, researchers have studied the comparative effects of face-to-face and electronic communication. Some have claimed that electronic communication is detrimental to outcomes while others have emphasized its advantages. For members of healthcare quality improvement (QI) collaboratives, a mix of both of types of communication is often used, due to geographical dispersion. This chapter examines the outcomes of a specific QI collaborative, the Empira Falls Prevention project in Minnesota, USA. Levels of electronic communication between collaborative members were found to be associated with a positive patient outcome, specifically a reduction in falls. Electronic and face-to-face communication differed in their association with success measures for the collaborative. The findings suggest that the two modes of communication can be leverage to attain maximum benefits from participating in a quality improvement collaborative.

Traditional expectations about healthcare continue to be challenged by the umbrella concerns about accountability and trust. The core of this challenge is two-fold: healthcare providers have seen the absolute trust placed into their intentions and practices erode through the quantification of quality and safety of care, and, the recipients of care have been empowered with timely and specific data to demand accountability rather than unquestionably trust providers. The purpose of this chapter is to review the

Preface

Complex quality issues, within complex systems, rarely have one cause. As a result, random activities with one piece of a process can provoke unexpected results. For example, technology solutions may improve some patient safety factors but may also cause unexpected problems. Therefore, although the vigorous pursuit of technology advancements is essential, the emergence of new interactions cannot be overlooked.

In this context, it is crucial to realize that we still cannot capture all the multidimensional variables that run parallel to, intersect with, diverge from and converge with the evolution of e-health. Small deviations are being carried through the interaction and result in a magnified impact, which is amplified when the incompatible worlds of the patient, family, and visitor meet the world of healthcare professionals. On the other hand, the quality movement needs to advocate the free flow of information in order to fertilize organizational learning and nourish worker intelligence (Wheatley, 1999).

However, information cannot be disentangled from e-health initiatives. Information technology provides alternative methods for making health information accessible to consumers. Furthermore, research shows an improvement of health awareness, high user satisfaction, evidence of greater benefit for under-served people and beneficial impact on health behavior (Gaston & Mitchell, 2005; Murray et al., 2005; Santo et al., 2005; Wofford et al., 2005).

However, do all these translate into a quality linkage of e-health?

Understanding the linkage between e-health and quality is a complicated task because no definitional consensus exists for either of these terms. The lack of shared definition can present challenges from both practical and academic perspectives (Pate & Turner-Ferrier, 2010; Kastania, 2010). Academically, the lack of shared definition can serve as a motivating force for a meaningful dialogue to promote knowledge. From a pragmatic point of view, different conceptualizations held by various stakeholders can also lead to a serious dialogue with the intention of arriving at a definitional resolution. On the other hand, the lack of consensus can cause inter, and intra-organizational dysfunctions, as organizations adhere to and try to leverage their positions for self-gain (Pate & Turner-Ferrier, 2010). Therefore, establishing a common language may serve as a powerful platform that enables e-health help organizations to achieve quality improvement more effectively.

However, what is clear about healthcare is that the interdependent and complex nature of healthcare delivery calls for structured ways to analyze the strategic goals, processes, technologies, outcomes, and other features of the healthcare system. Systems theory is a theoretical framework that serves as a starting point for this analysis (Austin & Boxerman, 1998; Ginter et al., 1998).

In its essence, systems theory provides a straightforward way of viewing the relationship between inputs and outputs. In its most basic form, system inputs are converted to and drive outputs, which, in turn, provides a feedback mechanism to the size and amount of inputs needed. On the other hand, Donabedian's (2005) well-known structure-process-outcome (SPO) framework provides a meaningful way of viewing the concept of quality. In this context, e-health technologies and supporting equipment clearly fall under the domain of structural measures of quality, which constitute 'input measures of an organization's capacity to permit or promote effective work' (Flood et al., 2000).

On empirical grounds, in a systematic review of the relationship between health information technology and quality, Chaudhry et al. (2006) found two main topics about the relationship. First, health information technology has been shown to increase adherence to clinical guidelines, based on the associated decision-making processes and functions, which are inherently built into adherence. Second, health information technology has also increased the ability of organizations to improve the quality of care by increasing monitoring through 'large scale screening and aggregation of data'.

On the other hand, the quality linkage of e-health can be traced in the patient safety and patient-centered care thinking. Patient safety could be described as a discipline that applies safety science methods to achieve reliable health care delivery. However, it is also thought as an attribute of the health care system that minimizes the incidence and impact of adverse events. Preliminary evidence of interaction with e-health could be found in safety culture, data mining, and medical simulation. Specifically, a prerequisite for the realization of the key dimensions of patient safety culture (Ginsburg et al., 2009; Singer et al., 2008) is the collection, analysis, and dissemination of information deriving from:

- Incidents and near misses.
- The adoption of the reporting, just, flexible and learning cultures (Ruchlin et al. 2004).

Data mining is becoming an increasingly indispensable tool in mining a broad range of health records (Norén et al., 2008). It can maintain quality assurance, simplify the automation of data retrieval, facilitate physician quality improvement (Johnstone et al., 2008), and accurately represent patient outcomes if combined with simulation (Harper, 2005). Recently, there is interest in switching to algorithms and database development for microarray data mining (Cordero et al., 2007). Finally, medical simulation bridges the knowledge gap by representing certain key characteristics of a physical system. Quality improvement, patient safety, and the evaluation of clinical skills have impelled medical simulation into the clinical arena (Carroll & Messenger, 2008) while there is conclusive evidence that simulation training improves provider self-efficacy and effectiveness (Nishisaki et al., 2007) and increases patient safety. It is also accepted that the process of iterative learning creates a much stronger learning environment, and computer simulators are an ideal tool for the evaluation of students' clinical skills (Murphy et al., 2007). Finally, a great potential of interaction has to be established through the assessment of biobanking, biochips, disease modeling, genomics, molecular imaging, nanotechnology, ontologies, and proteomics (Moumtzoglou, 2010).

Taking into account the patient-doctor encounter, as an element of a good outcome, we turn to the idea of patient-centeredness. Although definitions of patient-centered care vary, patient-centered care is the provision of care that is 'respectful of and responsive to individual patient preferences, needs and values and ensuring that patient values guide all clinical decisions' (IOM, 2001). In this context, Kilbridge (2002) suggested that twelve information technology applications, which involve the management of health care information, empower patients. These include:

1. Technologies which provide access to general and specific medical information.
2. Technologies capable of handling data entry and tracking of self-management data.

The applications included:

- Personal health records.
- Patient access to hospital information systems.
- Patient access to general health information.
- Electronic medical records (EMRs).
- Pre-visit intake.
- Inter-hospital data sharing.
- Information for physicians to manage patient populations.
- Patient-physician electronic messaging.
- Patient access to tailored medical information.
- Online data entry and tracking.
- Online scheduling.
- Computer-assisted telephone triage and assistance.
- Online access to provider performance data.

Finally, a key way to think e-health and educational linkage relates to the ways in which e-health applications and technologies can be introduced into educational settings taking into account the missing foci of healthcare delivery education.

Overall, if we also take into account that IOM (2003) suggested all health professionals be educated to deliver patient-centered care, a theoretical interaction between e-health and quality might be established.

Having said that, we have to admit that there is relatively little empirical evidence to substantiate many of the theoretical claims made about the linkage of quality and e-health, and a lack of robust research on the risks of implementing e-health technology (Black et al., 2011). The reasons are multi-faceted, including lack of primary research, methodological limitations, the inappropriate timeframe of the study, failure to involve patients, and inadequate attention to socio-technical factors.

However, despite the substantial gap in evidence, due to the theoretical linkage of quality and e-health, an evaluation framework of e-health has to be established, taking into account the six dimensions of quality, namely, patient safety, effectiveness, timeliness, patient-centeredness, efficiency and equitability.

ORGANIZATION OF THE BOOK

In chapter 1, Anastasius Moumtzoglou & Abraham Pouliakis argue that Population Health Management (PHM) aims to provide better health outcomes for preventing diseases, closing care gaps and providing more personalized care. Since the inception of the Pap test, cervical cancer (CxCa) decreased in countries applying screening programs, involving both prevention and treatment. In this chapter, the authors map a PHM roadmap to CxCa screening programs, examine the effect of supporting information technology systems, and propose a suitable architecture for implementation. Notwithstanding screening programs have a tight relation to PHM; the mapping reveals numerous interventions involving additional data sources, and timeless reconfiguration. They conclude that the use of open source platforms allows the implementation of IT systems supporting CxCa screening, when employed in a multitier web-based architecture.

In chapter 2, David Mendes, Manuel Lopes, Artur Romao & Irene Pimenta Rodrigues present a proposal to develop intelligent assisted living environments for home based healthcare. These environments unite the patient clinical history sematic representation with the ability to monitor the conditions of life and events recurring to a fully managed Semantic Web of Things (SWoT). Several levels of acquired knowledge and the case based reasoning that is possible by knowledge representation of the health-disease history and acquisition of the scientific evidence will deliver, through various voice based natural interfaces, the adequate support systems for disease auto management but prominently by activating the less differentiated caregiver for any specific need. With these capabilities at hand, home-based healthcare providing becomes a viable possibility reducing the institutionalization needs. The resulting integrated healthcare framework provides significant savings while improving the generality of health and satisfaction indicators.

In chapter 3, Wayne Usher identifies how Australian university students access and use various forms of technology (Web 1.0 – Internet, Web 2.0 – social media - SM) to retrieve personal health information. This chapter moves beyond Web 1.0, to present a theoretical basis for the claim, concerning the extent to which other forms of technology (e.g. Web 2.0 and wireless monitoring devices) have impacted on youth. What is more, attention will be directed towards outlining to what degree this has shaped their patterns of health information retrieval. Importantly, this chapter aligns with contemporary literature that suggests a need for further studies into the area of human - technology interactions, which promotes sustainable action plans and strategies that will create and encourage reform throughout e-health programs and interactive communication platforms. Given that Australian university students are prolific users of modern forms of communication technology and that youth, in general, characteristically undertake relatively high levels of risky health behaviors and unhealthy lifestyle choices, such a chapter would seem warranted.

In chapter 4, Athanasios Anastasiou, Kostas Giokas, Georgia Koutsouri & Dimitra Iliopoulou present the architecture and implementation of an automatic medication dispenser specifically for users who take medications without close professional supervision. By relieving the users from the error-prone tasks of interpreting medication directions and administrating medications accordingly, the device can improve the required level in compliance and prevent serious medication errors. By taking advantage of the scheduling flexibility provided by medication directions, the device makes the user's medication schedule easy to adhere and tolerant to tardiness whenever possible. This work is done collaboratively by the medication scheduler and dispenser controller in an action-oriented manner. An advantage of the action-oriented interface, between the components, is extensibility, as new functions can be added and existing ones removed with little or no need to modify the dispenser control structure. This chapter first describes the action-oriented design, principal components and hardware structures of the smart device. It then provides an overview of the heuristic algorithms used by the medication scheduler and their relative merits. The different available user options are presented depicting the user-specific operating modes of the device/service. The scope of the chapter is to describe the development of a smart electronic drug dispenser unit for the pharmaceutical adherence of patients.

In chapter 5, Vassilia Costarides, Apollon Zygomalas, Kostas Giokas & Dimitris Koutsouris argue that healthcare robotic applications are a growing trend due to rapid demographic changes that affect healthcare systems, professionals and quality of life indicators, for the elderly, the injured and the physically challenged. Current technological advances in robotic systems offer an exciting field for medical research, as the interdisciplinary approach of robotics in healthcare and specifically in surgery is continuously gaining ground. The chapter features a review of current applications, from external large scale robotic devices to nanoscale swarm robots programmed to interact on a cellular level.

In chapter 6, Konstantinos Bougoulias, Ioannis Kouris, Marios Prasinos, Kostas Giokas & Dimitris Koutsouris analyze the development of an Ob/Gyn EMR software for small Obstetrics and Gynecology organizations. The necessary gynecological information was gathered via research concerning the needs of the practice and was organized and categorized according to its importance to the clinicians. The user interface of the developed software provides access to obstetrics, gynecological, surgical, sterilization and PAP test data, along with video and image file storage capabilities. An integrated appointment scheduling module, as well as an expected labor day prediction module are also part of the application. The developed software is self-contained so that it can be installed on the clinician's computer or accessed within the clinic.

In chapter 7, Pedro Miguel Rodrigues, Diamantino Freitas, João Paulo Teixeira, Dílio Alves & Carolina Garrett present a new approach to detect early Alzheimer's disease Electroencephalogram temporal events to improve Alzheimer's disease (AD) early diagnosis. Using Self-Organized Maps (SOM), it was found that there are sequences of EEG energy variation, characteristic of AD, which appears with high incidence in Mild Cognitive Impairment (MCI) patients. Those AD events are related to the first cognitive changes in patients that interfere with the normal EEG signal pattern. Moreover, there are significant differences concerning the propagation time of those events between the study groups ($p=0.0082<0.05$). That means as AD progresses, the brain dynamics are progressively affected because AD causes brain atrophy.

In chapter 8, João Paulo Teixeira, Maria Goreti Fernandes & Rita Alexandra Costa present an algorithm to identify segments of silence or speech automatically. The algorithm was developed to measure the silence periods in spontaneous and read speech. These silence periods are one of the parameters used to know the degree of severity of stuttered speech. For this purpose, the three longer disfluent events (pauses or other disfluent events) and also the percentage of silence are useful. The algorithm is based on the evaluation of the energy and the zero crossing rate of the signal compared to the threshold values previously determined in silence. One experiment with eight subjects is described using the Stuttering Severity Instrument for Children and Adults – SSI and the percentage of silence in speech. It was concluded that the proportion of silence is good enough to separate stuttered from the normal speech but alone is not capable of measuring the degree of severity of the stuttered speech.

In chapter 9, Stelios Zimeras argues that segmentation is a powerful procedure that could be used to extract relevant information of the images based on advanced techniques (like active contours, region growing, Markov random fields, and medical atlas analysis). For the procedures, the main task is the contour, or volume or surface representation of specific parts of the organs that could be used for the benefit of the patients under doctor evaluation. So, in real cases, the proposed process must be quick, accurate and easy to implement. The segmentation of the organ is another problem that must be considered. In bronchus segmentation, a quick, efficient and easy to implement procedure is proposed based on the combination of boundary tracking and region growing techniques.

In chapter 10, Paula Estrella & Nikos Tsourakis acknowledge that when it comes to the evaluation of natural language systems, there is a lack of common evaluation methodologies, making the fair comparison of such systems a difficult task. Many attempts to standardize this process have used a quality model based on the ISO/IEC 9126 standards. The authors have used these standards for the definition of a weighted quality model for the evaluation of a medical speech translator, showing the relative importance of the system's features depending on the potential user (patient or doctor, developer). More recently, ISO/IEC 9126 has been replaced by a new series of standards, the 25000 or SQuaRE series, indicating that the model should be migrated to the new series to maintain compliance adherence to current standards. The chapter demonstrates how to migrate from ISO/IEC 9126 to ISO 25000 by using the authors' previous work as a use case.

In chapter 11, Anastasius Moumtzoglou argues that individualizing care must take into account the diversity of patient values and perspectives while attending to the specific needs of people must take into account the multifaceted nature of culture. Digital medicine enables digital proximity and self-care, challenges the traditional paternal model of medicine, reshapes the nature and expectations of health care delivery, emphasizes the active involvement of patients and has an enormous potential to empower patients. Moreover, the concepts of bio-objects, cultural competence, and patient-centered care could be apparently thought on a continuum with one pole representing the bio-objects and the other representing one of the health care quality dimensions, patient-centered care. All-embracing, digital medicine affects the core values of cultural competence, which are shared by patient-centered care, one of the health care quality dimensions.

In chapter 12, Alexandra Pomares-Quimbaya, Rafael A. González, Alejandro Sierra, Julián Camilo Daza, Oscar Muñoz, Angel García, Alvaro Bustamante, Olga Milena García & Wilson Ricardo Bohórquez contend that medical practice, monitoring and control guidelines enable standardization, assessment and quality improvement in healthcare. That often implies collecting and analyzing electronic medical records (EMRs) to calculate compliance metrics and support evidence-based decision-making. However, for these benefits to materialize, a set of challenges must be overcome, including the complexity required to represent guidelines in such a way that compliance can be automatically determined with the aid of software; the combination of both structured and unstructured (narrative text) data; and cultural or political barriers. In this chapter, the authors present a strategy to overcome these challenges using three case studies, in chronic diseases, for a developing country. As such, this work contributes to the use of ICT-supported medical guideline evaluation and a more reliable and context-dependent way of improving healthcare in developing countries.

In chapter 13, Bo Yu, Duminda Wijesekera & Paulo Costa argue that informed consents, either for treatment or sensitive information use/disclosure, that protect the privacy of patient/participant information subject to law that in certain circumstances may override patient wishes, are mandatory practice in healthcare. Similarly, for protecting and respecting research participants, informed consents are also a prerequisite for human subjects research. Although the healthcare industry has widely adopted Electronic Medical Record (EMR) systems, consents are still obtained and stored primarily on paper or scanned electronic documents. Integrating a consent management system for different purposes into an EMR system involves various implementation challenges. A case study, informed consent for genetic services, is used to show how genetic informed consents placed new challenges on the traditional ethical standards of informed consent, and how appropriate consents can be electronically obtained and automatically enforced using a system that combines medical workflows and hierarchically, ontologically motivated rule enforcement. Finally, the chapter describes an implementation that uses the open-source software-based addition of these components to an open-source EMR system, so that existing systems do not need to be scrapped or otherwise rendered obsolete.

In chapter 14, Priscilla A. Arling, Edward J. Miech & Greg W. Arling examine the outcomes of a specific QI collaborative, the Empira Falls Prevention Project in Minnesota, USA. Levels of electronic communication between collaborative members were found to be associated with a positive patient outcome, specifically a reduction in falls. Electronic and face-to-face communication differed in their association with success measures for the collaborative. The findings suggest that the two modes of communication can be leverage to attain maximum benefits from participating in a quality improvement collaborative.

In chapter 15, Vahé A. Kazandjian argues that traditional expectations about healthcare continue to be challenged by the umbrella concerns about accountability and trust. The core of this challenge is two-fold: healthcare providers have seen the absolute trust placed into their intentions and practices erode through the quantification of quality and safety of care, and, the recipients of care have been empowered with timely and specific data to demand accountability rather than unquestionably trust providers.

The chapter reviews the key dimensions of the operationalization of performance measurement and the translation of its findings to statements about quality and safety of care. The past four decades have seen the continuous discovery and refining of analytical tools to quantify what once was taken for granted: that patients always receive the best care possible. These tools have uncovered the probabilistic nature of medicine and the resulting nature of the relationships, outcomes have to processes. Hence the expectations of patients, payors of care and policy makers require being continuously modified to reflect the limitations of medicine and healthcare.

The education of various audiences as to what the measures mean not only is a necessary requisite for sound project design but also will determine how the accountability model is shaped in each environment based on the generic measurement tools results, local traditions of care and caring, and expectations about outcomes.

In chapter 16, Aleš Bourek predicts that future health systems, besides traditional areas defined and addressed since 1980, will face the advent of Proactive, Predictive, Prospective, Preventive, Participative and Personalized health care (HC). Reliable e-health platforms can help with these challenges. They should be designed and implemented in a way to help ordinary people achieve extraordinary results. Even the best projects addressing HC systems improvement are not automatically qualified for implementation unless adopted by policy makers. The introduction of strategies with a potential for healthcare systems improvement to policy makers is necessary but difficult because of the complexity of the addressed issue. Illustrated on four projects, selected from the 25 the author participated in, from 1993 to 2016, principles, processes and attitudes found beneficial for successful policy implementation in various healthcare environments are presented, to help with the integration of reliable electronic healthcare platforms into coming healthcare systems.

Anastasius Moumtzoglou
Hellenic Society for Quality and Safety in Healthcare, Greece & P. & A. Kyriakou Children's Hospital, Greece

REFERENCES

Austin, C. J., & Boxerman, S. B. (1998). *Information systems for health services administration* (5th ed.). Chicago, IL: Health Administration Press.

Black, A., Car, J., Pagliari, C., Anandan, C., Cresswell, K., Bokun, T., & Sheikh, A. et al. (2011). The Impact of eHealth on the Quality and Safety of Health Care: A Systematic Overview. *PLoS Medicine*, *8*(1), e1000387. doi:10.1371/journal.pmed.1000387 PMID:21267058

Carroll, J. D., & Messenger, J. C. (2008). Medical simulation: The new tool for training and skill assessment. *Perspectives in Biology and Medicine*, *51*(1), 47–60. doi:10.1353/pbm.2008.0003 PMID:18192765

Chaudhry, B., Jerome, W., Shinyi, W., Maglione, M., Mojica, W., & Roth, E. et al.. (2006). Systematic Review: Impact of Health Information Technology on Quality, Efficiency, and Costs of Medical Care. *Annals of Internal Medicine*, *144*(10), E12–W18. doi:10.7326/0003-4819-144-10-200605160-00125 PMID:16702590

Cordero, F., Botta, M., & Calogero, R. A. (2007). Microarray data analysis and mining approaches. *Briefings in Functional Genomics & Proteomics*, *6*(4), 265–281. doi:10.1093/bfgp/elm034 PMID:18216026

Donabedian, A. (2005, December). Evaluating the Quality of Medical Care.[A.B.]. *The Milbank Quarterly*, *83*(4), 691–729. Retrieved August 30 2009. doi:10.1111/j.1468-0009.2005.00397.x PMID:16279964

Gaston, C. M., & Mitchell, G. (2005). Information giving and decision-making in patients with advanced cancer: A systematic review. *Social Science & Medicine*, *61*(10), 2252–2264. doi:10.1016/j.socscimed.2005.04.015 PMID:15922501

Ginsburg, L., Gilin, D., Tregunno, D., Norton, P. G., Flemons, W., & Fleming, M. (2009). Advancing measurement of patient safety culture. *Health Services Research*, *44*(1), 205–224. doi:10.1111/j.1475-6773.2008.00908.x PMID:18823446

Ginter, P. M., Swayne, L. E., & Duncan, W. J. (1998).Strategic management of health care organizations (3rd ed.). Malden, MA: Blackwell Publishers, Inc. Harper, P. (2005).Combining data mining tools with health care models for improved understanding of health processes and resourse utilization. Clinical and Investigative Medicine, 28(6), 338-341.

Institute of Medicine. (2001). *Crossing the Quality Chasm: A New Health System for the Twenty- first Century*. Washington, WA: National Academy Press.

Institute of Medicine. (2003). *Health Professions Education: A Bridge to Quality*. Washington, WA: National Academy Press.

Johnstone, P. A., Crenshaw, T., Cassels, D. G., & Fox, T. H. (2008). Automated data mining of a proprietary database system for physician quality improvement. *International Journal of Radiation Oncology, Biology, Physics*, *70*(5), 1537–1541. doi:10.1016/j.ijrobp.2007.08.056 PMID:18037576

Kastania, A. N. (2010). Evaluation considerations for e-health systems. In A. Moumtzoglou & A. Kastania (Eds.), *E-Health Systems Quality and Reliability: Models and Standards*. Hershey, PA: IGI Global.

Kilbridge, P. (2002). *Crossing the Chasm with Information Technology: Bridging the Quality Gap in Health Care*. CA: California HealthCare Foundation.

Moumtzoglou, A. (2010). E-health as the realm of Healthcare Quality: A mental image of the future. In A. Moumtzoglou & A. Kastania (Eds.), *E-Health Systems Quality and Reliability: Models and Standards*. Hershey, PA: IGI Global.

Murphy, D., Challacombe, B., Nedas, T., Elhage, O., Althoefer, K., Seneviratne, L., & Dasgupta, P. (2007). Equipment and technology in robotics (in Spanish; Castilian). *Archivos Espanoles de Urologia*, *60*(4), 349–355. PMID:17626526

Murray, E., Burns, J., See Tai, S., Lai, R., & Nazareth, I. (2005). Interactive Health Communication Applications for people with chronic disease. *Cochrane Database of Systematic Reviews*, *CD004274*(4). doi:10.1002/14651858.CD004274.pub4 PMID:16235356

Nishisaki, A., Keren, R., & Nadkarni, V. (2007). Does Simulation Improve Patient Safety?: Self-Efficacy, Competence, Operational Performance, and Patient Safety. *Anesthesiology Clinics*, *25*(2), 225–236. doi:10.1016/j.anclin.2007.03.009 PMID:17574187

Norén, G. N., Bate, A., Hopstadius, J., Star, K., & Edwards, I. R. (2008). Temporal Pattern Discovery for Trends and Transient Effects: Its Application to Patient Records.*Proceedings of the Fourteenth International Conference on Knowledge Discovery and Data Mining SIGKDD 2008*, p. 963-971, Las Vegas NV. doi:10.1145/1401890.1402005

Pate, C., & Turner-Ferrier, J. (2010).Expoloring linkages between Quality, E-health and Healthcare Education. In: Moumtzoglou A. and Kastania A. (eds) E-Health Systems Quality and Reliability: Models and Standards, IGI Global, Hershey, P.A.

Ruchlin, H. S., Dubbs, N. L., & Callahan, M. A. (2004). The role of leadership in instilling a culture of safety: Lessons from the literature. *Journal of Healthcare Management*, *49*(1), 47–58. PMID:14768428

Santo, A., Laizner, A. M., & Shohet, L. (2005). Exploring the value of audiotapes for health literacy: A systematic review. *Patient Education and Counseling*, *58*(3), 235–243. doi:10.1016/j.pec.2004.07.001 PMID:16054796

Singer, S. J., Falwell, A., Gaba, D. M., & Baker, L. C. (2008). Patient safety climate in US hospitals: Variation by management level. *Medical Care*, *46*(11), 1149–1156. doi:10.1097/MLR.0b013e31817925c1 PMID:18953225

Wheatley, M. J. (1999). *Leadership and the new science: Discovering order in a chaotic world.* San Fransisco: Berrett-Koehler.

Wofford, J., Smith, E., & Miller, D. (2005). The multimedia computer for office-based patient education: A systematic review. *Patient Education and Counseling*, *59*(2), 148–157. doi:10.1016/j.pec.2004.10.011 PMID:16257619

Zinn, J. S., Shortell, S. M., & Scott, W. R. (2000). Organizational performance: Managing for success. In S. M. Shortell & A. D. Kaluzny (Eds.), *Health care management: Organization design and behavior* (4th ed., pp. 356–389). Albany, NY: Delmar.

Acknowledgment

I would like to thank all the authors for their diverse and outstanding contributions to this book.

Chapter 1
Population Health Management and Cervical Cancer Screening Programs:
Roadmap, Design, and Implementation of a Supporting IT System

Anastasius Moumtzoglou
Hellenic Society for Quality and Safety in Healthcare, Greece & P. & A. Kyriakou Children's Hospital, Greece

Abraham Pouliakis
National and Kapodistrian University of Athens, Greece

ABSTRACT

Population Health Management (PHM) aims to provide better health outcomes for preventing diseases, closing care gaps and providing more personalized care. Since the inception of the Pap test, cervical cancer (CxCa) decreased in countries applying screening programs, involving both prevention and treatment. In this chapter, we map a PHM roadmap to CxCa screening programs, examine the effect of supporting information technology systems, and propose a suitable architecture for implementation. Notwithstanding screening programs have a tight relation to PHM; the mapping reveals numerous interventions involving additional data sources, and timeless reconfiguration. Today, the use of open source platforms allows the implementation of IT systems supporting CxCa screening, when employed in a multitier web-based architecture.

INTRODUCTION

'Public health' connotes a relatively narrow field with activities carried out by agencies granted with official functions. 'Population health' a term with broader content, is related to a field relevant to the study of several important factors for health. As a result, it involves many terms, such as outcomes, disparities, determinants, and risk factors (Kindig, 2007)

DOI: 10.4018/978-1-5225-1724-5.ch001

Notwithstanding the term 'population health' combines the concepts of both health and population, every term has an essential meaning of its own. The population is related to a group of persons being organized into numerous different units of analysis. Similarly, the term health was defined in a negative manner, i.e. the absence of disease. Nowadays, the modern understanding stresses the positive aspects as well, and health is considered to be related to all life issues. Summarizing, today it is debated whether population health and public health are different or identical. Nevertheless, population health is defined as health outcomes and their distribution in a population (Kindig, 2007).

Population health management (PHM) has been defined as 'the technical field of endeavor which utilizes a variety of individual, organizational and cultural interventions to help improve the morbidity patterns (i.e., the illness and injury burden) and the health care use behavior of defined populations' (Hillman, 2002). It is differentiated from disease management because it includes (Howe & Spence, 2004)

- More chronic conditions and diseases.
- Uses a single point of contact and coordination and predictive modeling across multiple clinical conditions.

Moreover, PHM is considered a broader term than disease management, as it includes (Coughlin, Pope, & Leedle(Jr), 2006):

- Intensive care management for individuals at the highest level of risk.
- Personal health management for those at lower levels of predicted health risk.

At the provider level, Care Continuum Alliance (2012) highlights three components:

- The leadership and the central care delivery role of the primary care physician.
- The critical importance of patient activation.
- The capacity expansion of care coordination.

In this context, to successfully achieve all of these requirements, an organization should provide proactive, preventive and chronic care services to all managed patients. Additionally, this should take place both during encounters of patients with the healthcare system and in between. Therefore, providers should maintain regular contact with their patients and support them in the management of their health. Additionally, providers must manage patients at high risk, to prevent the deterioration of their health and avoid the development of complications. Finally, evidence-based protocols for the diagnosis and treatment of patients, in a consistent and cost-effective manner, are also required if for a provider-based PHM approach is followed.

Moreover, the Federal Agency for Healthcare Research and Quality (AHRQ) developed the concept of "practice-based population health" (PBPH) and defined it as "an approach to care that uses information on a group of patients within a primary care practice or group of practices, to improve the care and clinical outcomes of patients within that practice" (Cusack, Knudson, Kronstadt, Singer, & Brown, 2010).

To assist healthcare organizations to navigate the path toward the implementation of effective population health management solutions, in 2014, Sanders suggested a roadmap of 12 steps (Sanders, 2014):

- Organize accurate patient registries.
- Decide patient-provider acknowledgment.
- Define precise numerators in the patient registries.
- Continuously measure cost and clinical metrics.
- Adhere to clinical practice guidelines.
- Engage in risk-management outreach.
- Obtain external data.
- Exchange information with patients.
- Educate and engage with patients.
- Develop and adhere to complex clinical practice guidelines.
- Coordinate between patient and care team.
- Track-specific outcomes.

Obviously, the implementation of health IT is among the essential components and requirements for planning and implementing PHM. The adoption of Electronic Health Records is just the first step toward the creation of the requisite infrastructure. A wide range of other IT applications to automate PHM, track results and engage the patients in their health care is required. Additionally, IT systems should repeatedly be evaluated because of: rapid technological changes, new government regulations and new approaches to patient management.

AHRQ recommends health IT tools for the stratification and monitoring of populations, as follows:

- Target patients being in greatest need of health services by stratifying the patients and narrowing subpopulations.
- Make patient related data actionable by generating alerts to the patients.
- Make data actionable by generating alerts towards health providers, about patient care needs.

Cervical cancer (CxCa) is one of the most common cancers among women with age between 14 and 44 years. Moreover, it is the third cause of death related to cancer, following breast and lung cancer (Jemal et al., 2011). The Human papillomavirus (HPV) is responsible and strongly associated to CxCa. From the more than 100 HPV types, thirteen are found to be highly oncogenic and accountable for the development of CxCa (Malik, 2005; McCance, 1988; J. S. Smith et al., 2007). HPVis mainly sexually transmitted, affects millions of women worldwide, and moreover, it is very common in the young population (approximately 70% of women will be infected during their lifetime). HPV infection is usually transient, as regresses, but, an infection by high-risk HPV type/s and a compromised immune system constitute a fundamental factor for cervical intraepithelial neoplasia (CIN) or cancer (Riou et al., 1990; Wentzensen & Klug, 2008).

As many years are required for the development of precancerous lesions and subsequent progression to cancer (Ferenczy & Franco, 2002; Koshiol et al., 2008; Schlecht et al., 2001), there is adequate time for preventive actions. Therefore, CxCa prevention is an exciting application topic for PHM methodologies, being by nature compliant with PHM concepts, because it involves prevention and treatment. Additionally, there are high-risk patients, for example, patients with compromised immune system (immunosuppressed patients, patients with transplantations and patients with HIV).

The objective of the chapter is threefold:

- Present basic concepts of CxCa screening programs, according to the European Guidelines (European Commission. Directorate-General for Health and Consumer Protection, 2008).
- To provide an update (Moumtzoglou & Pouliakis, 2015) of the mapping of PHM principles to CxCa screening programs
- To present the design of an Information Technology (IT) system supporting CxCa screening at national level focusing on open source tools as well as stability and reliability.

BACKGROUND

The evolution of thinking about population health which accounts for a natural history of the field of public health and health promotion has been traced by Hayes and Dunn (1998),Glouberman and Hayes (1998), and McGrail et al. (1998).

Public health addresses environmental conditions that exert widespread effects on the health of populations, as it has been defined as ‘fulfilling society’s interest in assuring conditions in which people can be healthy (Institute of Medicine (U.S.). Committee for the Study of the Future of Public Health., 1988). Public health interventions include:

- Sanitation.
- The protection of drinking water.
- Mass immunization against vaccine-preventable diseases.
- Control of microbiological, radiological, and chemical hazards.

The World Health Organization (1986) defined health promotion as the process of enabling people to increase control over, and to improve their health, focusing less on physical factors and more on lifestyle. Health promotion addressed people in their social and cultural contexts and sought to involve them as active players in their health. Population health has been defined as “a conceptual framework for thinking about why some populations are healthier than others, as well as the policy development, research agenda, and resource allocation that flow from it” (Young, 1998). It focuses on the health outcomes of a group of individuals, their distribution within the group, and the multiple determinants that contribute to physical, mental, and social health outcomes (Dunn & Hayes, 1999; Misra, Guyer, & Allston, 2003; Strike, Goering, & Wasylenki, 2002). Population health is inherently cross-sectoral, requiring a comprehensive understanding of the complex pathways through which policies and interventions in all sectors may adversely or positively impact on health and its underlying determinants.

The distinction between public and population health continues to be a point of discussion (Kindig, 2007). Whereas public health focused traditionally on environmental factors that influence disease, population health allows for all of the factors affecting the health of populations. The IOM (2002) foresees closer linkages between the fields of public and population health, suggesting that public health can be enriched by the incorporation of population health principles. Health promotion and population health are intrinsically linked and have been collectively referred to as “population health promotion” (Hamilton & Bhatti, 1996).

Following the initial contributions of Lalonde (1974) and Epp (1986), the underlying philosophy of the population health approach began to take shape in Canada. The concept facilitates the identification of courses of action in health improvement and provides a greater understanding of what contributes to sickness and death. Moreover, it envisions four broad influences on health:

- Human biology.
- Environment.
- Lifestyle.
- Health care organization.

Lalonde (1974) rated the first three categories as being of equal importance as health care organization. However, the model was criticized for overly stressing the role of personal responsibility. Epp (1986) proposed a new approach:

- Emphasizing health inequities.
- Suggesting the increase of prevention efforts.
- Enhancing people's ability to cope with the disease.

The Canadian Institute for Advanced Research carried the concept of population health forward by offering evidence for each of the health determinants while Evans and Stoddart (1990) developed a population health framework based on the determinants of health and their interactions.

The Federal/Provincial/Territorial Advisory Committee on Population Health (1994) built on the work of the Canadian Institute for Advanced Research and presented another interpretation of health determinants and the method by which they should be evaluated. Five categories of determinants underpin the health of a population:

- Personal health practices.
- Individual capacity and coping skills.
- Social and economic environment.
- Physical environment.
- Health services.

In a subsequent revision in 1996 they acknowledged the importance of biology and genetic endowment as health determinants (Health Canada, 1996). Edwards and McDowell (1998) developed a five-stage framework that describes the academic field of population health. The sequence identifies population health issues, analyzes their causes and determinants, designs interventions, implements effective health care delivery systems and builds evidence-based health policy. These stages are put into practice under three integrating themes which include:

- Risk assessment.
- Multiple interventions.
- Evidence-based policy.

Since the foundations of cytopathology by G. Papanicolaou in 1928 (Papanicolaou, 1928) and the proposal of the worldwide known Pap test for preventing cervical cancer (CxCa) (Diamantis, Magiorkinis, & Koutselini, 2014; Papanicolaou & Traut, 1941), Pap test was (Brown, Bradbury, & Kraushaar,

1949; Hollenbeck, 1957) and still is the most valuable tool for cervical cancer prevention (Zhao et al., 2015). It is performed by extracting painlessly cells from the cervix, and evaluating them on glass slides via a microscope. This assessment is a task that requires effort and can be accomplished by well-trained cytopathologists or cytotechnologists.

Due to the nature of CxCa and its progressive evolution, screening programs can effectively prevent this disease (Papanicolaou & Traut, 1941; Syrjanen et al., 2010). This can be achieved only if screening is well organized, including quality control and quality assurance procedures. Moreover, this can be effective if the program is compliant with the PHM principles. The prevalence of cervical cancer, after the application of organized CxCa screening programs, via the methods introduced by George Papanicolaou, was decreased by 75% between 1955 and 1992. Unfortunately, there are still many deaths. In Europe, each year more than 50,000 women develop CxCa, and about 50% (25,000) die from this disease. The American Cancer Society data indicate that 12,200 new CxCa cases were expected in the United States in 2010 resulting in 4,210 deaths (American Cancer Society, 2010). In the UK, approximately 7-8% of the screened population have an abnormal smear (Paraskevaidis, Kyrgiou, & Martin-Hirsch, 2007); from these women, roughly 1.5-2% will harbor a high-grade lesion and 5% a low-grade lesion. Women with high-grade lesions require medical treatment (surgical operation) and women with low-grade lesions require at least frequent monitoring and follow-up as a low-grade lesion may regress or progress to high grade. CxCa screening is by nature compliant to the three integrating themes proposed by Edwards and McDowell (Edwards & McDowell, 1998), women are assessed for risk to harbor or develop the disease, there is a cyclic process including multiple interventions and the policy is evidence-based because in all countries that screening programs are applied CxCa incidence has dropped by 70%.

MAPPING POPULATION HEALTH MANAGEMENT ROADMAP INTO CERVICAL CANCER SCREENING PROGRAMS

In this section, we analyze the potential application of the PHM roadmap (Sanders, 2014), on a point by point basis, in CxCa screening programs. The primary source of information is the European Guidelines for quality assurance in CxCa screening (European Commission. Directorate-General for Health and Consumer Protection, 2008). Many of the proposed procedures in the guidelines are compliant with the PHM roadmap. However, there are cases that gaps were found. In this case, we highlight them and propose solutions, based on PHM principles and IT solutions.

At an operational level, a CxCa screening program should be centralized. Ideally, an IT system should serve the entire population of a country. The primary reason is that women under control may change their residence (Pouliakis, Karakitsou, Iliopoulou, Koutsouri, & Karakitsos, 2013). Web-based ICT systems can be used nationwide and may provide high security and adequate flexibility. However, continuous support is required if the deployment is for the first time. On the other side, a single point of control, as required by PHM, creates a burden in a single place. Solutions to overcome this limitation exist. For instance, hierarchical approaches may provide centralized control and simultaneously decentralized user training and support (Pouliakis & Karakitsos, 2012). That can reduce the workload of central offices and provide more personalized support, as required by the PHM principles.

The process of a CxCa screening program has a well-known and organized workflow (Figure 1); this process can be formulated as follows (Athanasiadi et al., 2014; Pouliakis, Iliopoulou, & Karakitsou, 2012):

Figure 1. Workflow of the screening process

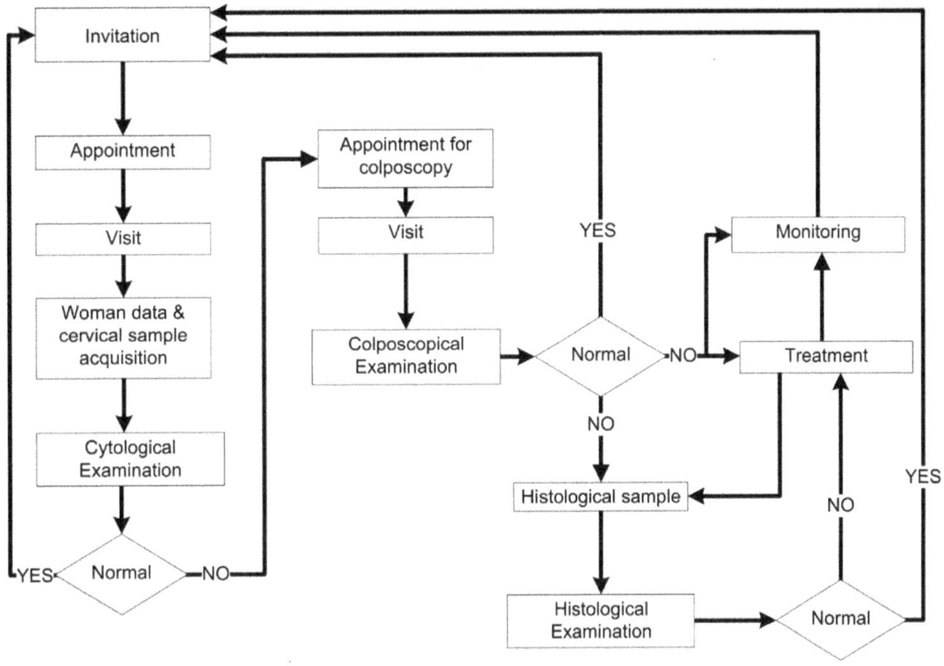

- During specific time intervals and depending on the woman health status of cervix and age, each woman is invited for the Pap test. This invitation is expected to motivate women to book a meeting to a health center and finally visit it for the Pap smear.
- During this visit, a specialist (usually a midwife or a gynecologist or eventually a nurse) records the woman's updated contact details, demographic data as well as her medical history. Additionally, a cervical cytological sample is obtained and sent to a specialized cytopathology laboratory.
- In the cytopathology laboratory, the sample is prepared (i.e. glass slide preparation, if required and staining) and subsequently is assigned to a specialized cytopathologist (in some countries nonmedical specialists – screeners are employed) for the Pap test. The result of this analysis is then sent back to the health center that the woman visited her family doctor, and in some cases the patient.
- The result of the Pap examination is necessary for the subsequent woman management. According to this outcome, the time that the next invitation will be sent to the woman is decided. Moreover, it is determined if it is necessary to perform additional examinations. For example, to repeat the Pap test in a short period or to perform a colposcopic examination, sometimes including a biopsy. An abnormal result of the Pap smear poses different requirements for the woman management. Usually, the process points towards a review by a certified colposcopist (gynecological subspecialty) or to repeating the Pap test in a short time (usually six months). In the first case, a new visit to the colposcopy clinic is arranged. If there is a normal result, the woman can be assigned to the usual cycle of invitations. However, in the case that the colposcopy result is abnormal a new sample, this time, a tissue sample from the cervix (i.e. biopsy) is obtained and subsequently sent to a histology laboratory for further examination.

- The result of the histological examination is then sent both to the health center that treats the woman and to the colposcopy clinic.
- If there are abnormal histological results, the colposcopy clinic is set accountable for the care of the woman (i.e. becomes the Accountable Care organization-ACO according to PHM) and her treatment. If the histopathology result is within the normal limits, then the woman may return to the standard cycle and wait for the next invitation for the Pap test. In an abnormal result, a new visit to the colposcopy clinic for treatment should be arranged, or a more frequent test Pap cycle can be applied. After surgical treatment, close monitoring for several years is required. In some cases, colposcopy is followed by immediate treatment (see and treat strategy).

This process is subsequently mapped to the 12 steps of the PHM roadmap; additional requirements are highlighted, and the design of an IT system to support such operations is proposed (Moumtzoglou & Pouliakis, 2015).

Organize Accurate Patient Registries

Each CxCa screening program starts with the definition of the population that should be under control (Athanasiadi et al., 2014; European Commission. Directorate-General for Health and Consumer Protection, 2008; Pouliakis et al., 2012). In fact, CxCa screening programs define, within the country, catchment areas. These are smaller geographical regions, used for finer control and precise management of the population and the screening project. That poses an additional requirement to store information relevant to the location of each patient; thus, GIS related information such as woman's address, including postal code and even GIS coordinates could be useful. The largest registry, therefore, is the population registry. Linkage of the IT system supporting the screening program to the national population registry is, therefore, an option. However, there are cases that such records are not always complete. A more practical solution could be the linkage with the registry of the social security number, which additionally provides a unique identification number for each person. This identification number is usually linked to the medical records of the women that, in fact, could be distributed in several hospitals around the country. The later facilitates the implementation of PHM concepts towards distributed, but accessible patient records.

The ICT system is required be linked to numerous other registries (Figure 2), depending on the availability of such systems, while the preferred method is to connect them, at a national level; otherwise, data should be stored and maintained within the CxCa screening program ICT system. As mentioned, the primary interconnection is with the population registry, since the country population is dynamic and always changing, and the participating women ages evolve, it is more practical to obtain demographic data from external records rather that maintain such data within the ICT database. Therefore, the ICT system would be more efficient if it accesses population information from databases relevant to new births, relocations, and changes in communication details (if available). In cases that population registries do not include death records, a linkage to appropriate registries is additionally required. A third, but crucial link is to cancer registry; thus, information related to CxCa (or cancers having as a primary source the cervix) can be retrieved. Nowadays, there are registries related to neoplastic diseases as well; in this manner, High-grade Squamous Intraepithelial Lesion (HSIL) diagnoses (a CxCa precursor) can be forwarded to keep up to date those registries.

Considering technology, there are numerous technologies available to communicate and exchange data. However, it is important to know which system initiates such data exchange; it is preferable that

Figure 2. Interconnection of the Screening Program ICT system with other systems. Lower part: linkage requirements due to the screening program, upper part: additional requirements due to PHM (Moumtzoglou & Pouliakis, 2015)

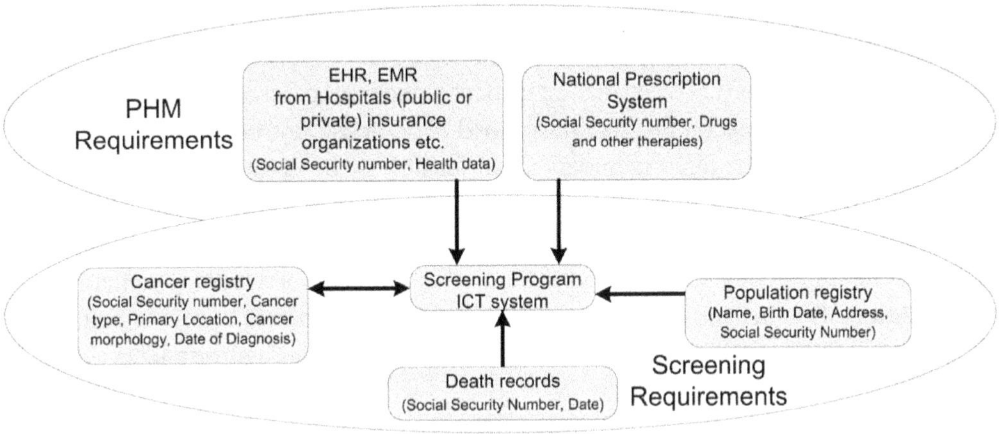

this communication be initiated immediately by the system that holds the new data or requests data from another system. For example, when a new cervical neoplastic case is found, it is the cancer registry that will initiate the communication and 'push' this information to the screening system (or make it available on request). In contrast, if the screening system has the capability to store locally histological results, it is the screening system that will initiate this communication and feed the data to the cancer registry. Of course, data integrity checks have to be performed automatically by a specialized algorithm; in cases of deviations or compromised data, human operators should be alerted and take action. Additionally, security of all communication channels has to be fulfilled by the use of adequate strength encryption algorithms and access control mechanisms.

The PHM requirements for sharing of information relevant to patients' health problems, medications, results from laboratory tests, and procedures, add another layer of information. Now (due to PHM requirements) it is necessary to have a more holistic and patient-centric approach; thus, it is not only the three links (population, death and cancer registries) required by CxCa screening programs that should be maintained. Additional links to obtain complete medical records, usually dispersed in numerous places, and should be held as well (see Figure 2 upper part). For example, links with systems storing prescription data and hospitals or insurance organizations maintaining EHRs. This requirement poses additional difficulties because the increased sources of data increase the need for data integrity checks and maintenance. Thus, data providers have to improve data integrity by increasing the amount of data provided preferably in discrete form (i.e. use formalization as much as possible and agree in advance the values of the various fields), and by the use of standards for data structures.

Decide Patient-Provider Acknowledgment

Identifying and defining the attributed providers, for each woman, seems to be a relatively easy process for a first look. The responsible team for every woman according to the CxCa screening workflow (Figure 1) is composed of the following team members:

- The midwife, nurse or gynecologist that performs a physical examination (macroscopic view) and obtains the cervical cytological material/sample.
- The cytopathologist that performs the Pap test.

In abnormal cytological cases the gynecologist involved in colposcopy that will treat the woman. Moreover, in extreme situations (i.e. when malignant or precancerous cases are found), the histopathologist and a surgeon, usually the gynecologist that performed the colposcopy, become members of this team.

Algorithms determining the team members seem feasible to be created and integrated into the IT system supporting the CxCa screening process because each health center (where the woman appears for test Pap or treatment) has associations with one or more cooperating cytopathology laboratories as well as one or more colposcopy clinics or outpatient offices. That is a necessity to handle the cervical samples and additionally to instantly arrange meetings for women requiring gynecological consideration. These associations can be used to propose automatically and even assign providers and clinicians to manage women.

PHM requirements, pose a requirement in the long term, to analyze patient visit patterns to physicians, in order to extract financial indices and evaluate performance. However, women participating in CxCa screening programs sometimes may have their own preferences to particular doctors (especially gynecologists). Moreover, an assignment to a particular doctor may be established or forced through the insurance organization that has a special contract with specific physicians. These two examples, exemplify this task of PHM requirement, even for women participating in a screening program Thus, although an IT system may have the potential to suggest and assign specific doctors, in reality, women may visit other health professionals. Under such conditions, the analysis of visit patterns faces difficulties. The most difficult issue is perhaps the collection of visit details of women to individual physicians, in public or private hospitals, or even physician offices. A potential solution appears to be the proposed link to the prescription systems (Figure 2), where those data are stored. Alternatively (or cooperatively), the establishment of legal frameworks, requiring recording of all visits and patient management actions to centralized systems for the entire population of a country could be of help.

Define Precise Numerators in the Patient Registries

This PHM requirement is pivotal in achieving physician involvement in patient management, as well as effectiveness. This requirement is relevant to the capability of the IT system to identify large cohorts of the participating women with some unique features. There are various reasons for a patient to be a part of particular groups and, unable to comply fully with medical protocols. This includes:

- Language and communication difficulties (for example, emigrants or patients with cognitive problems).
- Physical inability.
- Economic issues.
- Refusal to participate despite knowing the underlying danger.
- Religion reasons.
- Medication contradictions.
- Geographic reasons.
- Transportation barriers.

The European guidelines (European Commission. Directorate-General for Health and Consumer Protection, 2008) have already anticipated those situations, and have proposed guidance to handle them:

- Women with disabilities should not be excluded from screening because they are at equal risk to the rest of the population.
- Assessment of women having individual needs should be performed.
- Women who never had a sexual activity are at low risk (as HPV is mainly sexually transmitted); however, because this is subject to change, all women should be invited irrespective of their sexual history.
- Hysterectomised women are excluded only if surgery was not connected with cervical neoplasia. However, if the cervix is still in place, these women should be screened, because they can develop CxCa.
- Health professionals should be sensitive and trained to handle educational, linguistic and religion characteristics of women.

A structure to support such requirements in IT systems (Athanasiadi et al., 2014; Pouliakis, Athanasiadi et al., 2014; Pouliakis et al., 2012; Pouliakis, Margari et al., 2014) has already being proposed. The required data can be relatively easily obtained from participating women during their first visit, and stored in the database of the IT system supporting the CxCa screening program. However, this is only a part of the information that can be available for women as numerous other valuable data may be obtained from interconnected systems:

- Ethnicity can be provided from population or social security number registries.
- Mortality can be provided from death records or other sources that have such data.
- Women with hysterectomy can be identified from EHRs and women that had cervical cancer from cancer registries or registries of pre-neoplastic diseases, although such data can be provided by these women during their visits for screening.

As guidelines may change in time, an IT system compliant with the PHM roadmap should have a flexible architecture in many terms:

- Easily configurable to present new data.
- Linkage to new databases to retrieve information in a friendly and not time-consuming method.
- Reconfigurable algorithms identifying the population of particular groups.
- Alert generation and forwarding to appropriate health providers.
- Support to facilitate escalation of procedures when deviations occur.

This process can be summarized as follows:

- Data acquisition.
- Operation of algorithms to determine particular women and assignment of these to strata (by flagging) relevant to their risk level.
- Identify a responsible clinician and assign tasks.
- Alert both the woman and the physician.

- Follow the process according to already specified guidelines for patient management
- In the case of deviations alert and escalation procedures according to a specific workflow.

Continuously Measure Cost and Clinical Metrics

This activity of the roadmap is relevant to metrics of clinical outcomes as well as cost-effectiveness. According to the European Guidelines, the CxCa screening programs have challenges; there are multiple actors involved: patients, health specialists of different disciplines, technical specialties such as computer scientists and professionals from health and management authorities. CxCa screening programs have a nationwide scale, thus affect a substantial part of the population. According to the European Guidelines, the IT is essential for managing the screening program and for preferably automatic computation of numerous indicators. These can be used to measure the clinical effectiveness (Arbyn et al., 2007) of the screening method (Table 1).

Within the CxCa screening program, there are numerous indicators already specified by the guidelines (European Commission. Directorate-General for Health and Consumer Protection, 2008). A design of an IT system having the potential to extract automatically such indices has also been presented as well in the literature (Athanasiadi et al., 2014). The grouping of these indices falls into three categories: Screening intensity, Screening tests performance and diagnostic assessment and treatment. Unfortunately, the prerequisites and costs of the various activities within a CxCa screening program may vary substantially because they are dependent on screening technologies (for example, conventional vs. liquid based cytology tests have different costs); moreover, a different organization of the activities and a possible redistribution of resources within the healthcare system additionally affect the final costs. For example, differences in sample taking (midwives vs. physicians), in sample pre-processing (conventional vs. liquid-based smear or HPV test), screening personnel (cytopathologists vs. screeners), the volume and distribution of tests, the excess consumption of tests and/or treatment, affect the cost per woman and thus the cost-effectiveness measures (Hristova & Hakama, 1997).

In summary, the European guidelines do already provide a plethora of metrics for the clinical/health performance. However, there are no defined metrics for cost effectiveness. The PHM roadmap, under these conditions, adds another layer of metrics, i.e. the financial layer besides the clinical layer. IT systems supporting the CxCa screening program should be designed in advance in order to support such functionality. IT systems seem to face many difficulties in the analysis of cost metrics due to frequent changes. One solution would be to enter data to other systems; that will be responsible for cost related metrics calculations. Additionally, models for the financial layer must be continuously evaluated and

Table 1. Indicators of the effectiveness of cervical cancer screening methods (ranking)

1. Reduction of mortality (i.e. gained life-years due to screening)
2. Reduction of morbidity (i.e. lesions identified in early stage)
3. Reduction of cancer incidence
4. Reduction of incidence of CIN3 or worst (CIN3+)
5. Increased detection rates for CIN2+ or CIN3+
6. Increased test positivity with increased, similar, or minor reduction of positive predictive value

adaptable to changes this is due to advances in medical technology, changes in medical practices and frequently government regulations. Thus, IT systems either for the screening program or the cost metrics should have the capability to be easily adaptable/configurable to keep up with upgrades promptly.

Adhere to Clinical Practice Guidelines

PHM systems do pose requirements for the management of the population cohorts. Hopefully, CxCa screening programs have long-term well-established procedures for women management by a few characteristics; these include the age, Pap test outcome, colposcopy outcome, and histology results. The workflow described in Figure 1 is a relatively good mapping of the employed algorithms and their influence on the design of IT systems. The vast majority of screened women have a negative Pap test, and they will be screened after three to five years (according to the EU guidelines). The screening age starts at 25 or 30 years and ends to 60 or 65 years. Furthermore, there are guidelines from numerous organizations (Ebina et al., 2015; Massad, 2003; R. A. Smith, Brooks, Cokkinides, Saslow, & Brawley, 2013), and these are adopted, especially for the management of abnormal cases.

Irrelevant of the complexity of guidelines, they are well-designed algorithms that are easily implementable in any IT system. The difficulty on the part of the roadmap is related to the adaptation of IT systems to changes. Clinical practice guidelines are (not surprisingly) different from country to country; because they are associated with the availability of financial and human resources; and are sometimes revised frequently (Vassilakos, Catarino, Frey Tirri, & Petignat, 2015). The second reason for changes is the evolution of new tests. For example, there are numerous studies evaluating HPV DNA or RNA testing as biomarkers that have a role in disease diagnosis (Basu et al., 2016; Coquillard, Palao, & Patterson, 2011; Duvlis et al., 2015; Monsonego et al., 2012; Wentzensen, Schiffman, Palmer, & Arbyn, 2016). These new tests claim to replace the traditional Pap test or drastically change screening intervals and patient management as well. Moreover, there are algorithms for patient triage based on the cumulative evaluation of many biomarkers (Bountris et al., 2014; Karakitsos et al., 2012; Kyrgiou et al., 2016; Pouliakis, Karakitsou et al., 2014; Spathis et al., 2012). Irrelevant of the reasons, IT systems should be easily modifiable to support these different algorithms and patient management. An attractive approach seems to be the use of pluggable algorithms; having the capability to evaluate the status of each woman and produce an appropriate recommendation for the next management step (or steps). Moreover, this approach would lead to personalized management. Technological solutions do exist; for example, the web services approach provides a secure method, and there are open source projects for their implementation (The Apache Software Foundation, 2016c).

Engage in Risk-Management Outreach

As already mentioned an IT system supporting PHM should be capable of identifying and evaluating large portions of the population with distinctive characteristics (see the section: Define precise numerators in the patient registries). Such functionality is relevant to the patient data stored in the CxCa screening IT system registry. This step of the roadmap is beyond the registered patients; over time as patient-related data become richer and new risk groups may be identified. In this situation, the goal is to identify individuals proactively before they become members of the registry (i.e. to find women before they become patients).

The CxCa screening process is by its design related to this target, as Pap test, detect women before they develop the disease (i.e. when a non-cancerous lesion is detected); thus, there is the opportunity to act proactively either by close monitoring or by cure in the pre-neoplastic stage. The population involved in the CxCa process is enormous affecting all women in a country at the age of 20+. Additionally, the proposed data exchange schemes with population registries augment this data set to all females from their birth date, because they should be invited at the appropriate age. Thus, CxCa screening systems engage women before they become patients and fulfill this requirement by the concept.

In this aspect it is important to develop (and put in practice) predictive modeling algorithms that forecast which patients are likely to have the disease and, therefore, they may cause significant health costs. Algorithms to identify such cases even when there are missing data have been reported in the literature (Bountris et al., 2014; Karakitsos et al., 2012; Karakitsos et al., 2011; Kitchener et al., 2014; Komoto, Nishiwaki, Okamura, Tanaka, & Takebayashi, 2014; Kyrgiou et al., 2016; Pouliakis, Karakitsou, et al., 2014). Studies to relate CxCa with diet (Tomita et al., 2010; Ziegler et al., 1991), sexual behaviour (Natphopsuk et al., 2012; Price, Easton, Telljohann, & Wallace, 1996; Reiter, Katz, Ferketich, Ruffin, & Paskett, 2009; A. M. Smith et al., 2011) smoking (Natphopsuk et al., 2012), partner sexual behaviour (Niruthisard & Trisukosol, 1991) hygiene and other venereal diseases (Herrero et al., 1990) have been reported . Therefore, IT systems adapted to the PHM requirements should be capable of embedding intelligent algorithms within a fast changing environment and leading towards their continuous evaluation in large datasets. Under these conditions automated alert mechanisms should be in place, and moreover management algorithms should be supported by the system along with their close monitoring, in order to identify a population at risk even when there is no Pap test data. Obviously, the difficulty is to collect those personal data, online questionnaires publicly available may facilitate this process. However, women filling such questionnaires and have high-risk results should be facilitated immediately to arrange a Pap test meeting, i.e. by a few mouse clicks. The already proposed concept of pluggable algorithmic components in the IT system seems to be of interest in this case.

Obtain External Data

The PHM roadmap proposes the use of data stored outside the hospitals managing patients; this is due to the shift of healthcare from clinics to homes. CxCa screening is an extremely distributed process, engaging an organization body composed of health centers, cytopathology and histopathology laboratories and colposcopy/gynecology clinics distributed at a country level, either public and/or private. This part of the roadmap is translated to the solution of the problem of the acquisition of data outside of the organization body that handles a patient. Important data for the CxCa screening process are related to demographic information, educational status, nutrition, sexual lifestyle and habits, vaccination status and even financial status. A part of those data cannot be acquired from external sources but should be provided by the women during their visits. In contrast, this information may be available from national registries especially those of educational and financial status. The barrier for such implementations and interconnections is not technological. The process is complicated at the managerial level due to the business processes, the government regulations, the relationships among data holders, and the agreements for data sharing. Technologies, such as Web services, and mediation systems to databases, import directly database dumps, HL7 interconnections can be used to retrieve such data.

Exchange Information with Patients

Although the roadmap considers information exchange with the patients to be a low ranked step, in CxCa screening, it is fundamental. This is mainly happening because the screening process (in organized screening but not in opportunistic screening) is based on invitations (Figure 1). Therefore, it is crucial to organize well-established communication channels with participating women. IT systems supporting this process can have relatively easy functionalities to generate messages and moreover dispatch them electronically to participating women. Such methods include interfaces with e-mail systems (via well-established and secure protocols such as POP3 and SMTP) and SMS dispatch systems to incorporate the handheld device. User preferences should be respected. Thus, messages can be sent to women according to their preferences on the communication means. Other methods involve the generation of printable invitation letters to be dispatched via regular mail, especially for older women that are not familiar with digital technology. Fortunately, as the millennium population prevails, digital communication will prevail over traditional means. An advantage of electronic communication is their capability to supply delivery confirmation. In contrast, regular mail not only has an associated time delay but requires registered letters; this adds more cost to the screening program. Other communication methods may involve social networks and a tight cooperation and well-defined software interfaces with such service providers and systems.

PHM requirements pose even more intensive communication needs with women; the use of voice and video communication channels are of interest. To fulfill such requirements, women's records should contain extensive details for communication media, enhanced with IP-based communication tools. This anytime and anyplace communication tools can increase patient engagement and can improve health outcomes. Moreover, it is not only the one-way communication (health professional - woman) that requires enhancements; communication initiated by women have to be facilitated too. For this purpose call centers capable of all traditional and modern communication types may be operational, in order to receive requests and route them to specialized personnel. Finally, tracking of all communication activities should be maintained, as it is crucial to perform data analysis and improve this essential requirement.

Educate and Engage with Patients

The exponential growth of knowledge has nowadays made the health information complicated. Such complication generates confusion to women and leads to difficulties in the process of decision-making (Arkin, 1999). As already proposed in the previous section, there should be well-established communication channels which can be exploited for educational functions. For effectiveness reasons, the IT systems that support this process should allow tailoring of information provided to women according to their profiles and preferences; this is dependent on their educational background, age, language barriers, religion, and medical status. For instances, the educational material targeted to a mid-aged woman with CIN1 is not the same to the information that should be provided to educate a young pregnant woman harboring CIN2. The solution to this comes through patient stratification into groups, and the creation of appropriate educational material for each case, tailored for personal use. A model of building educational materials in a hierarchical method could be of interest. The use of multimedia content (according to the digital profile of the woman and preferences) is today preferable, because:

- Can be relatively cost efficient to be produced.
- Can be distributed via the Internet with minuscule cost.

- Can educate women in a shorter time than traditional leaflets.
- It is available on the mobile device and can be consumed immediately upon arrival.

Multimedia material coupled with the GIS capabilities of mobile devices is nowadays capable of containing useful links to arrange, immediately, meetings at the nearest available medical center as the modern mobile device is aware of the owner location. Summarizing, the communication facilities coupled with the profile of each woman and the use of intelligent algorithms may be used to tailor educational material and have a significant effect on the CxCa screening process through patient education and engagement.

Develop and Adhere to Complex Clinical Practice Guidelines

CxCa screening has well-established workflow and guidelines because it has evolved and matured since the fifties (Papanicolaou & Traut, 1941). Specifically, there are:

- Established protocols for reporting cervical pathology (the Bethesda classification system which has evolved) (Henry, 2003; Nayar & Wilbur, 2015; Solomon & Nayar, 2004).
- Existing tiered and stratified classification system for reporting histological and colposcopic outcomes.
- Guidelines according to HPV infection status, vaccination, age, pregnancy and cervical medical history.

As mentioned in section "Adhere to basic, clinical practice guidelines" medical protocols and guidelines should be embedded into the IT system, but this PHM requirement increases complexity. One important factor is that HPV infection (the cause of CxCa) is in the majority of cases transient. When there are more complex situations, for patients with co-morbidities (for example, immunosuppressed patients and women harboring HIV) there should be a different management approach. Today, there are not clinical protocols that account for patients with comorbidities. Usually, physicians are using their own approach to treating women or chain many protocols together. It is expected that guidelines will evolve because the medical literature becomes more focused and protocols to handle such complex situations will become available. Thus, IT systems supporting CxCa screening can have two roles in this environment:

- Collect data for women, either via the medical history provided during visits or from relevant registries.
- Alert physicians and enlist women in such groups, in order to be managed appropriately.

Moreover, by these two functions, useful data can be collected and via their analysis guidelines can be produced. Such guidelines should be 'pluggable' in the form of new algorithms (via the pluggable algorithm procedure).

To the authors' opinion, CxCa screening programs optimized for comorbidities and the relevant complex protocols will have a competitive advantage and will differentiate health providers both in cost and clinical effectiveness.

Coordinate Between Patient and Care Team

Modern medicine requires that each patient be at the center of a plan supported by many specialists, i.e. patient-centered care (Dalal et al., 2016; Gans, 2016; Sklar, 2016; Zhang et al., 2016). In CxCa screening, the vast majority is healthy women and not patients, which are examined at regular intervals for preventive medicine reasons. In cases of deviations (i.e. women not coming for their Pap test), they should be alerted in an appropriate manner and moreover motivated to return to the regular plan (an escalation procedure may be required, for instance, to start with a reminder e-mail or SMS and even be called by a health professional). In cases of women harboring cervical lesions, the supporting team is augmented and composed at least of two persons: the midwife, which has a close relationship with every woman and the gynecologist/colposcopic. In more severe situations, additional medical specialties are involved (histopathologist and surgeon). Modern medicine and PHM require that the team be well-organized and all actors (including the woman) well-coordinated and communicate. Therefore, the availability of communication tools and their capabilities, the completeness of patient data, convenient access to all data and additionally a tracking system capable of detecting deviations from targets are crucial.

Time is heavily involved because it is crucial for the patient's health; thus, the IT system seems to require project management functionalities. If this concept is applied, every woman is a separate project. This should have (as every other project): targets, tasks, milestones, risk management, and resources. Thus, modern IT systems supporting CxCa screening seem to require project management functionalities.

Track Specific Outcomes

Data analysis is a major PHM requirement which aims to the objective measurement and monitoring of specific results, for example, related to mortality, health status/morbidity, prevalence, patient experience, and costs. All of these are the cornerstone to the evaluation of efficiency and quality. As mentioned, EU guidelines have already provided detailed tables to measure the project results for the clinical aspect and not for the patient satisfaction and costs. Entities related to the implementation of such an IT system targeted to CxCa screening have been proposed as well (Athanasiadi et al., 2014). PHM pushes CxCa screening programs further; because the requirements for such analyses are not known in advance, i.e. during system design.

Fulfillment of this requirement seems to be out of the implementation scope of an IT system that supports CxCa screening, as the end users are management bodies (for example, the ministry of health). To support such functionality, rule engines can be used to integrate the numerous data types required to perform the analysis, and OLAP (on-line analytical processing) techniques are of interest to performing data mining and producing the required reporting. In that sense, the IT system should support random queries of stored information or information that has the capability to fetch and communicate/extract the data for further processing by external systems.

DESIGN AND IMPLEMENTATION OF AN IT SYSTEM SUPPORTING CxCa SCREENING

In this section, the various aspects of a system software architecture supporting CxCa screening programs as well as implementation details are presented. Special consideration is given on the reliability of the system.

System Design

The semantics of the IT system include: the patient (i.e. women that participate in the screening program) along with numerous contact details, the second semantic is the visit, being linked to invitations appointments and a multitude of information such as demographic data, medical history, biological samples and examinations such as cytological, colposcopic, histological and if required therapies. The third entity is the user linked with as roles, rights and work institute.

Numerous requirements are adopted from the European Guidelines (European Commission. Directorate-General for Health and Consumer Protection. & International Agency for Research on Cancer., 2008) as well as from the PHM requirements. According to these, the information system should be designed completely to support all the aspects and the workflow of the screening process and enable monitoring and evaluation. These functionalities include:

- Identify the target population that should participate in the screening program; this database includes the entire target population.
- Identify individual women in the target population, that are not screened or already screened, and identify women in special target groups.
- Produce and store invitations to be sent to the women in order to: i) invite/remind to visit a health center for the Papanicolaou test, and to re-attend for screening at the appropriate interval ii) support early recall, if required due to woman's characteristics; for example when being in a higher risk group.
- Recording the screening findings and identify further actions required.
- Monitor if recommended actions have been fulfilled by the women, and get information for further management.
- Provide follow-up for patients that have been treated.
- Identify cancers and deaths in the participating population.
- Permit linkage of individual screening episodes, and cancers and pre-cancerous lesions for quality assurance purposes and provide feedback to laboratories and clinicians.

Cytopathology laboratories are crucial in this process; laboratories are equipped with their own information systems which facilitate their internal workflow and support accreditation purposes (Pouliakis, Athanasiadi et al., 2014; Pouliakis, Margari et al., 2014).

Institutes, Actors, and Hierarchy

As depicted in Figure 1, there are many places involved in this process. In the proposed architecture, these places are called "institutes." The term involves all places that a system user may reside, i.e. health centers, cytopathology laboratories, colposcopy clinics, histopathology laboratories, etc.

Health centers are the first level handling the women. A health center is a part of a larger structure; actually health centers may be considered remote branches of hospitals and each health center is managed by a single hospital. Since health centers are places that women may book appointments and additionally medical tasks there are performed, it is required to have the personnel for secretary support as well as medical and/or paramedical personnel.

Similarly to colposcopy clinics is the second level for management; women visit colposcopy clinics for additional examinations and therapeutic measures if required, a colposcopy clinics are located to hospitals that are responsible for their management and are staffed by personnel for secretary support as well as medical and paramedical staff.

At the third level two types of laboratories are involved: cytopathology and histopathology, performing test Papanicolaou examinations and histological examinations respectively. These places are not visited by women but operate in the business to the business manner with the health centers and colposcopy clinics. For these laboratories secretary support to handle bureaucratic procedures related to examination results, specialized medical personnel for examination of the received samples and medical technicians for sample preparation is required.

The hierarchical organization of these institutes is depicted in Figure 3. Institutes belong to organizations; i.e. hospitals that manage health centers colposcopy clinics, and cytopathology and histopathology laboratories. At a higher level of the hierarchy is the management authority being responsible for many hospitals in a specific geographic region. According to the European Guidelines screening programs have catchment areas according to specific geographical borders and population limits. For such implementation, each management authority is responsible for a single catchment area.

Additionally, there are other actors not appearing in the workflow diagram (Figure 1), i.e. personnel for technical support, such as users' management, for example, user creation and assignment of rights and personnel accessing quality indicators and statistics for a single catchment area or at the national level.

Patient Entity Model

Due to PHM requirements, each patient should be accurately identifiable and moreover has much information related to communication capabilities and preferences. According to the proposed design (Figure 4), a patient should be linked with numerous telephone numbers, addresses, e-mails, insurance (either private or public) as well as identification data such as police ID card number, passport number, VAT number, Social Security Number etc. (these numbers identify uniquely each patient and split information of the same person to various databases or even to the same database). As mentioned in the PHM

Figure 3. Hierarchy of organizations involved in the CxCa screening process

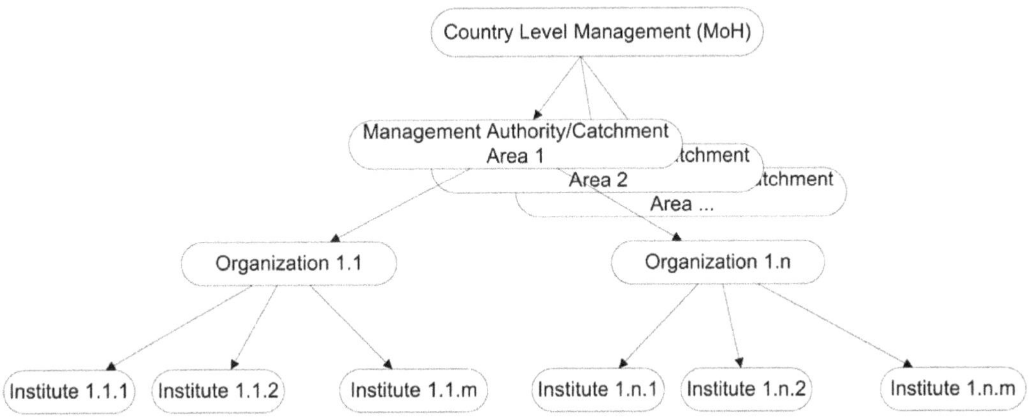

Figure 4. Patient model

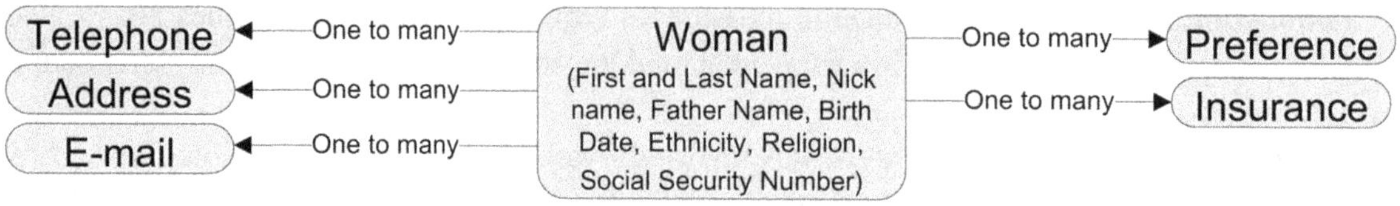

requirements, information should be tailored to patient profile and preferences. Thus, there should be taken special consideration to record the preferences, especially for methods that prefer to be informed for invitations, appointments, as well as the availability of Papanicolaou test results.

Visit Entity Model

Vast amounts of data relevant to the medical record as well as other personal information, such as demographic data of participating women, are created during their visits. In order to extract quality indices of the system, visits are linked to appointments which may be triggered by an invitation (see Figure 5). In detail, during visits, demographic information, the medical history record and medical information generated during the visit (or related to the visit) are registered. Specifically, the macroscopic view of the cervix, the result of the colposcopic examination and a biological sample, either cellular of tissue according to the intended test (Pap test or histological examination) are extracted. These data are mapped in the entity relation diagram of Figure 5.

User Entities and Their Roles

The user model (Figure 6) is not related to the patient. However, it is crucial for the system operation. Similarly to the patients, users have several contact details such as telephone numbers and e-mail addresses. The user "belongs" to one or more institutes (as a single user may visit several places for work duties) and may have one or multiple roles This is due to their job duties, but for system flexibility as well; for example, a midwife working in a remote health center with a limited number of participating women may act as secretary as well.

User rights are defined by their roles and are defined according to the CRUD operations (*C*reate, *R*ead, *U*pdate, *D*elete) on the patient and other system records as these are stored in the system database. For example, secretaries may have Create, Read, and Update rights on patient entities but no permission for Delete operations. Similarly, doctors may have Read and Update rights to such entities but no Delete and Create. Via this modular methodology defining CRUD operations for all system entities role rights can be identified and managed. Finally, a logging system of all user actions, a table that stores each CRUD operation on each specific system entity is required.

For the implementation of the workflow, a variety of user roles is required. That is essential to have a system capable of handling the processes and ensuring that each person has all the rights required to perform the assigned tasks, without compromising security. According to the role rights and the specific user various system, functionalities may be available or locked.

Figure 5. Visit model

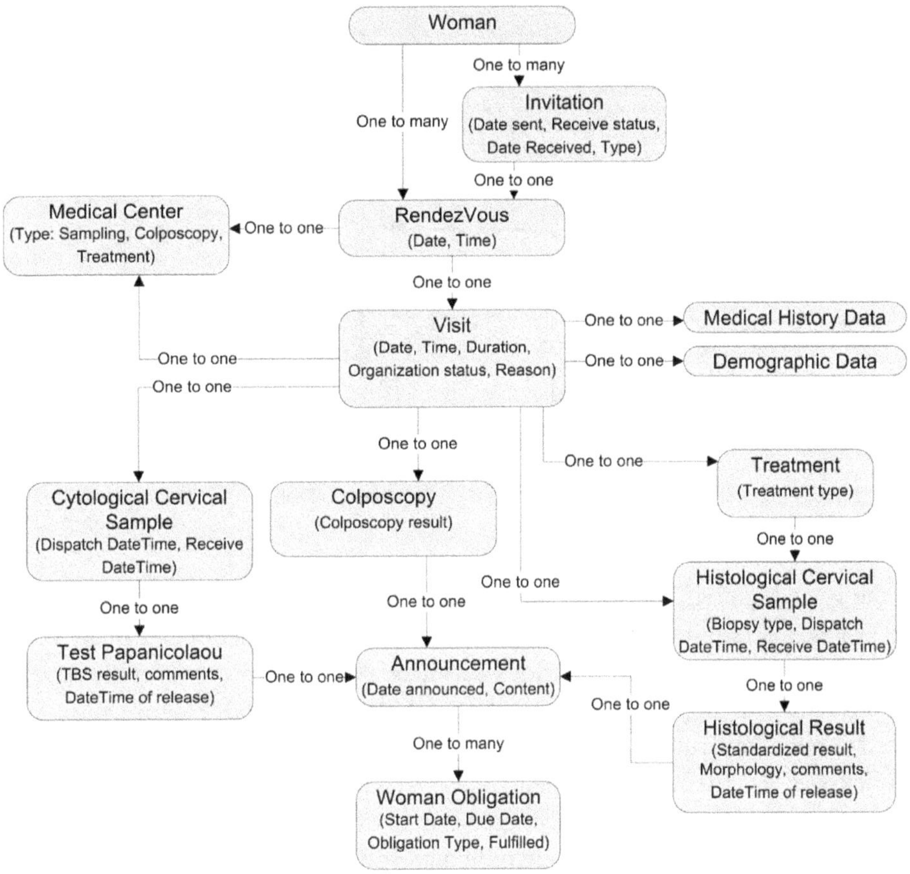

Figure 6. User model

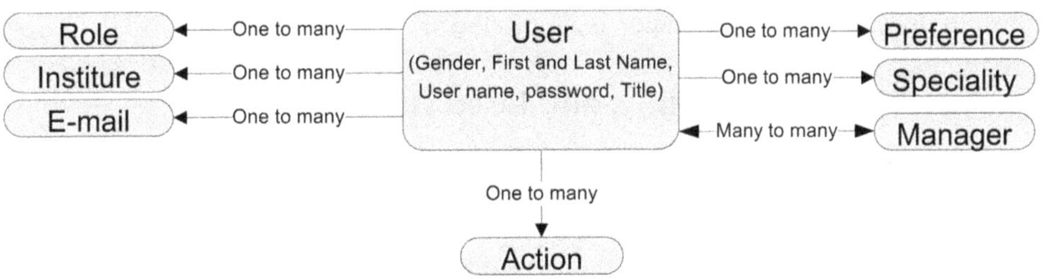

Implementation Via Open Source Platforms

Modern multiuser systems are based on a multi-tier web based system (Figure 7). Open source tools are capable of providing the required functionality and additionally to handle scalability and security. In such systems, the first tier is the web browser located on the user client machine; the second tier is the application server responsible for fulfilling requests from clients and providing responses and the third tier is the database server responsible to reliably store data and supply them to the application server

Figure 7. Architecture of a multitier system

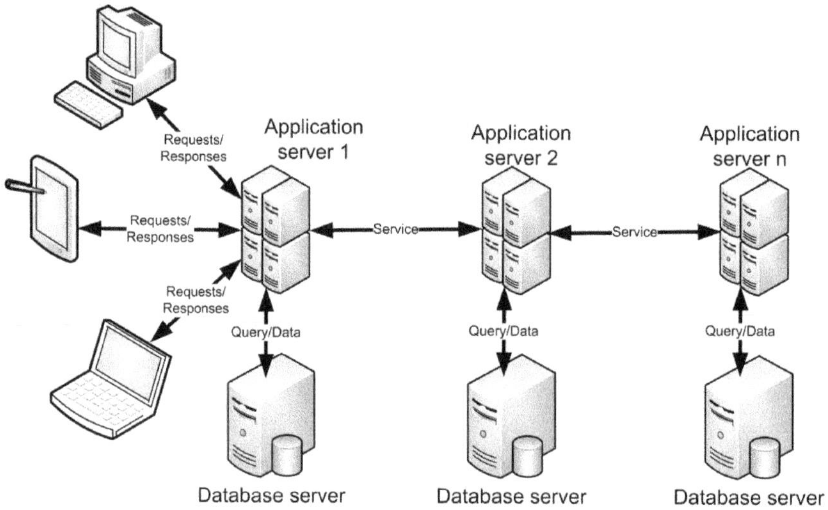

according to the issued queries. Data exchange for the purpose of PHM requirements and integration with other IT systems is required between the CxCa screening IT system and many other application servers in order to provide and request various services. For example, to provide new records in the cancer registry system or to apply for the patient record from a hospital.

Experience from the implementation of a prototype IT system to support the Greek CxCa screening program (Pouliakis et al., 2012) via the open source Apache Tomcat application server (The Apache Software Foundation, 2016b) and the MySQL community database server (Oracle Corporation, 2016b), proved that these two tools are adequate to handle data from hundreds of thousands of women and simultaneously support several tenths of users. The user interface is accessed via web browsers, is generated on the application server side and based on the Java programming language. Thus, changes to the system functionality can be performed on a single side and are immediately available to the end users. Therefore, system updates and maintenance is facilitated.

Reliability: Availability, Scalability, and Load Handling

Availability is the ability of a system to cope with and recover from failures of the host servers; either because of hardware reasons or due to failure of the operating system and the application software. High availability systems should be operational and reliable either when such failures occur or when hardware and other activities are required due to planned maintenance. Such activities should be transparent to the end users and may not cause downtime. High availability is crucial for a CxCa screening program smooth operation as it serves numerous users and participating women. Improvements for high availability may be performed by hosting the application server and database server in high availability machines or server farms having more than one network connections.

Scalability refers to the capability of a system to scale and handle the processing and communication load in order to adequately serve the users. This is translated to load sharing across multiple machines. In early stages of the CxCa IT system operation, the number of users is relatively low. At this stage, a single machine hosting both the Tomcat Application server and the MySQL database server is adequate. However in a large scale system operation, the computing and communication load becomes high, and an action plan should be available in order to maintain the system reliability. An escalation plan may have various steps, and the approach may be different depending on the following requirements:

- Split of the application server and the database server into two separate servers, as, in this case, their communication load between the application server and database server is increased, a high-speed connection (usually via a local area network) should be maintained between these two hardware components
- Additional escalation to support the load and increase system reliability may be performed by further split either of the application server or the database server or both
- Split the application server to numerous physical or virtual servers. The Tomcat application server by design supports load balancing, clustering and therefore mechanisms for failover (Lin, Funk, Curwen, & Maucherat, 2016; Sicard, Noel De Palma, & Hagimont, 2016; Viswanathan, 2001). The proposed solution is a creation of a server farm composed of many computers; this will not only distribute user load but additionally handle hardware of software failure in one or more computers. It also enables maintenance activities without user disruption. Application of load balancing or software connectors depends on the implementation of the solution (The Apache Software Foundation, 2016a).
- On the database server tier, the MySQL database is well known and already deployed for numerous applications which demand high availability. The MySQL system may support database replication as well as and geographically redundant, multi-server solutions. According to the MySQL 5.7 user guide, the uptime can be up to 99.999% (Oracle Corporation, 2016a) using the commercialized cluster edition.

CONCLUSION

Population health management requires healthcare providers to develop new skills and new infrastructure for delivering care promising a holistic approach and more personalization. In this context, mapping the population health management roadmap into the cervical cancer screening programs reveals the essentiality of a radical redesign for the following reasons:

- The number of data sources in cervical cancer screening programs should increase regarding their number and the complexity of data. However, the challenge is not technical as there are well-known and secure protocols to exchange information. The major issue is data integrity, automated translation in a standardized format and agreements between data owners.
- The IT systems should be easily reconfigurable to handle new data and incorporate new algorithms required at various levels. For example, protocols to apply and to identify patients in different risk groups.
- Data provisioning to external systems becomes more complicated, as reporting requirements and especially cost metrics is not included. Methods for self-describing data would be more efficient to fulfill this necessity.

Technology is not a barrier to the implementation of such systems, as open source platforms when employed in a multitier web-based architecture, nowadays have the capability to synthesize reliable, scalable and fail-safe IT systems capable of holding enormous amounts of data and serving simultaneously the number of users required to perform the CxCa screening process.

Concluding, CxCa screening programs, and the relevant information structure have already incorporated, by design and their nature, many principles required by PHM. However, there is a lack of support for many requirements. Adaptation of such IT systems, to be fully compliant to PHM needs, requires radical redesign, numerous interconnections to external sources of data and communication-related services, as well as continuous support and evaluation by the interested stakeholders.

REFERENCES

Arbyn, M., Herbert, A., Schenck, U., Nieminen, P., Jordan, J., McGoogan, E., & Martin-Hirsch, P. et al. (2007). European guidelines for quality assurance in cervical cancer screening: Recommendations for collecting samples for conventional and liquid-based cytology. *Cytopathology*, *18*(3), 133–139. doi:10.1111/j.1365-2303.2007.00464.x PMID:17573762

Arkin, E. B. (1999). Cancer risk communication-what we know. *Journal of the National Cancer Institute. Monographs*, *1999*(25), 182–185. doi:10.1093/oxfordjournals.jncimonographs.a024200 PMID:10854479

Athanasiadi, E., Pouliakis, A., Bilirakis, E., Fragoulakis, V., Bilirakis, C., & Karakitsos, P. (2014). Quality Indicators for Cervical Cancer Screening Programs: The Role of Computerized Systems.[IJRQEH]. *International Journal of Reliable and Quality E-Healthcare*, *3*(4), 19–37. doi:10.4018/ijrqeh.2014100102

Basu, P., Banerjee, D., Mittal, S., Dutta, S., Ghosh, I., Chowdhury, N., & Ratnam, S. et al. (2016). Sensitivity of APTIMA HPV E6/E7 mRNA test in comparison with hybrid capture 2 HPV DNA test for detection of high risk oncogenic human papillomavirus in 396 biopsy confirmed cervical cancers. *Journal of Medical Virology*, *88*(7), 1271–1278. doi:10.1002/jmv.24453 PMID:26693677

Bountris, P., Haritou, M., Pouliakis, A., Margari, N., Kyrgiou, M., Spathis, A., & Koutsouris, D. D. et al. (2014). An intelligent clinical decision support system for patient-specific predictions to improve cervical intraepithelial neoplasia detection. *Biomed Res Int*, *341483*. doi:10.1155/2014/341483 PMID:24812614

Care Continuum Alliance. (2012). *Advancing the Population Health Improvement Model.* Retrieved from http://www.fiercehealthit.com/story/hennepin-health-project-looks-build-countywide-ehr-program-national-implica/2012-01-10

Coquillard, G., Palao, B., & Patterson, B. K. (2011). Quantification of intracellular HPV E6/E7 mRNA expression increases the specificity and positive predictive value of cervical cancer screening compared to HPV DNA. *Gynecologic Oncology*, *120*(1), 89–93. doi:10.1016/j.ygyno.2010.09.013 PMID:20950847

Coughlin, J. F., Pope, J. E., & Leedle, B. R. Jr. (2006). Old Age, New Technology, and Future Innovations in Disease Management and Home Health Care. *Home Health Care Management & Practice*, *18*(3), 196–207. doi:10.1177/1084822305281955

Cusack, C. M., Knudson, A. D., Kronstadt, J. L., Singer, R. F., & Brown, A. L. (2010). *Practice-Based Population Health: Information Technology to Support Transformation to Proactive Primary Care*. Retrieved from https://pcmh.ahrq.gov/sites/default/files/attachments/Information%20Technology%20to%20Support%20Transformation%20to%20Proactive%20Primary%20Care.pdf

Dalal, A. K., Dykes, P. C., Collins, S., Lehmann, L. S., Ohashi, K., Rozenblum, R., & Bates, D. W. et al. (2016). A web-based, patient-centered toolkit to engage patients and caregivers in the acute care setting: A preliminary evaluation. *Journal of the American Medical Informatics Association*, *23*(1), 80–87. doi:10.1093/jamia/ocv093 PMID:26239859

Dunn, J. R., & Hayes, M. V. (1999). Toward a lexicon of population health. *Canadian Journal of Public Health*, *90*(Suppl 1), S7–S10. PMID:10686751

Duvlis, S., Popovska-Jankovic, K., Arsova, Z. S., Memeti, S., Popeska, Z., & Plaseska-Karanfilska, D. (2015). HPV E6/E7 mRNA versus HPV DNA biomarker in cervical cancer screening of a group of Macedonian women. *Journal of Medical Virology*, *87*(9), 1578–1586. doi:10.1002/jmv.24199 PMID:25880030

Ebina, Y., Yaegashi, N., Katabuchi, H., Nagase, S., Udagawa, Y., Hachisuga, T., & Yoshikawa, H. et al. (2015). Japan Society of Gynecologic Oncology guidelines 2011 for the treatment of uterine cervical cancer. *International Journal of Clinical Oncology*, *20*(2), 240–248. doi:10.1007/s10147-015-0806-7 PMID:25800808

Edwards, N., & McDowell, I. (1998). *Proposal for a Population Health PhD Program submitted to the Ontario Council of Graduate Studies*. Ottawa, Canada: University of Ottawa, Institute of Population Health.

Epp, J. (1986). *Achieving Health for All: A Framework for Health Promotion*. Ottawa, Canada: Minister of Supply and Services Canada.

European Commission. Directorate-General for Health and Consumer Protection. (2008). *European guidelines for quality assurance in cervical cancer screening*. Retrieved from http://bookshop.europa.eu/en/european-guidelines-for-quality-assurance-in-cervical-cancer-screening-pbND7007117/

European Commission. Directorate-General for Health and Consumer Protection., & International Agency for Research on Cancer. (2008). European guidelines for quality assurance in cervical cancer screening. Office for Official Publications of the European Communities.

Evans, R. G., & Stoddart, G. L. (1990). Producing health, consuming health care. *Social Science & Medicine*, *31*(12), 1347–1363. doi:10.1016/0277-9536(90)90074-3 PMID:2126895

Federal/Provincial/Territorial Advisory Committee on Population Health. (1994). *Strategies for Population Health: Investing in the Health of Canadians*. Ottawa, Canada: Minister of Supply and Services Canada.

Ferenczy, A., & Franco, E. (2002). Persistent human papillomavirus infection and cervical neoplasia. *The Lancet Oncology*, *3*(1), 11–16. doi:10.1016/S1470-2045(01)00617-9 PMID:11905599

Gans, D. N. (2016). Patient-centered care: A short-term investment for a long-term return. *MGMA Connexion*, *16*(2), 22–23. PMID:27049157

Glouberman, S., & Hayes, M. (1998). *Population Health, Sustainable Development and Policy Futures. A think piece for Health Canada*. Ottawa, Canada: Canadian Policy Research Networks.

Hamilton, N., & Bhatti, T. (1996). *Population Health Promotion: An Integrated Model of Population Health and Health Promotion*. Ottawa, Canada: Health Canada.

Hayes, M., & Dunn, J. (1998). *Population Health in Canada: A Systematic Review*. Ottawa, Canada: Canadian Policy Research Networks.

Health Canada. (1996). *Towards a common Understanding: Clarifying the Core Concepts of Population Health - A Discussion*. Ottawa, Canada: Health Canada.

Henry, M. R. (2003). The Bethesda System 2001: An update of new terminology for gynecologic cytology. *Clinics in Laboratory Medicine, 23*(3), 585–603. doi:10.1016/S0272-2712(03)00053-2 PMID:14560530

Herrero, R., Brinton, L. A., Reeves, W. C., Brenes, M. M., Tenorio, F., de Britton, R. C., & Rawls, W. E. et al. (1990). Sexual behavior, venereal diseases, hygiene practices, and invasive cervical cancer in a high-risk population. *Cancer, 65*(2), 380–386. doi:10.1002/1097-0142(19900115)65:2<380::AID-CNCR2820650234>3.0.CO;2-9 PMID:2295062

Hillman, M. (2002). *Testimony before the Subcommittee on Health of the House Committee on Ways and Means, Hearing on Promoting Disease Management in Medicare*. Retrieved 10 June, 2015, from http://waysandmeans.house.gov/Legacy/health/107cong/4-16-02/4-16hill.htm

Howe, R., & Spence, C. (2004). Population Health Management: Healthways PopWorks (Vol. 2). HCT Project. Retrieved from http://mthink.com/article/population-health-management-healthways-popworks/

Hristova, L., & Hakama, M. (1997). Effect of screening for cancer in the Nordic countries on deaths, cost and quality of life up to the year 2017. *Acta Oncologica (Stockholm, Sweden), 36*(Suppl 9), 1–60. PMID:9143316

Institute of Medicine. (2002). *The Future of the Public's Health in the 21st Century*. Washington, DC: National Academy Press.

Institute of Medicine (U.S.). Committee for the Study of the Future of Public Health. (1988). The future of public health. Washington, DC: National Academy Press.

Jemal, A., Bray, F., Center, M. M., Ferlay, J., Ward, E., & Forman, D. (2011). Global cancer statistics. *CA: a Cancer Journal for Clinicians, 61*(2), 69–90. doi:10.3322/caac.20107 PMID:21296855

Karakitsos, P., Chrelias, C., Pouliakis, A., Koliopoulos, G., Spathis, A., Kyrgiou, M., & Paraskevaidis, E. et al. (2012). Identification of women for referral to colposcopy by neural networks: A preliminary study based on LBC and molecular biomarkers. *Journal of Biomedicine & Biotechnology, 303192*. doi:10.1155/2012/303192 PMID:23093840

Karakitsos, P., Pouliakis, A., Meristoudis, C., Margari, N., Kassanos, D., Kyrgiou, M., & Paraskevaidis, E. et al. (2011). A preliminary study of the potential of tree classifiers in triage of high-grade squamous intraepithelial lesions. *Analytical and Quantitative Cytology and Histology, 33*(3), 132–140. PMID:21980616

Kindig, D. A. (2007). Understanding population health terminology. *The Milbank Quarterly, 85*(1), 139–161. doi:10.1111/j.1468-0009.2007.00479.x PMID:17319809

Kitchener, H., Canfell, K., Gilham, C., Sargent, A., Roberts, C., Desai, M., & Peto, J. (2014). The clinical effectiveness and cost-effectiveness of primary human papillomavirus cervical screening in England: Extended follow-up of the ARTISTIC randomised trial cohort through three screening rounds. *Health Technology Assessment*, *18*(23), 1–196. doi:10.3310/hta18230 PMID:24762804

Komoto, S., Nishiwaki, Y., Okamura, T., Tanaka, H., & Takebayashi, T. (2014). Effect size and cost-effectiveness estimates of breast and cervical cancer screening reminders by population size through complete enumeration of Japanese local municipalities. *BMC Public Health*, *14*(1), 43. doi:10.1186/1471-2458-14-43 PMID:24433346

Koshiol, J., Lindsay, L., Pimenta, J. M., Poole, C., Jenkins, D., & Smith, J. S. (2008). Persistent human papillomavirus infection and cervical neoplasia: A systematic review and meta-analysis. *American Journal of Epidemiology*, *168*(2), 123–137. doi:10.1093/aje/kwn036 PMID:18483125

Kyrgiou, M., Pouliakis, A., Panayiotides, J. G., Margari, N., Bountris, P., Valasoulis, G., & Paraskevaidis, E. et al. (2016). Personalised management of women with cervical abnormalities using a clinical decision support scoring system. *Gynecologic Oncology*, *141*(1), 29–35. doi:10.1016/j.ygyno.2015.12.032 PMID:27016226

Lalonde, M. (1974). *A New Perspective on the Health of Canadians. A Working Document*. Ottawa, Canada: Minister of Supply and Services Canada.

Lin, P., Funk, T., Curwen, M., & Maucherat, R. (2016). *So You Want High Performance*. Retrieved March 28, 2016, from http://tomcat.apache.org/articles/performance.pdf

Malik, A. I. (2005). The role of human papilloma virus (HPV) in the aetiology of cervical cancer. *JPMA. The Journal of the Pakistan Medical Association*, *55*(12), 553–558. PMID:16438278

Massad, L. S. (2003). Guidelines for cervical cancer screening from the american cancer society: The Earth is moving. *Journal of Lower Genital Tract Disease*, *7*(2), 87–88. doi:10.1097/00128360-200304000-00002 PMID:17051050

McCance, D. J. (1988). Human papillomavirus (HPV) infections in the aetiology of cervical cancer. *Cancer Surveys*, *7*(3), 499–506. PMID:2854000

McGrail, K., Ostry, A., & Thomas, V. (1998). *Determinants of Population Health: A Synthesis of the literature*. Paper prepared for the National Research and Development Program, Ottawa, Canada.

Misra, D. P., Guyer, B., & Allston, A. (2003). Integrated perinatal health framework. A multiple determinants model with a life span approach. *American Journal of Preventive Medicine*, *25*(1), 65–75. doi:10.1016/S0749-3797(03)00090-4 PMID:12818312

Monsonego, J., Hudgens, M. G., Zerat, L., Zerat, J. C., Syrjanen, K., & Smith, J. S. (2012). Risk assessment and clinical impact of liquid-based cytology, oncogenic human papillomavirus (HPV) DNA and mRNA testing in primary cervical cancer screening (the FASE study). *Gynecologic Oncology*, *125*(1), 175–180. doi:10.1016/j.ygyno.2012.01.002 PMID:22233689

Moumtzoglou, A., & Pouliakis, A. (2015). Mapping Population Health Management Roadmap into Cervical Cancer Screening Programs. *International Journal of Reliable and Quality E-Healthcare*, *4*(3), 1–18. doi:10.4018/IJRQEH.2015070101

Natphopsuk, S., Settheetham-Ishida, W., Sinawat, S., Pientong, C., Yuenyao, P., & Ishida, T. (2012). Risk factors for cervical cancer in northeastern Thailand: Detailed analyses of sexual and smoking behavior. *Asian Pacific Journal of Cancer Prevention*, *13*(11), 5489–5495. doi:10.7314/APJCP.2012.13.11.5489 PMID:23317205

Nayar, R., & Wilbur, D. (2015). *The Bethesda system for reporting cervical cytology: definitions, criteria, and explanatory notes* (2nd ed.). New York: Springer. doi:10.1007/978-3-319-11074-5

Niruthisard, S., & Trisukosol, D. (1991). Male sexual behavior as risk factor in cervical cancer. *Journal of the Medical Association of Thailand*, *74*(11), 507–512. PMID:1800607

Oracle corporation. (2016a). *MySQL 5.7 Reference Manual*. Retrieved from http://dev.mysql.com/doc/refman/5.7/en/ha-overview.html

Oracle corporation. (2016b). *MySQL web site*. Retrieved May 5, 2016, from http://www.mysql.com/

Papanicolaou, G., & Traut, H. (1941). The diagnostic value of vaginal smears in carcinoma of the uterus. *American Journal of Obstetrics and Gynecology*, *42*, 193–206.

Pouliakis, A., Athanasiadi, E., Karakitsou, E., Archondakis, S., Mourtzikou, A., Stamouli, M., & Karakitsos, P. et al. (2014). ISO 15189:2012 Management Requirements for Cytopathology Laboratory Information Systems. *International Journal of Reliable and Quality E-Healthcare*, *3*(3), 37–57. doi:10.4018/ijrqeh.2014070103

Pouliakis, A., Iliopoulou, D., & Karakitsou, E. (2012). Design and Implementation Issues of an Information System Supporting Cervical Cancer Screening Programs. *Journal of Applied Medical Sciences*, *1*(1), 61–91.

Pouliakis, A., & Karakitsos, P. (2012). *Advantages Of A Hierarchical Software Deployment Strategy For The Hellenic Cervical Cancer Prevention Screening Program*. Paper presented at the 37th European Congress of Cytology, Dubrovnik-Cavtat, Croatia.

Pouliakis, A., Karakitsou, E., Chrelias, C., Pappas, A., Panayiotides, I., Valasoulis, G., & Karakitsos, P. et al. (2014). The Application of Classification and Regression Trees for the Triage of Women for Referral to Colposcopy and the Estimation of Risk for Cervical Intraepithelial Neoplasia: A Study Based on 1625 Cases with Incomplete Data from Molecular Tests. *Biomed Res Int*, *2014*, 914740. PMID:26339651

Pouliakis, A., Karakitsou, E., Iliopoulou, D., Koutsouri, G., & Karakitsos, P. (2013). *Roaming Women In The Hellenic Population Based Cervical Cancer Screening Program. Secure Access Of Medical Records And High Flexibility*. Paper presented at the 18th International Congress of Cytology, Paris, France.

Pouliakis, A., Margari, N., Spathis, A., Kottaridi, C., Stamouli, M., Mourtzikou, A., & Karakitsos, P. et al. (2014). ISO 15189:2012 Technical Requirements for Cytopathology Laboratory Information Systems. *International Journal of Reliable and Quality E-Healthcare*, *3*(3), 58–80. doi:10.4018/ijrqeh.2014070104

Price, J. H., Easton, A. N., Telljohann, S. K., & Wallace, P. B. (1996). Perceptions of cervical cancer and Pap smear screening behavior by women's sexual orientation. *Journal of Community Health*, *21*(2), 89–105. doi:10.1007/BF01682301 PMID:8728358

Reiter, P. L., Katz, M. L., Ferketich, A. K., Ruffin, M. T., & Paskett, E. D. (2009). Measuring cervical cancer risk: Development and validation of the CARE Risky Sexual Behavior Index. *Cancer Causes & Control*, *20*(10), 1865–1871. doi:10.1007/s10552-009-9380-5 PMID:19543986

Riou, G., Favre, M., Jeannel, D., Bourhis, J., Le Doussal, V., & Orth, G. (1990). Association between poor prognosis in early-stage invasive cervical carcinomas and non-detection of HPV DNA. *Lancet*, *335*(8699), 1171–1174. doi:10.1016/0140-6736(90)92693-C PMID:1971033

Sanders, D. (2014). *A Landmark, 12-Point Review of Population Health Management Companies* (Executive Report). Retrieved from https://www.healthcatalyst.com/landmark-review-of-population-health-management-companies

Schlecht, N. F., Kulaga, S., Robitaille, J., Ferreira, S., Santos, M., Miyamura, R. A., & Franco, E. L. et al. (2001). Persistent human papillomavirus infection as a predictor of cervical intraepithelial neoplasia. *Journal of the American Medical Association*, *286*(24), 3106–3114. doi:10.1001/jama.286.24.3106 PMID:11754676

Sicard, S., De Palma, N., & Hagimont, D. (2016). *J2EE Server Scalability through EJB Replication*. Retrieved April 30, 2016, from http://sardes.inrialpes.fr/papers/files/06-Sicard-SAC.pdf

Sklar, D. P. (2016). Giving Voice to Patient-Centered Care. *Academic Medicine*, *91*(3), 285–287. doi:10.1097/ACM.0000000000001080 PMID:26907893

Smith, A. M., Heywood, W., Ryall, R., Shelley, J. M., Pitts, M. K., Richters, J., & Patrick, K. et al. (2011). Association between sexual behavior and cervical cancer screening. *Journal of Women's Health*, *20*(7), 1091–1096. doi:10.1089/jwh.2010.2585 PMID:21682554

Smith, J. S., Lindsay, L., Hoots, B., Keys, J., Franceschi, S., Winer, R., & Clifford, G. M. (2007). Human papillomavirus type distribution in invasive cervical cancer and high-grade cervical lesions: A meta-analysis update. *International Journal of Cancer*, *121*(3), 621–632. doi:10.1002/ijc.22527 PMID:17405118

Smith, R. A., Brooks, D., Cokkinides, V., Saslow, D., & Brawley, O. W. (2013). Cancer screening in the United States, 2013: A review of current American Cancer Society guidelines, current issues in cancer screening, and new guidance on cervical cancer screening and lung cancer screening. *CA: a Cancer Journal for Clinicians*, *63*(2), 88–105. doi:10.3322/caac.21174 PMID:23378235

Solomon, D., & Nayar, R. (2004). *The Bethesda system for reporting cervical cytology: definitions, criteria, and explanatory notes* (2nd ed.). New York: Springer. doi:10.1007/978-1-4612-2042-8

Spathis, A., Kottaridi, C., Chranioti, A., Meristoudis, C., Chrelias, C., Panayiotides, I. G., & Karakitsos, P. et al. (2012). mRNA and DNA detection of human papillomaviruses in women of all ages attending two colposcopy clinics. *PLoS ONE*, *7*(11), e49205. doi:10.1371/journal.pone.0049205 PMID:23166611

Strike, C., Goering, P., & Wasylenki, D. (2002). A population health framework for inner-city mental health. *Journal of Urban Health*, *79*(4), S13–S20. doi:10.1093/jurban/79.suppl_1.S13 PMID:12473695

The Apache Software Foundation. (2016a). *The Apache Tomcat Connectors / mod_jk - ISAPI redirector - NSAPI redirector*. Retrieved May 9, 2016, from http://tomcat.apache.org/connectors-doc/index.html

The Apache Software Foundation. (2016b). *Apache Tomcat web site*. Retrieved May 8, 2016, from http://tomcat.apache.org/

The Apache Software Foundation. (2016c). *Welcome to the Apache Web Services™ Project*. Retrieved 4th May, 2016, from https://ws.apache.org/

Tomita, L. Y., Longatto Filho, A., Costa, M. C., Andreoli, M. A., Villa, L. L., Franco, E. L., & Cardoso, M. A. (2010). Diet and serum micronutrients in relation to cervical neoplasia and cancer among low-income Brazilian women. *International Journal of Cancer*, *126*(3), 703–714. doi:10.1002/ijc.24793 PMID:19642096

Vassilakos, P., Catarino, R., Frey Tirri, B., & Petignat, P. (2015). Cervical cancer screening in Switzerland: Time to rethink the guidelines. *Swiss Medical Weekly*, *145*, w14112. doi:10.4414/smw.2015.14112 PMID:25664576

Viswanathan, V. (2001). *Load Balancing Web Applications*. Retrieved from http://onjava.com/pub/a/onjava/2001/09/26/load.html

Wentzensen, N., & Klug, S. J. (2008). Early detection of cervical carcinomas: Finding an overall approach. *Deutsches Ärzteblatt International*, *105*(37), 617–622. doi:10.3238/arztebl.2008.0617 PMID:19471627

Wentzensen, N., Schiffman, M., Palmer, T., & Arbyn, M. (2016). Triage of HPV positive women in cervical cancer screening. *Journal of Clinical Virology*, *76*(Suppl 1), S49–S55. doi:10.1016/j.jcv.2015.11.015 PMID:26643050

WHO. (1986). *Ottawa Charter for Health Population*. Retrieved from http://www.who.int/healthpromotion/conferences/previous/ottawa/en/

Young, T. K. (1998). *Population health: concepts and methods*. New York: Oxford University Press.

Zhang, J., Chen, Y., Ashfaq, S., Bell, K., Calvitti, A., Farber, N. J., & Agha, Z. et al. (2016). Strategizing EHR use to achieve patient-centered care in exam rooms: A qualitative study on primary care providers. *Journal of the American Medical Informatics Association*, *23*(1), 137–143. doi:10.1093/jamia/ocv142 PMID:26568605

Ziegler, R. G., Jones, C. J., Brinton, L. A., Norman, S. A., Mallin, K., Levine, R. S., & Hoover, R. N. et al. (1991). Diet and the risk of in situ cervical cancer among white women in the United States. *Cancer Causes & Control*, *2*(1), 17–29. doi:10.1007/BF00052357 PMID:1873430

KEY TERMS AND DEFINITIONS

Cytopathology: A specialty of medicine related to the study and diagnosis of diseases by the examination of cells.

Health Promotion: The process of enabling people to increase control over, and to improve their health, focusing less on physical factors and more on lifestyle.

Information Technology: The use of computers, storage media, networks and any other physical devices, infrastructure and processes in order to create, store, retrieve, secure, process and exchange all electronic data in any form.

Population Health: A term with broader content, which is related to a field relevant to the study of several important factors for health. As a result, it involves many terms, such as outcomes, disparities, determinants, and risk factors.

Population Health Management: The aggregation of patient information (data) across multiple resources related to health information, the analysis of the data into a single patient record, and the outcome of the actions of health care providers which can improve clinical and economic outcomes.

Public Health: A term which connotes a relatively narrow field with activities carried out by agencies granted with official functions.

Quality Control (QC): The set of processes by which entities review the quality of all factors involved in product, service or activity, during QC processes, the products, services, and activities are tested or validated in order to reveal defects and problems, before their release.

Chapter 2

Healthcare Computer Reasoning Addressing Chronically Ill Societies Using IoT:

Deep Learning AI to the Rescue of Home-Based Healthcare

David Mendes
DECSIS, Portugal

Artur Romão
DECSIS, Portugal

Manuel Lopes
Universidade de Évora, Portugal

Irene Pimenta Rodrigues
Universidade de Évora, Portugal

ABSTRACT

The authors present a proposal to develop intelligent assisted living environments for home based healthcare. These environments unite the chronical patient clinical history sematic representation with the ability of monitoring the living conditions and events recurring to a fully managed Semantic Web of Things (SWoT). Several levels of acquired knowledge and the case based reasoning that is possible by knowledge representation of the health-disease history and acquisition of the scientific evidence will deliver, through various voice based natural interfaces, the adequate support systems for disease auto management but prominently by activating the less differentiated caregiver for any specific need. With these capabilities at hand, home based healthcare providing becomes a viable possibility reducing the institutionalization needs. The resulting integrated healthcare framework will provide significant savings while improving the generality of health and satisfaction indicators.

DOI: 10.4018/978-1-5225-1724-5.ch002

INTRODUCTION

The societal and epidemiological conditions in developed countries have progressed in such a way that the current Public Health Systems are not adequate any longer. There is an urgent need for systems to attend the chronic conditions instead of the acute events that the health systems were designed for in the middle of the XX century. In order to develop the requirements of these next generation public healthcare systems, formal ways of evaluation and scoring have to be set up that need to take advantage of some of the emerging technological breakthroughs at hand. Among these we aimed our work at joining the capabilities of having computable extended health/disease process knowledge enriched by IoT enabled ambient assisted living to acquire large numbers of health related events at population scale. Two sections in this paper are related to the different aspects of this question. First the Clinical Knowledge representation for reasoning and acquisition based in NLP (Natural Language Processing) and second the several questions that need to be addressed when applying the IoT and SWoT (Semantic Web of Things) in the healthcare process and the public system. Regarding the Clinical KR, we found that the problem known as "Knowledge Acquisition Bottleneck" (Wong, Liu, & Bennamoun, 2012) is currently the major obstacle for the development of adequate representations of medical knowledge computable representations, namely ontologies in the specific domain and in particular in the healthcare sub domain. Trying to devise a valid solution to that problem in order to enable clinical automatic reasoning either in a local, distributed or Semantic Web fashion, different sub problems had to be addressed and solutions found are proposed and summarized in "Our Solution" section.

The particular solution illustrated here is the extension of the usual DRS (Discourse Representation Structure) that usually handles single texts and our proposal that we named CIDERS (Clinical Integrated Discourse Enhanced Representation Structure) which has the extended capability of representing the whole discourse of a patient's clinical history.

First of all, we introduce the scientific question of overcoming the KAB problem and explain why it is so hard to overcome.

Next the solution proposed is detailed in its various problems, and pragmatic approaches taken for the problem's different facets.

The fourth section briefly explains the rationale behind CIDERS and why it may be a natural extension of the application of ACE tools in our work.

In the fifth section, we present the results obtained so far and explain the promising applicability to different clinical realities with expectable similar results.

We develop then the second issue addressed in this paper that is the utilization of the IoT related technologies in Ambient Assisted Living, with all the underlying issues and possible problems that have to be circumvented and propose ways of pragmatically handle them when needed and possible. We introduce the notions of emerging Intelligent Homes (vs. Smart Homes), and finally in the last section some conclusions are drawn and summarized from the various sections of the present paper.

NOMENCLATURE

AAL: Ambient Assisted Living
ACE: Attempto Controlled English
AI: Artificial Intelligence

BAN: Body Area Network
CAT: Computer Aided Translation
CIDERS: Clinical Integrated Discourse Extended Representation Structure
CNL: Controlled Natural Language
CORE: Clinical Observations Recording and Encoding
CPR: Computer Based Patient Record Ontology
CQA: Clinical Question Answering
DO: Disease Ontology
DR: Discourse Reasoning
DRS: Discourse Representation Structure
EHR: Electronic Health Record
FOL: First Order Logic
GS: Gold Standard
ICF: International Classification of Functionality
IE: Information Extraction
IoT: Internet of Things
KAB: Knowledge Acquisition Bottleneck
KR: Knowledge Representation
LAN: Local Area Network
MEMS: Micro-Electro Mechanical Systems
NLP: Natural Language Processing
OGCP: Ontology for General Clinical Practice
OGMS: Ontology for General Medical Science
OWL2: Web Ontology Language Version 2
SNOMED-CT: Systematized Nomenclature of Medicine - Clinical Terms
SOAP: Subjective, Objective, Assessment, Plan
TM: Translation Memories
WAN: Wide Area Network
WBAN: Wireless Body Area Network
WHO: World Health Organization
WS: Web Services
WSD: Word Sense Disambiguation

HEALTH-DISEASE PROCESS KNOWLEDGE REPRESENTATION

The Problem of Clinical Knowledge Acquisition

In the KR community of the AI science domain, recent developments are sprouting that lead to the establishment of expressive ontologies based in OWL2 as the foundation for distributed reasoning in complex domains in the Semantic Web (D. Mendes, Rodrigues, & Baeta, 2013). This approach has revealed a serious problem when trying to represent highly specialized and complex domains of science, namely the medical domain that is the "*Knowledge Acquisition Bottleneck*" (Wong et al., 2012). The ontology creation and development has traditionally been in charge of multidisciplinary domain experts that have to master both their particular scientific field and the ontology engineering novel techniques. These experts are very few and they are normally engaged in defining the ontological terminological structures of their domain ontologies, the TBox, and cannot be worried with the ABox to enrich the ontologies into KBs that can be automatically reasoned upon.

The Possible Solutions

The diverse solutions that appeared in the literature involve some form of automated acquisition trying to relieve the Domain Experts from the heavy burden. This is not obvious how to accomplish. We evaluated literature from the early (Studer, Fensel, Decker, & Benjamins, 1999) to the current methodological review (Zouaq & Nkambou, 2010) that focuses particularly on automatic methods for ontology learning from texts as they summarize the state of the art in natural language processing techniques, statistical and machine learning techniques for ontology extraction. The current methodologies are focused on the paradigm of domain modeling. They shift the workload for the domain experts, from the direct acquisition to the modeling, but fail to realize that a feasible solution lies in a two-step approach like ours. In our case we have a machine learning phase to tutor the model from some source reports, and then use the *Gold Standard*, partially enriched ontology, to trigger the automatic ontology learning from the full set of texts that represent the reasoning domain (D. Mendes et al., 2013).

Our Solution

To be able to use the reasoning techniques and methodologies that represent the state-of-the-art in the Artificial Intelligence domain we made a thorough inventory of biomedical ontologies currently available in OWL2 format. It was found that no solution for complete Clinical Practice representation is available with enough expressiveness in its foundation for exact clinical reasoning, and we introduced the OGCP presented in the next section (D. J. M. Mendes, Rodrigues, Baeta, & Solano-Rodriguez, 2015). Formal ontologies make the semantics of terms and relations explicit such that automated reasoning can be used to verify the consistency of knowledge. To express the richness of medical knowledge without any loss of intending meaning, a broad set of ontological relations, only expressible in OWL2 using *role-chains*, for instance, have to be part of our TBox and it will have a *SHOIN DL*. While this level of representational capability is compulsory for clinical reasoning there is also an important constraint relating to the usability of our ontology that is the need to have a near real-time classification complexity because it has to be very responsive in the interactive sessions that the doctors will use when using natural language questioning. We have to use pragmatic solutions to these real constraints and *OGCP* is formed of a dual capability because the ABox only possesses *EL++ DL* expressiveness. We use the ELK (Kazakov, Krötzsch, & Simančík, 2013) consequence based reasoner that has polynomial time response to classify on-the-fly the CNL assertions introduced interactively by the users.

Our pragmatic approach rests on the evidence that to overcome the *KAB* the tools available to the public, in general, have to be supportive in nature like:

- Being based on natural language interaction,
- Responsive in order to be accepted by the clinical community as a working tool, and
- Scientifically extremely accurate and self-evident because not even the slightest chance of error is acceptable in the medical domain and especially in healthcare.

Moreover, we accept as evidence that natural language is the *Lingua Franca* for communication among physicians, and we have to gather information in computable form from text that they traditionally use to pass their information. Thus, we can conform the scope of our work in:

1. Develop an Ontology suitable to model the healthcare processes accurately.
2. Develop a process for automatic acquisition of the ontology ABox from text.
3. Use this framework as support for natural language *CQA* to be used as an *AI* professional aid.

OGCP Ontology

Taking into account the considerations introduced in (Meystre, Savova, Kipper-Schuler, & Hurdle, 2008; Spasic, Ananiadou, McNaught, & Kumar, 2005) and more recently illuminated by the developments in technology and tooling as referred in (I. Yoo et al., 2012) we directed our efforts to finding the adequate ontology that does not fall short in particular issues of different medical specialties. To accomplish a successful work the resulting ontologies have to attain the sort of user-friendliness, reliability, cost-effectiveness, and breadth of coverage that is necessary to ensure extensive usage as introduced by (B Smith & Brochhausen, 2010). Considering that the amount of Clinical data digitally preserved in natural language texts is colossal and ever increasing, numerous problems have to be solved as reviewed by (Liu, Hogan, & Crowley, 2011; Meystre et al., 2008). Most of the clinical data is in text form coming either from typing entry, transcription from dictation or speech recognition applications. Accurate coding is necessary for comparability, auditability and last but not least important, accountability. We intend to figure out a *"picture of Healthcare provisioning"* through clear identification of the meaning of the available data and not only by the capability of cataloging and codifying that huge amount of data.

Ultimately none of the currently existing proposed ontology structures is appropriate for clinical practice knowledge representation and we introduce OGCP. The ontology alignment in our OGCP is not an issue as it results of the hard labor of the OBO Foundry (Courtot, Mungall, Brinkman, & Ruttenberg, 2011) that has established inter-operable biomedical ontologies since the advent of the Gene Ontology that dates back to 2001. All their work has been supported by the Ontological Realism philosophical principles since 2007 (Barry Smith et al., 2007).

We adopt the SNOMED-CT CORE subset as terminological source due to its full coverage, acceptance and applicability to our specific case. We explored thoroughly the CPR ontology (Ogbuji, 2011) and found it to be an adequate framework for full breadth coverage of the clinical practice but was lacking, however, the ontological relations needed to enforce any model of disease. CPR can be seen as an extensible framework to be heavily structured further by any suitable modeling upper ontologies like those that the *OBO Foundry* mandates. With the CPR as a healthcare provisioning representation support we still had to enforce any existing model for medical science, and we had the OGMS complemented with the DO to do so as a general practice model.

We have developed a full workflow to extract the "clinical process automatically" from SOAP reports. IE typically requires some "pre-processing" such as spell checking, document structure analysis, sentence splitting, tokenization, WSD, part-of-speech tagging, and some form of parsing namely for identification of strings representing quantities or abbreviations, as in laboratory results, for instance. The telegraphic form that is common to clinicians also poses some constraints to the usual NLP techniques used in other

Figure 1. Ontological structure of OGCP

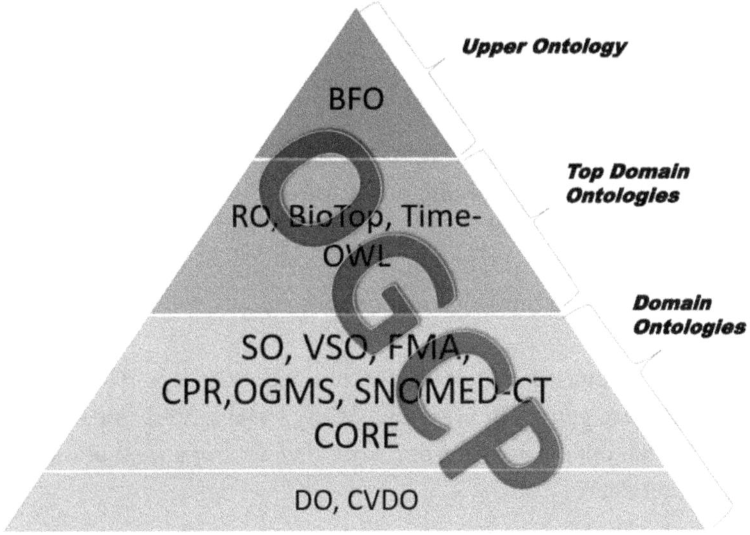

fields. We used this to our advantage tutoring a controlled translation to enforce GS TM that enables the subsequent automatic acquisition from the widely available text notes thus surpassing the KAB problem.

SOAP Reports

The SOAP note was first conceived by *Dr. Lawrence Weed, MD* in the 1970s, under the acronym Problem Oriented Medical Record (POMR). At the time, there was not an objective method of documentation, which led to physicians making unscientific decisions about patient treatment. SOAP notes gave physicians rigor, structure, and a way for practices to communicate with each other. In the early 1970s, the adopters of SOAP notes were able to retrieve all patient records for a given medical problem. Before Electronic Medical Record (EMR) software, providers had trouble accessing needed charts. Before standardized SOAP notes, providers communicated with each other in unstructured formats, leaving patient care up to a great chance. A SOAP note is a documentation method employed by healthcare providers to create patient's chart.

There are four parts of a SOAP note: Subjective, Objective, Assessment, and Plan:

- **Subjective:** Describes the patient's current condition in narrative form. This section usually includes the patient's chief complaint, or reason they came to the physician. It is normally the place for the symptoms brought in by the patient and includes:
    - Onset (when and mechanism of injury if applicable),
    - Chronology (better or worse since onset, episodic, variable, constant, etc.),
    - Quality (sharp, dull, etc.),
    - Severity (usually a pain rating),
    - Modifying factors (what aggravates/reduces the complaint activities, postures, drugs, etc.),
    - Additional symptoms (un/related or significant symptoms of the chief complaint), and
    - Treatment (has the patient seen another provider for this symptom?).

- **Objective:** Documents objective, repeatable, and traceable facts about the patient's status. Associated with signs including:
    - Vital signs,
    - Findings from physical examinations, such as posture, bruising, and abnormalities,
    - Results from laboratory, and
    - Measurements, such as age and weight of the patient.
- **Assessment:** The Physicians medical diagnoses for the medical visit on the given date of a written note.
- **Plan:** This describes what the health care provider will do to treat the patient, ordering labs, referrals, procedures performed, medications prescribed, etc.

This clinically oriented structuring is well known and widely accepted in the healthcare community, and text sources based on it are generally available. Many EHR systems provide a software module to create them. It represented an opportunity for our work developing a methodology to enrich our ontology from such an important source.

Tutoring Process

The first step in developing the automatic acquisition is a preparation process where the system is taught using some similar SOAP texts on how to properly identify and classify all the different segments. This preliminary phase needs to be done for every clinical reality that is to be subjected afterward of KB creation, for a specific doctor, a given service, a period or anything intended. For this preliminary step to be accomplished, we took inspiration for the supervised training in the development of a GS clinical annotated corpus presented in (Roberts et al., 2009). In fact, the set of the resulting TM obtained can be seen as a GS for the accurate clinical term identification. The process can be pictured like this:

Figure 2. Supervised translation memory(ies) (TM) training

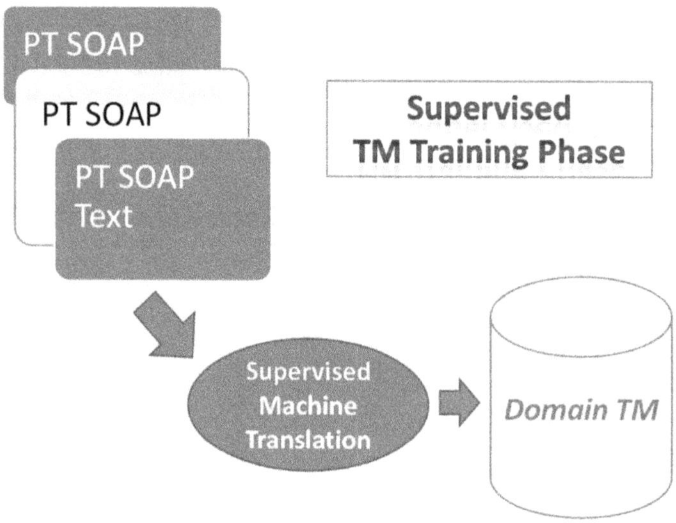

The learning process is based on the refinement of the Translation Memory(ies) (*TM*) applied to that specific acquisition. It can be seen as a "manual translation tutoring" although the focal point is not really the translation from different "natural languages" to English but, in fact, from the original controlled technical jargon to "specialized English". After the tutoring incremental process, the found acronyms, named entities, and clinical terms are ready to be adequately tagged in the process presented ahead in the next section for the correct Ontology Driven (OD) annotation.

The Automatic ABox Population Task

After using a relatively small, although representative, set of training SOAP reports the automatic process for the elicitation of the clinical reality represented by assertion facts into a fully enriched KB is possible and very effective. This high quality level is perceived by the users when interactively interrogating and enhancing the ontology but also by the preliminarily indicative, very good indices of recall, precision and F-Measure that are currently undergoing the process of comparative testing.

The novel scientific advance that enables these promising results is the dual *DL* expressiveness of our OGCP based KB. The ABox of the KB is *EL++* which is very effective computationally both in the acquisition and the classification processes.

Before entering the explanation of the pipeline proposed for automatic acquisition from texts the used tools and methodologies have to be presented. Both the Attempto Controlled English (ACE) set of CNL tools and Protégé views accessible through the ACE view plugin and the bag of Apache ecosystem of tools for NLP are used in this work. ACE is a precisely defined subset of English that can automatically and unambiguously be translated into FOL. Thus, it is both human and machine understandable. Teaching the construction and interpretation rules takes about two days (N. E. Fuchs & Schneider, 2006). ACE appears perfectly natural, but it is, in fact, a formal language. ACE texts are computer-processable and can be unambiguously translated into DRS. DRS derived from ACE texts have been translated into various other languages, for instance into FOL and for stable model semantics. The Attempto project (Kaljurand & Fuchs, 2007) developed a bidirectional translation of ACE into and from OWL2. This tool can be used whether locally, via the Protégé plugin, via a WS or through a Web Interface. We have been using it extensively through its various incarnations in our ontology modeling efforts. In concrete terms we used the ACE Plugin to derive all the inferable consequence rules for the TBox of our OGCP ontology in order for the posterior usability of the consequence driven reasoner ELK that operates over the less expressive acquired EL++ ABox.

We take advantage of the semi-structure of the SOAP reports to perform the population of the leaf-nodes of the KB with ontologically rich nodes. Clinical concept acquisition encompasses, in our view, the application of the notion of non-taxonomic roles extraction, which is ontological relations, from the sources. This theme has been extensively discussed in literature. Without non-taxonomic roles, ontology generation boils down to generating taxonomies that miss a lot of crucial semantic information compared to ontologies (Petrova et al., 2015), so we retrieve the ontological relations using this novel mechanism.

DR is built by the ACE Parser according to all the learned cases, the ABox, and using the OGCP KB available to build "on-the-fly" the Clinical Integrated Discourse Extended Representation Structure (CIDERS).

Figure 3. Knowledge base (KB) enrichment through interrogation

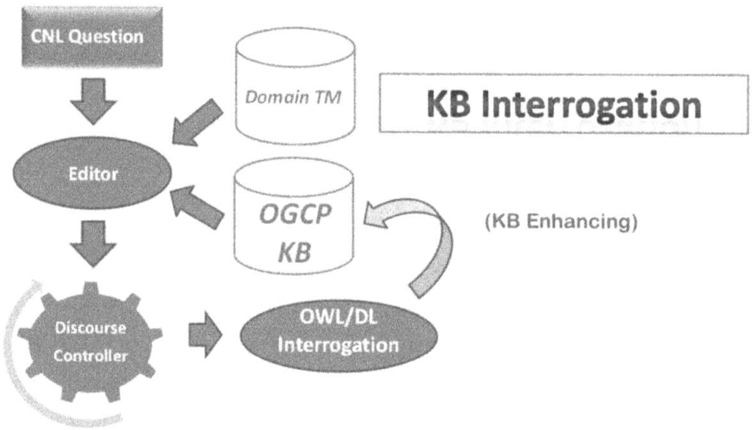

Interactive Extended DRS Aware Enrichment through CQA

All the possible consequences inferable from our base OGCP ontology, without any assertions included yet, are already incorporated because we used the mainstream Pellet or Hermit reasoners to develop all the consequence rules. This was a necessity for the ELK reasoner to have all the rules already "at hand" in order to expand only those EL facts collected in the ABox without compromising the scientific foundation of clinical reasoning. When using the, more than enough, SNOMED-CT CORE subset of clinical terms, full classification of the KB is done is some seconds and all the consequences were previously expanded so that the ELK reasoner only classifies the ABox when interactively the clinician poses *CNL* questions. *The answers are then provided in acceptable negligible time delays in commodity laptops.* We wrap-up here some achieved controlled results.

Q: What is the patient's personal history?
A: Hypertension for 15 years; Diabetes Mellitus type 2 for ten years; Cholecystectomy 2 years ago; Diabetic father; Obese BMI 26,5; Abdominal perimeter 106 cm.

This is a direct expression of the entailment of having several PH entries. The OWL verbalizer just tries to present the best possible, with higher usage evaluation in the trained expression in the time framing of the represented events in the OWL-Time properties related to that patient.

Q: What is the suggested diagnosis?
A: Laboratory routines: lipid profile; HgA1c; Rx thorax; ECG in rest; Echocardiogram; Effort test (Effort proof or Cardiac scintigraphy);

Suggested diagnosis triggers the mark words Suggested and diagnosis. With Suggested, ELK rules are automatically generated that try to satisfy the set of inferences that are consistent with the KB for every patient that has the same, or non-contradictory set of conditions modeled by CVDO on top of OGMS. Diagnoses suggested then are all those already part of the historical practice (ABox Clinical Integrated

Discourse Extended Representation Structure (CIDERS)) or enforced by the underlying ontological framework. The verbalizer then proceeds as in the previous example.

Q: What is the immediately recommended therapy assuming that AHT and Diabetes are not controlled?
A: Rich fiber and vegetable diet; polifraccionate and hiposaline; IECA or ARA II; Calcium Antagonist; Metformine; Estatine;

Here we have the most challenging inferencing situation. The sole generation of hypothesis based on the set of assertional *EL++* facts is not enough to sustain the question any longer. Rules generated in this situation explore the additional VNN ¬controlled(Diabetes) and ¬controlled (AHT) to trigger further rules in order to generate all the consequences consistent with the new negated hypotheses (that have to be syntactically pre-processed).

These are, of course, highly controlled results that are only possible, so far, under the interactive set of Protégé and the set of plugins detailed above.

CIDERS

The ACE web service that we use to automatically generate the DRS is fed with the extended scope conformed by the *"OWLification"* of the subsequent texts acquired, so far. All the acquired texts represent the known clinical history. The DRS forming abilities of the Web Service explained in (N. E. E. Fuchs, Kaljurand, & Kuhn, 2008) are thus enhanced to consider all the texts for word sense and discourse disambiguation, ellipsis and anaphora resolution,

The domain of discourse gets narrower as more and more texts are fed to the ontology ABox, and this renders the DRS more accurate as the ontology is enriched with more detailed clinical historical facts.

CIDERS can then be considered as an OWL clinical history that can be verbalized. This verbalization and OWL formalization functions as a discourse controller for Question/Answering enrichment and Clinical Decision Support System processes.

IoT TO THE RESCUE FOR INTELLIGENT LIFE EVENT ACQUISITION

Using the IoT in the Healthcare Process

The Internet of Things (IoT) is finding its most promising field of application in the development of AAL tools (Atzori, Iera, & Morabito, 2010). It is becoming gradually evident that the assistance needs for older adults have to rely upon automatization technologies to assist traditional human caregivers. These emerging widespread technologies available in "Smart Homes" can in fact enable less differentiated caregivers to provide assisted help. Hetero caregivers (formal and informal), if supported by technology can deliver better assistance if duly directed by evidence based AI tooling. This capability is especially evident in the vulgar case of multi-morbidity which is the most common situation amongst aging adults. The interactions of diverse drugs, therapies and other caregiving details that arise when co-morbidities are present, can be handled in an integrated form if a computer based Intelligent Healthcare Supervisor is monitoring and acting in the living environment. This assisted living environment comprises a multi-tier area network consisting of Body Area Network (BAN), the LAN and ultimately the WAN. In our case we suggest the usage of a highly secure hybrid cloud for the Docker/Container based virtualization to provide the needed distributed persistence where the reasoning is to be based upon. The reasoning capabilities, tightly related to the scope of the clinical knowledge (automatically) reflected upon, range from very severe alarms that trigger rules in the BAN like a heart failure, for instance, to evidence based reasoning available in a supercomputing framework that can reason over the overall clinical history and living conditions acquired that trigger highly sophisticated caregiving suggestions.

Event Acquisition in Assisted Living Environments

As seen in the previous section, our proposed systems possess the capability of reasoning about the health/disease process of a person due to the CIDERS representation acquired. This clinical history can be reasoned upon and continuously enhanced through the monitoring of the daily events and activities. To implement a controlled living environment, the usual approach is to augment a home with various types of sensors and actuators. These Smart Homes gather knowledge in order to provide comfort for the residents but can be used as well to assess the cognitive and physical health of those residents. Both the living conditions and the bodily signs and symptoms need to be controlled.

Sensor Enabling the Person and the Environment

Sensors are tending to be non-intrusive wearable and mobile. Most prominent emerging technologies range from MEMS to epidermal electronics that enable new health related sensors. Non-invasive sensors in form of patches, small holter-type and body worn devices as well as smart garments monitor health signals. Blood glucose and pressure as well as cardiac activity can be measured using wearables that use infrared, optical and oscillometric sensing. Table 1 summarizes typical wearable and mobile sensors (Memon, Wagner, Pedersen, Beevi, & Hansen, 2014):

WBANs enable wireless communication around a human body. Several technologies have been proposed to achieve energy efficient communication including (Ylisaukko-oja, Vildjiounatie, & Mantyjarvi, 2004) or (H.-J. Yoo & Bae, 2013). More recently, using the body tissue as transmission medium is being proposed. From the foundational thesis by Wegmüller (Wegmüller, 2007) to the more recent works like (Bae, Cho, Song, Lee, & Yoo, 2012; Vallejo, Recas, del Valle, & Ayala, 2013).

The amount and quality of continuous monitoring data is getting to paramount levels to what is duly considered Big Data and has to be handled as such. The huge data gathering can be pictured as an upward flow from the BAN to the WAN according to the architecture suggested in the beginning of this section. Caregiving rules activation represent the opposite flow of data/information/knowledge in a downward direction.

Healthcare Process Activation Ruling

For the upward flow of knowledge, a minimal set of information is collected to generate axioms in the Functionality Ontology (OF) developed to model the WHO International Classification of Functionality (ICF) (WHO, 2001). This information set on the inabilities to accomplish everyday living chores generates, when verified in relation with the healthcare process knowledge, the latest scientific evidence and the actual case based living conditions, the advising for the least differentiated caregiver. As an example

Table 1. Wearable and mobile sensors

Sensor	Measurement	Data Rate
Accelerometer	Acceleration	High
Gyroscope	Orientation	High
Glucometer	Blood Glucose	High
Pressure	Blood Pressure	Low
CO_2	Respiration	Very Low
ECG (Electrocardiography)	Cardiac Activity	High
EEG (Electroencephalography)	Brain Activity	High
EMG (Electromyography)	Muscle Activity	Very High
EOG (Electrooculography)	Eye Movement	Very High
Pulse Oximeter	Blood Oxygen Saturation	Low
GSR (Galvanic Skin Response)	Perspiration	Very Low
Thermal	Body Temperature	Very Low
Civet Fluximeter	Urine Flow	Very Low

Figure 4. Knowledge flow in intelligent assisted living

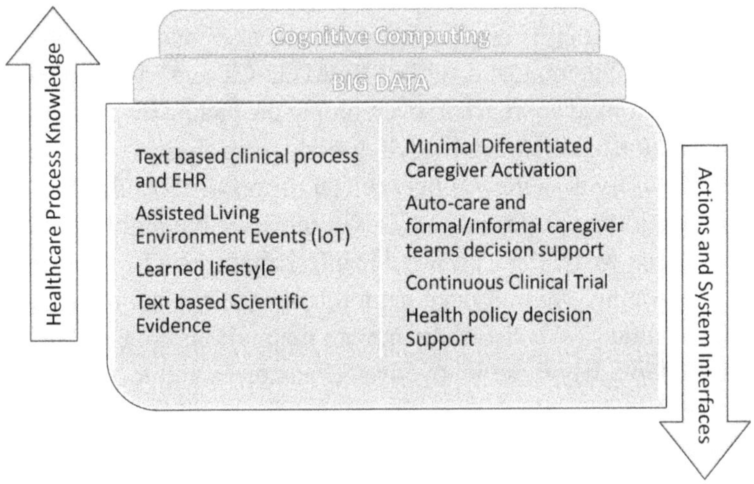

we usually use the simple reminder of an automatic phone call to the informal caregiver that some medication has to be taken at a certain hour. Also a record of the therapeutic adherence is maintained in the extended healthcare process in an effort to strengthen this adherence in the aged population.

From Smart Homes to Intelligent Homes

Apart from providing the connected reality to the physical world of the old person, the Smart Home is now able to provide counseling and support for the healthcare activities that have to be part of the daily lives of the elder. This is made through natural interfaces that expand the Smart Phone personalities into a truly health assistant. Different issues and obstacles to ICT adherence for elder people are addressed in literature from preliminary works (Loader, Hardey, & Keeble, 2008), going through important developments (Cocosila & Archer, 2010; Haux, Howe, Marschollek, Plischke, & Wolf, 2008) and policy conforming documents in the European reality (European Union, 2010) redounding in more recent overviews of the problem (Erden, Velipasalar, Alkar, & Cetin, 2016; Heart & Kalderon, 2013; Kozar-Westman, Troutman-Jordan, & Nies, 2013; Li, Lu, & McDonald-Maier, 2015; Memon et al., 2014; Mowafey & Gardner, 2013; Rashidi & Mihailidis, 2013). In our work developments we take in consideration the myriad of issues when developing natural interfaces directed to the diverse caregivers ranging from the auto-care to specialized professional teams. The domiciliation of care renders huge savings as has been already demonstrated (Fillmore, DuBard, Ritter, & Jackson, 2014) while, simultaneously, improves the perceived quality of care and raises globally the health indicators. This is all made possible by Healthcare Intelligent Homes that can contribute to resolve the chronically ill society that we live in.

CONCLUSION

We presented our proposal for an extended Discourse Representation Structure that is part of a knowledge representation infrastructure directed to QA interactive clinical decision support systems. These systems are enabling the usage of highly optimized distributed consequence based reasoners that were referred in the literature only in 2011. With these very recent developments it is possible to validate a controlled size knowledge base that is created by automatically populating a proposed ontology that relies on extensive, and very solid, foundations like SNOMED-CT and FMA among other OBO Foundry ontologies. We demonstrate a solid approach to overcoming the "Knowledge acquisition Bottleneck" by using an automated acquisition of very tractable KB directly from clinical text reports based on the well-known SOAP methodology. Dividing the KB between an expressive foundation (*SHOIN*) that relies on the coordination of OBO foundry ontologies and a less expressive but highly effective in computational characteristics (EL++) ABox we render a knowledge infrastructure with very interesting properties for CP representation and reasoning. We introduce natural language clinical reasoning aids that are based on such breakthrough techniques. We also show how to maintain the size of the OGCP ontology very limited in order to be able to apply these innovative AI advances and techniques in commodity hardware. Logical inferencing and clinical facts entailment that are possible through this novel capability is an interesting contribution to the application of AI to healthcare. We these tools at hand we delve into the field of Intelligent Ambient Assisted Living fueled by the IoT and raise the veil in our proposal for homes that can contribute significantly to a new wave of caregiving facilities that provide better quality of life for our elder population.

ACKNOWLEDGMENT

Acknowledgments are to be issued to DECSIS and Universidade de Évora that funded this project works.

REFERENCES

Atzori, L., Iera, A., & Morabito, G. (2010). The Internet of Things: A survey. *Computer Networks*, *54*(15), 2787–2805. doi:10.1016/j.comnet.2010.05.010

Bae, J., Cho, H., Song, K., Lee, H., & Yoo, H. J. (2012). The signal transmission mechanism on the surface of human body for body channel communication. *IEEE Transactions on Microwave Theory and Techniques*, *60*(3), 582–593. doi:10.1109/TMTT.2011.2178857

Cocosila, M., & Archer, N. (2010). Adoption of mobile ICT for health promotion: An empirical investigation. *Electronic Markets*, *20*(3-4), 241–250. doi:10.1007/s12525-010-0042-y

Courtot, M., Mungall, C., Brinkman, R. R., & Ruttenberg, A. (2011). Building the OBO foundry - One policy at a time. In *CEUR Workshop Proceedings* (Vol. 833, pp. 377–380).

Erden, F., Velipasalar, S., Alkar, A. Z., & Cetin, A. E. (2016). *Sensors in Assisted Living*. Retrieved May 30, 2016, from https://www.researchgate.net/profile/Fatih_Erden2/publication/297659778_Sensors_in_Assisted_Living_A_survey_of_signal_and_image_processing_methods/links/56e18f9508ae40dc0abf5111.pdf

European Union. (2010). *ICT & Ageing-European study on users, markets and technologies*. European Commission. Retrieved from http://scholar.google.com/scholar?hl=en&btnG=Search&q=intitle:ICT+&+Ageing+European+Study+on+Users+,+Markets+and+Technologies+Final+Report#0\nhttp://scholar.google.com/scholar?hl=en&btnG=Search&q=intitle:ICT+&+Ageing-European+Study+on+Users,+Markets+and+T

Fillmore, H., DuBard, C. A., Ritter, G. A., & Jackson, C. T. (2014). Health care savings with the patient-centered medical home: Community Care of North Carolina's experience. *Population Health Management*, *17*(3), 141–148. doi:10.1089/pop.2013.0055 PMID:24053757

Fuchs, N. E., & Schneider, G. (2006). Attempto Controlled English Meets the Challenges of Knowledge Representation, Reasoning, Interoperability and User Interfaces. American Association for Artificial Intelligence.

Fuchs, N. E. E., Kaljurand, K., & Kuhn, T. (2008). *Discourse representation structures for ace 6.0*. Department of Informatics, University of Zurich. Retrieved from http://citeseerx.ist.psu.edu/viewdoc/download?doi=10.1.1.148.6989&rep=rep1&type=pdf

Haux, R., Howe, J., Marschollek, M., Plischke, M., & Wolf, K. (2008). Health-enabling technologies for pervasive health care: On services and ICT architecture paradigms. *Informatics for Health & Social Care*, *33*(2), 77–89. doi:10.1080/17538150802127140 PMID:18604752

Heart, T., & Kalderon, E. (2013). Older adults: Are they ready to adopt health-related ICT? *International Journal of Medical Informatics*, *82*(11), e209–e231. doi:10.1016/j.ijmedinf.2011.03.002 PMID:21481631

Kaljurand, K., & Fuchs, N. E. (2007). *Verbalizing OWL in Attempto Controlled English* (Vol. 258). OWLED.

Kazakov, Y., Krötzsch, M. R., & Simančík, F. (2013). The Incredible ELK. *Journal of Automated Reasoning*, *53*(1), 1–61. doi:10.1007/s10817-013-9296-3

Kozar-Westman, M., Troutman-Jordan, M., & Nies, M. A. (2013). Successful aging among assisted living community older adults. *Journal of Nursing Scholarship, 45*(3), 238–46. http://doi.org/<ALIGNMENT.qj></ALIGNMENT>10.1111/jnu.12027

Li, R., Lu, B., & McDonald-Maier, K. D. (2015). Cognitive assisted living ambient system: A survey. *Digital Communications and Networks*, *1*(4), 229–252. doi:10.1016/j.dcan.2015.10.003

Liu, K., Hogan, W. R., & Crowley, R. S. (2011). Natural Language Processing methods and systems for biomedical ontology learning. *Journal of Biomedical Informatics*, *44*(1), 163–179. doi:10.1016/j.jbi.2010.07.006 PMID:20647054

Loader, B. D., Hardey, M., & Keeble, L. (2008). Health informatics for older people: A review of ICT facilitated integrated care for older people. *International Journal of Social Welfare*, *17*(1), 46–53. doi:10.1111/j.1468-2397.2007.00489.x

Memon, M., Wagner, S., Pedersen, C., Beevi, F., & Hansen, F. (2014). Ambient Assisted Living Healthcare Frameworks, Platforms, Standards, and Quality Attributes. *Sensors (Basel, Switzerland)*, *14*(3), 4312–4341. doi:10.3390/s140304312 PMID:24599192

Mendes, D., Rodrigues, I. P., & Baeta, C. F. (2013). Enrichment/Population of customized CPR (Computer-based Patient Record) ontology from free-text reports for CSI (Computer Semantic Interoperability). *International Journal of E-Health and Medical Communications*. Retrieved from http://www.ejhi.net/ojs/index.php/ejhi/article/view/194

Mendes, D. J. M., Rodrigues, I. P., Baeta, C. F., & Solano-Rodriguez, C. (2015). Extended Clinical Discourse Representation Structure for Controlled Natural Language Clinical Decision Support Systems. *International Journal of Reliable and Quality E-Healthcare*, *4*(2), 1–11. doi:10.4018/IJRQEH.2015040101

Meystre, S. M., Savova, G. K., Kipper-Schuler, K. C., & Hurdle, J. F. (2008). Extracting information from textual documents in the electronic health record: A review of recent research. *Yearbook of Medical Informatics*, 128–144. Retrieved from http://www.ncbi.nlm.nih.gov/pubmed/18660887 PMID:18660887

Mowafey, S., & Gardner, S. (2013). Towards ambient intelligence in assisted living: The creation of an Intelligent Home Care. *Science and Information Conference*. Retrieved from http://ieeexplore.ieee.org/xpls/abs_all.jsp?arnumber=6661717

Ogbuji, C. (2011). A Framework Ontology for Computer-Based Patient Record Systems. In *Proceedings of the ICBO: International Conference on Biomedical Ontology* (pp. 217–223).

Petrova, A., Ma, Y., Tsatsaronis, G., Kissa, M., Distel, F., Baader, F., & Schroeder, M. (2015). Formalizing biomedical concepts from textual definitions. *Journal of Biomedical Semantics*, *6*(1), 22. doi:10.1186/s13326-015-0015-3 PMID:25949785

Rashidi, P., & Mihailidis, A. (2013). A Survey on Ambient-Assisted Living Tools for Older Adults. *IEEE Journal of Biomedical and Health Informatics*, *17*(3), 579–590. doi:10.1109/JBHI.2012.2234129 PMID:24592460

Roberts, A., Gaizauskas, R., Hepple, M., Demetriou, G., Guo, Y., Roberts, I., & Setzer, A. (2009). Building a semantically annotated corpus of clinical texts. *Journal of Biomedical Informatics*, *42*(5), 950–966. doi:10.1016/j.jbi.2008.12.013 PMID:19535011

Smith, B., Ashburner, M., Rosse, C., Bard, J., Bug, W., Ceusters, W., & Lewis, S. et al. (2007). The OBO Foundry: Coordinated evolution of ontologies to support biomedical data integration. *Nature Biotechnology*, *25*(11), 1251–1255. doi:10.1038/nbt1346 PMID:17989687

Smith, B., & Brochhausen, M. (2010). Putting Biomedical Ontologies to Work. *Methods of Information in Medicine*, *49*(2), 135–140. doi:10.3414/ME9302 PMID:20135080

Spasic, I., Ananiadou, S., McNaught, J., & Kumar, A. (2005). Text mining and ontologies in biomedicine: Making sense of raw text. *Briefings in Bioinformatics*, *6*(3), 239–251. doi:10.1093/bib/6.3.239 PMID:16212772

Studer, R., Fensel, D., Decker, S., & Benjamins, V. R. (1999). Knowledge engineering: Survey and future directions. Lecture Notes in Computer Science, 1570, 1–23. http://doi.org/ doi:<ALIGNMENT.qj></ALIGNMENT>10.1007/10703016_1

Vallejo, M., Recas, J., del Valle, P. G., & Ayala, J. (2013). Accurate human tissue characterization for energy-efficient wireless on-body communications. *Sensors (Basel, Switzerland)*, *13*(6), 7546–7569. doi:10.3390/s130607546 PMID:23752565

Wegmüller, M. S. (2007). Intra-Body Communication for Biomedical Sensor Networks. *ETH*, (17323). http://doi.org/<ALIGNMENT.qj></ALIGNMENT>10.3929/ethz-a-005479240

WHO. (2001). The International Classification of Functioning. *Disability and Health. World Health Organization*, *18*, 237. doi:10.1097/01.pep.0000245823.21888.71

Wong, W., Liu, W., & Bennamoun, M. (2012). Ontology learning from text: A look back and into the future. *ACM Comput. Surv.*, *44*(4), 20:1–20:36. http://doi.org/<ALIGNMENT.qj></ALIGNMENT>10.1145/2333112.2333115

Ylisaukko-oja, A., Vildjiounatie, E., & Mantyjarvi, J. (2004). Five-Point Acceleration Sensing Wireless Body Area Network - Design and Practical Experiences.*Eighth International Symposium on Wearable Computers*. doi:10.1109/ISWC.2004.22

Yoo, H.-J., & Bae, J. (2013). Low energy wireless body area network systems. In *Wireless Symposium (IWS), 2013 IEEE International* (pp. 1–2). http://doi.org/ doi:10.1109/IEEE-IWS.2013.6616846

Yoo, I., Alafaireet, P., Marinov, M., Pena-Hernandez, K., Gopidi, R., Chang, J. F., & Hua, L. (2012). Data Mining in Healthcare and Biomedicine: A Survey of the Literature. *Journal of Medical Systems*, 1–18. PMID:21537851

Zouaq, A., & Nkambou, R. (2010). A Survey of Domain Ontology Engineering: Methods and Tools. *Advances in Intelligent Tutoring Systems*, 103–119. http://doi.org/<ALIGNMENT.qj></ALIGNMENT>10.1007/978-3-642-14363-2_6

KEY TERMS AND DEFINITIONS

CIDERS: A knowledge representation of the health-disease process that is acquired from text based sources of the clinical history.

Clinical Question Answering: The utilization of progressively more complex clinical questions posing by the users to assist in the deep learning question answering by the computer systems.

Deep Learning: Using an ontology framework for computer systems to be able of reasoning with the exact semantic meaning of the general available knowledge.

Health-Disease Process: The lifetime span of the health process that is subjected to care by the self, informal caregivers or formal health and emergency professionals.

Least Differentiated Caregiver: When applying the scalable model of caregiving based on the International Classification of Functionality emerges the possibility of pinpointing the exact caregiver for any given health event or need that can deliver the adequate response with the lower cost associated.

Wireless Body Area Network: The utilization of virtually noninvasive sensors to collect and monitor numerous health related signals and deliver them through a gateway to higher levels of knowledge aware reasoning systems.

Chapter 3
E-Health:
Modern Communication Technology Platforms for Accessing Health Information

Wayne Usher
Griffith University, Australia

ABSTRACT

This chapter will identify how Australian university students access and use various forms of technology (Web 1.0 – Internet, Web 2.0 – social media - SM) to retrieve personal health information. This chapter will move beyond Web 1.0, to present a theoretical basis of claim, concerning the extent to which other forms of technology (e.g. Web 2.0 and wireless monitoring devices) have impacted on youth. What is more, attention will be directed towards outlining to what degree this has shaped their patterns of health information retrieval. Importantly, this chapter aligns with contemporary literature that suggests a need for further studies into the area of human - technology interactions, which promotes sustainable action plans and strategies that will create and encourage reform throughout e-health programs and interactive communication platforms. Given that Australian university students are prolific users of modern forms of communication technology and that youth, in general, characteristically undertake relatively high levels of risky health behaviours and unhealthy lifestyle choices, such a chapter would seem warranted.

INTRODUCTION

There is limited rigorous cross sectional research, investigating and comparing Australian university students' and their technology usage to access health information. What is more, research outlining contrasting patterns of Web 1.0, Web 2.0 and wireless monitoring device adoption by university students to address chronic disease (CD) is narrow. Therefore, this chapter builds on past and presents contemporary research that outlines how modern forms of communication technologies are impacting on individuals' health information access, implementation and health care delivery into the early 21st century. Hence, a broad objective of this chapter is to address how emerging health technologies have the potential to manage CD and heighten health information access and dissemination. A more specific objective is to demonstrate how technologies, such as the Internet/World Wide Web (Web 1.0), social media (SM - Web

DOI: 10.4018/978-1-5225-1724-5.ch003

2.0), and various wireless mobile monitoring devices / platforms, are being collectively harnessed and have the potential to address Australia's CD epidemic, especially amongst youth.

The chapter is organized as follows. First, a synopsis of the current university students and Australia's CD epidemic is presented. Within this section it will be highlighted as to what are the major contributing risk factors and CD conditions represented both globally and nationally. Second, a summary of major technology (Web 1.0) innovations and university students' will be presented with further attention given to user trends. This section will draw on research by Usher et al., (2015) which goes to provide evidential baseline data concerning the current landscape as it stands. Such approaches are legitimised by drawing on past and contemporary research. Third, the remaining body of this section describes and discusses past research in the area of Web 1.0 and university students' usage trends and access to technology for the purpose of health information retrieval.

The fourth section gives reference to potential future research directions, with specific attention given to outlining how Web 2.0 technologies have created a new healthcare ecosystem. Emphasis is directed towards outlining how new communication technologies have heightened an active pre-eminence of health content creation, accessibility, delivery and adoption over passive content consumption. This section concludes by presenting how that enabling technologies, such as Web 2.0, offer for the first time the potential for individuals to be connected into a healthcare ecosystem that can deliver actionable information in a timely manner, overcoming the barriers of multiple data silos across many platforms.

Lastly, the chapter concludes by offering a glimpse into future possibilities surrounding emerging strategies, technologies and potential recommendations to heighten the uptake as to the sustainability of e-health and how they could potentially provide a framework that legitimizes university students' participation in discourses around health information access and implementation.

BACKGROUND

University Students and Australia's Chronic Disease Epidemic

University students typically enter a dynamic transitional period of new independence from their parents that is characterised by rapid, interrelated changes in body, mind, and social relationships (Pullman et al., 2009). Arnett (2000) has distinguished the period between ages 18 and 25 as a phase of "emerging adulthood," a liminal period between adolescence and adulthood. Although the university years are often viewed as a key phase for personal growth and development, they also represent a period of increased risk for injury, morbidity, and mortality associated with multiple health behaviours (Binkowska-Bury & Januszewicz, 2010). More precisely, many university students fail to meet recommended nutritional guidelines, have decreased physical-activity (Lowery et al., 2000; Hendricks et al., 2006; Reddy et al.,. 2011) and many first-year boarding university female students are significantly more likely to start binge eating (Barker, 2007).

Australian university students are becoming less physically active and have increasingly adopted a sedentary lifestyle centered on computer use and television viewing (Alricsson et al., 2008), leading to increased health risks. Correspondingly, chronic diseases are currently contributing to around 70% of the total burden of illness and injury experienced by the Australian population, with the expected proportion to increase to 80% by 2020 (Department of Health and Ageing, 2008). There are 8 identified health areas which contribute significantly to the burden of illness and injury in Australia, identified as National Health Priority Areas, these being:

1. Arthritis,
2. Musculoskeletal conditions,
3. Asthma,
4. Cardiovascular health,
5. Diabetes mellitus,
6. Injury,
7. Obesity, and
8. Mental health.

With a chronic disease epidemic emerging throughout the Australian population, Yee et al., (2008) argued that current health care delivery, management and education models pertaining to chronic disease and addressing health inequalities will not meet future demands, and that productivity and efficiency of future healthcare and education will be sustainable only if organisations leverage advances in technology (i.e. the Internet). As health provision moves into the early 21st century, it is important for health care providers to adopt new initiatives in an attempt to cater to modern health problems, chronic diseases, and escalating health care costs (Towards a National PHC Strategy, 2008; World Health Organisation, 2010). Such ideologies are underpinned by the perception that healthy lifestyles depend on the early adoption of healthy living habits and readily accessible information; unhealthy lifestyles among youths are strongly linked to unhealthy habits in adulthood (Lowery et al. 2000; Landsberg et al. 2010).

As young people are seen to be in a unique stage of knowledge absorption and personality shaping and are prolific in their technology usage (Anderson, 2001; Bernhardt & Hubley, 2001), it would seem appropriate that early intervention programs should be aimed at combining young peoples' health awareness and communication networks as a strategy for combating Australia's growing illness epidemic. Thus, the understanding and evaluation of healthy lifestyles and knowledge management via modern communication networks (i.e. the Internet) among university students are essential for the promotion of their healthy growth and for guiding early preventative programs. Furthermore, Landsberg et al. (2010) identifies that the university environment is an ideal and cost-effective means of developing healthy lifestyles.

MAIN FOCUS OF THE CHAPTER

Internet (Web 1.0) and University Students

With the advent of the Internet (Web 1.0), has come an increase in information retrieval. From its earliest conception and implementation, Web1.0 technology has become the information *ether* to which has permeated every aspect of society, with an unprecedented impact on the Australian healthcare industry. Kamel Boulos & Wheeler (2007) identified that the Internet has been presented as an enabler in health information retrieval and health care, for patients, organizations, clinicians and lay persons. What is more, such an invention as Web 1.0 has provided the necessary e-platform for creating and sustaining positive behavioural changes in patients suffering from CD (Ritterband, Thorndike, Cox, Kovatchev, & Gonder-Frederick, 2009). They go on to comment that:

Website use leads to behaviour change via different mechanisms of change (e.g., knowledge and motivation). Behaviour change impacts physiology and target behaviours to bring about symptom improvement, and treatment maintenance helps users maintain these gains. (p.20).

Usher (2009) supports such claims by identifying that individuals who access, understand and use health websites that possess a high degree of reliability, interactivity and are user-friendly, demonstrate a higher degree of self-efficacy when it comes to their individual health literacy levels.

Web 1.0 Usage Trends Amongst University Students

It is a given that university students use the Internet (Anderson, 2001). University students continue to be early adopters of new Internet tools and applications in comparison to general Internet-using populations (Johnson-Yale *et al.,* 2009). A recent report indicated that American college students were heavy users of the Internet, with 74% of the students surveyed reportedly using the Internet for "four or more hours per week" (Pew Internet & American Life Project, 2009). The Internet is increasingly becoming part of our lives, its use being centered on the younger age-group of citizens between 15 and 24 (90.3%) and between 25 and 34 years of age (78.3%) are Internet users. Correspondingly, as access improves into the early 21st century, people will increasingly use the Internet to find health information (Fox & Jones, 2009; Uden-Kraan, 2009). Research has indicated that between the years 1998–2005, the number of Australian households, with access to the Internet, rose from 1,098,000 to 4,039,000, a rise of 268% (ABS, 2005). Similarly, a recent Nielsen's Internet & Technology Report (2010) indicates that the average Australian Internet user spent 17.6 hours per week online throughout 2009, up from 16.1 hours in 2008. Consequently, with such exponential growth and access to the Internet, it is expected that online health information access and use will steadily grow throughout all Australian demographics; especially with university students. Furthermore, numerous publications (Nöthlings et al., 2010; Hu et al., 2011; Reddy et al., 2011) have shown that healthy lifestyle practices and readily accessible information / education do reduce disease occurrence and mortality rates.

Cain et al., (2009) posit that the transformation of health information dissemination is mirrored in the steady increase in access and usage demonstrated by individuals when concerned with the Internet. Commonly cited estimates over the years have suggested that more than half (Brodie et al., 2000; Fox et al., 2000) and as much as 80% of young adults with Internet access have used it for health care purposes. In a similar study, it was found that more than 60% reported that they frequently searched the Internet for information and that they used various search engines and multiple websites to find health information (Escoffery et al., 2005). For the past 20 years we have been immersed in what has been termed the 'information age', during which the availability of information of all types, including health information, has been greatly improved by the advent of computers and the Internet (Fox & Jones, 2009; Hitlin & Rainie, 2005).

Global and US health website traffic rankings reveal that individuals are increasingly accessing the Internet to find relevant and timely health information (eBizMBA – Rank, 2010), (See Table 1).

Table 1. Top six most popular health websites (2010) – Visitors / month

Website Name	URL	Visitors / Month
Yahoo!Health	http://health.yahoo.com	21 500 000
National Institute of Health	http://www.nih.gov/	20 000 000
WebMD	http://www.webmd.com/	19 500 000
Medicine Net	http://www.medicinenet.com/script/main/hp.asp	10 500 000
MayoClinic	http://www.mayoclinic.com/	7 000 000
Drugs	http://www.drugs.com/	6 000 000

Source: *eBizMBA Rank* – http://www.ebizmba.com/articles/health-websites.

Numbers vary and none are very accurate, but it is estimated that there are over 100,000 health-related websites on the Internet today (Risk & Dzenowagis, 2001), whilst health topics most often explored by young adults (17 – 25 years of age) include sexually transmitted diseases, diet, fitness and exercise and sexual behaviour (Borzekowski, 2001; Korp, 2006). From an American perspective, 80% of adults now have an 'always present' connection via wireless devices (Nielsen's Internet & Technology Report, 2010), with such increased Internet availability changing the behavior of health care consumers (Fox & Jones, 2009; Pew Internet & American Life Project, 2009).

The phenomena of modern communication technologies (i.e. the Internet) have been extensively researched throughout the world; especially undertaken in the United States and in European countries (Steptoe et al. 2002; American College Health Association, 2007; Laska et al. 2009), however, there is limited rigorous cross sectional research, investigating and comparing Australian university students' e-health knowledge management. From such an identified research gap, this study sought to determine the level of online health information usage trends by Australian university students.

METHOD

Data Collection

The survey was developed using the Lime Survey (www.limesurvey.org) on-line tool supported by the Griffith University Survey Research Centre. The survey was designed to collect both quantitative and qualitative empirical data and was hosted on the Griffith University website (Gold Coast campus, Australia). The survey was promoted via Facebook and 2 broadcast emails to students' email accounts who were attending Griffith University, Gold Coast, Australia (Arts, Education & Law). Questions were developed to achieve the stated research aim of the project. Ethics approval for the research was obtained through the Griffith University Office of Ethics (GU Ref No: EDN/18/11/HREC).

The main criterion to be included in the analysis was that participants needed to be currently living in Australia and they were a university student (either full or part time). A total of 365 responses was initially collected. Nevertheless, only 275 responses were included for analysis, with 90 responses being excluded due to either not meeting the selection criterion, limited detail associated with demographics or not a full survey completion.

Data Analysis

Data analysis was undertaken using Statistical Package for the Social Sciences (SPSS) (PASW18). Initial data preparation involved the development of 1 integrated SPSS file to incorporate all responses from the pilot and final survey undertaken. Initial data analysis used Frequencies to provide a profile of respondents by demographic characteristics (e.g. gender, age, course major, states where live) and questions relating to health / medical information used. Qualitative data were classified into groups and data analysis using Frequencies were performed. Chi-square tests were undertaken to assess factors that may differentiate females and males. Statistically significant differences were reported using $p < 0.05$.

RESULTS

Demographics of Participants

Two hundred and seventy-five (275) responses were received, with 82.5% of responses from female participants and 17.5% by male participants. The average of age of respondents was 24.45 (SD = 8.19). Participants were enrolled in a wide range of university programs, in which most of them majored in Education (41.1%), followed by Law / Criminology (13.5%) and Business (13.1%). Ninety-eight percent of participants lived in Queensland while 2.2% lived in New South Wales and 0.4% lived in Victoria. Table 2 summarizes the demographics of the participants, who are currently an Australian citizen and enrolled as a university student (either full time or part time).

Trends of Online Health / Medical Information used Amongst Australian University Students

A question was proposed to participants in an attempt to ascertain whether they have ever used the Internet to access health / medical information. Among the 275 participants, 90.2% of them revealed that they have used the Internet for finding such information, while 9.8% indicated they had never done so. For the latter group of participants, 50.0% of them stated the reasons as to why they have never used the Internet to search for health / medical information. These included that they: 1) perceived the Internet as an unreliable source (50.0%), 2) did not see the need for it (37.5%), 3) had no interest or curiosity for the topic (8.3%) and 4) never thought of searching the Internet for such a topic (4.2%).

For participants (n = 248) who stated they have used the Internet as a means for sourcing health / medical information, they were then asked to rank the top 3 ways they used the Internet to find such information. The top 3 methods were:

1. A random search engine (Google, AltaVista, Yahoo) (83.3%),
2. A referral from media communications (television, magazine, radio, and social media) (27.0%), and
3. A referral from a friend (26.5%) (See Table 3).

Table 2. Demographic information of participants

	N	%
Gender		
Female	227	82.5
Male	48	17.5
Course Major		
Education	113	41.1
Law/Criminology	37	13.5
Journalism	10	3.6
Arts/Design	14	5.1
Music	9	3.3
Psychology	6	2.2
Sociology	3	3.0
Media/Communication	20	7.3
Photography	5	1.8
Environmental Science	1	0.4
Languages/Linguistics	4	1.5
Business	36	13.1
	17	6.2
States Where Live		
NSW	6	2.2
QLD	268	97.5
VIC	1	0.4
	M	**SD**
Age	24.45	8.19

Table 3. Top 3 ways to search for health/medical information (Total response number for top 1 = 242, top 2 = 218, top 3 = 204)

	1st Method		**2nd Method**		**3rd Method**	
	N	**%**	**N**	**%**	**N**	**%**
A random search engine	**204**	**83.3**	12	5.2	13	5.8
A referral from family member	13	5.3	51	21.9	43	19.0
A referral from friend	1	0.4	31	13.3	**60**	**26.5**
A referral from lecturer	1	0.4	10	4.3	4	1.8
A referral from health professional	12	4.9	59	25.3	43	19.0
A referral from media	2	0.8	**63**	**27.0**	57	25.2
A referral from book	1	0.4	2	0.9	0	0
Other way	11	4.5	3	1.3	2	0.9
None	0	0	2	0.9	4	1.8

Participants, who stated they have accessed online health / medical information (n = 248), were also asked to indicate how often they would search the Internet for health / medical information and how much time they spent reading it once they accessed the information. Interestingly, data from this study revealed that the majority of respondents searched for health information:

1. Every few months (44.6%),
2. At least once per month (15.7%) and
3. A few times per month (11.2%).

Further data also indicated that once they accessed the information, they would mostly spend:

1. More than 1-15 minutes (40.9%),
2. More than 15-30 minutes (33.1%) and
3. More than 30-60 minutes (19.4%) reading the information.

In addition, participants were asked to rank, from 6 core health categories (See Table 4), the top 3 types of health information they would mainly access and read from the Internet.

Among the 248 participants in the group (who had previously used online information), only 244 of them responded to this question. Table 4 identifies that the top 3 rankings were: 1) specific diseases (n = 97, 39.8%), 2) medical treatment (n = 62, 25.4%) and 3) health services (n = 52, 21.3%). Qualitative data identified those participants who indicated 'other information' revealed a curiosity about symptoms, diagnosis, nutrition / dietary, pregnancy and personal health issues.

Related to the 6 core health categories, participants were then asked to elaborate on each health category, providing further specific detail. On each of the 6 health categories, participants provided specific information which was then grouped into smaller categories, upon which the top 3 most often stated were chosen. The top 3 most often searched health topics, from each of the 6 core health categories, resulted in 18 sub-categories (See Table 5).

Table 4. Top 3 types of health/medical information university students mainly access and read (total response number for top 1, top 2, top 3 each = 244)

	1st Type		2nd Type		3rd Type	
	N	%	N	%	N	%
1. Specific Diseases	<u>97</u>	<u>39.8</u>	36	14.8	32	13.1
2. Medical Treatment	49	20.1	<u>62</u>	<u>25.4</u>	43	17.6
3. Natural Therapy	34	13.9	42	17.2	18	7.4
4. Pharmaceutical Drugs	9	3.7	32	13.1	25	10.2
5. Health Services	18	7.4	42	17.2	<u>52</u>	<u>21.3</u>
6. Mental Health	23	9.4	18	7.4	31	12.7
Other	14	5.7	5	2.0	20	8.2
None	0	0	7	2.9	23	9.4

Table 5. Top 3 most frequent stated specific health information for the six groups

	N	%
1. Specific Diseases		
1.Sexual transmitted disease	**17**	**11.9**
2.Cancer	**17**	**11.9**
3.Mental illness	10	7.0
2. Medical Treatment		
4.Treatment for skin problems	6	5.2
5.Treatment for flu/cold	5	4.3
6.Treatment for cancer	4	3.5
3. Natural Therapy		
7.Natural medicine/remedies	**14**	**18.2**
8.Dietary tips	7	9.1
9.Herbal remedies	5	6.5
4. Pharmaceutical Drugs		
10.Pain killers	5	9.8
11.Drugs for respiratory problems	4 (each)	7.8 (each)
(e.g. asthma /anti-anxiety drugs)	3	5.9
12.Anti-depressants		
5. Health Services		
13.Medical services	**47**	**56.0**
14.Mental health services	6	7.1
15.Naturopath/ women health services	4 (each)	4.8 (each)
6. Mental Health		
16.Unipolar disorder (depression)	**28**	**43.1**
17.Anxiety disorders	**13**	**20.0**
18.Eating disorders	4	6.2

From these 18 sub-categories the top most often searched for information were issues pertaining to:

1. Mental health (depression and anxiety) (63.1%),
2. Medical services (56%),
3. Natural medicine / remedies (18.2%),
4. Sexually transmitted diseases (11.9%), and equally
5. Cancer (11.9%).

Participants were also asked about whether they had a favorite health website they used to obtain health / medical information (n = 226, 91.1%). Six percent (6.2%) of them said yes, while 93.8% said no to this question. For those who responded yes, they mostfrequently used such sites as 'Better Health' (a general health website -www.betterhealth.vic.gov.au), 'Beyond Blue' (a mental health website -www. beyondblue.org.au), and 'HealthInsite' (a general health website - www.healthinsite.gov.au).

Chi square analyses (with Yates continuity correction) were performed for gender and the question of whether they have ever searched for online health / medical issues. However, no significant difference was demonstrated between gender and history of health/medical information search ($X^2 = .91$, $p = .34$, phi = .07). Chi square analyses were also undertaken for gender across questions about the top 1 way of searching health / medical information, the top 1 information that most often being accessed, frequency of online health / medical information used and whether they have a favorite website for health / medical issues. Similarly, no significant results were found.

DISCUSSION OF RESULTS

This study opens a small window through which we can begin to study the opinions that Australian university students hold pertaining to the Internet and how they relate to it for health inquires. This Australian study mirrors similar earlier research by Kenneth (2005) and Fox & Raine (2006) upon which they conclude that the Internet is having a powerful influence on young adults, with 80% of those with Internet access, going online at least once a month for health information and that this information influenced their decisions about how to treat a specific disease (70%). Results from this study identify that every few months (44.6%), 90.2% of participants used the Internet for accessing health information and mostly spent more than 1-15 minutes reading (40.9%) about specific diseases (39.8%).

Interestingly, a majority of participants (n = 226, 91.1%) indicated that they *did not* have a favourite health website that they used to access health information and that a random Internet search (Google, AltaVista, Yahoo) (n = 204, 83.3%) was the main way that they obtained health information. Similarly, in a recent study, it was found that almost all of the respondents (n = 8,353) used search engines to find and access online health information (Head & Eisenberg, 2011). Boyer and Geissbuhler (2006) offer a possible explanation for such online information search behavior by stating that it seems that these mechanisms prevail mainly because they are easy, accessible, fast and contain a great deal of information. Hence, a recommendation from this study is to design avenues that will assist university students to develop critical appraisal skills associated with the retrieval, evaluation, and implementation of online health information. This is, perhaps, an initial step in improving the acceptance and adoption of e-health knowledge management by university students in a broader context (Mitra et al., 2005).

Furthermore, this study recommends that student health services should provide links that would direct university students to reliable health websites that address their identified health concerns. Issues related to the credibility of information on health websites are crucial considerations for students (Escoffery et al., 2005) and that the main problems reported in the search for e-health were the ignorance of good web pages (64.8%) and the lack of confidence or search skills (23.2%) (Head & Eisenberg, 2011). Similarly, Wood (2004) asserts that once university students have found information on the web, they lack the skills to critically analyse the information they have found, making the assumption that 'all information is equal, truthful, and has the same value'. He also found that students do not understand or appreciate the reasons for, and necessity of, accurately crediting the information source.

For those who had a favorite health website (6.2%), they most frequently used such sites as 'Better Health' (www.betterhealthvic.gov.au), 'Beyond Blue' (www.beyondblue.org.au) and 'HealthInsite' (www.healthinsite.gov.au). A closer inspection of these health websites revealed that they maintain and display many of the components that increase a health website's reliability levels (authority, accuracy, objectivity, currency, intended audience, coverage, confidentiality and justifiability) (Usher, 2009). Furthermore, these identified websites are Government designed, advertised and supported portals. These websites are becoming a more frequent and acceptable form of information exchange and health care delivery across all sectors of the health care landscape (Nielsen's Internet & Technology Report 2010). A further recommendation from this study would be to increase university students' knowledge pertaining to a health website's reliability components so as to encourage future access to reliable health websites. Increased levels of reliability are a major factor in, and motivation for, current and future Internet trends and patterns of online health information usage (Usher, 2009).

Another important consideration necessary for interpreting results from this study is the disproportional gender ratio of participants (female 227, 82.5% and male 48, 17.5%), whereby it could be assumed that the results obtained from this study is gender specific. Therefore, further research and cross-gender studies should be undertaken to determine e-health knowledge management trends by male university students, thus providing a heightened holistic approach to e-health care delivery (Horgan, et al., 2010; Head & Eisenberg, 2011; Jimenez-Pernett & de Labry-Lima, 2010). Current research supports such a recommendation stating that young men use the Internet more intensively for downloading news and entertainment, while young women use the Internet predominately for information about education and health-related information (ONS, 2009). Similarly, Escoffery et al. (2005) found differences in Internet use for health information by gender and by level of Internet experience.

Participants (n = 244) ranked 6 core health categories with further elaborations generating 18 subsequent sub-categories. Interestingly, these correspond with a number of Australia's identified National Health Priority Areas. Given these results, further research is warranted in an attempt to investigate the development and implementation of early preventative programs for Australian University students that address such issues as:

1. Mental health (depression and anxiety),
2. Medical services,
3. Natural medicine / remedies,
4. Sexually transmitted diseases, and
5. Cancer.

Justification for such a recommendation is supported by current research by Stallman (2011), who identifies that mental illness among Australian university students is five times higher than in the general population. Furthermore, it is understood that depression is commonly linked with a range of other health risk behaviours that Australian university students engage in, such as tobacco use, illicit drug use, alcohol misuse and dependence, eating disorders and obesity (MHS in Australia, 2010).

LIMITATIONS

The study had some limitations associated with the survey instrument, the major limitation being the initial online data collection method (LimeSurvey). There was an inability (due to an unbiased e-mail alert) to collect / identify equal sample sizes from male and female participants, resulting in a higher participation rate from Australian female University students. However, it was an expectation that given the nature of many of the University programs (i.e. Bachelor of Primary Education); a higher female participation rate was expected.

Secondly, the identified participation rates were only achieved via an email broadcast to Griffith University students (Arts, Education and Law). Due to regulations and privacy restrictions, only 2 e-mails were sent. This limited level of survey notification would have significantly affected participation rates. Future recommendations would include a need to establish a more concentrated avenue/s for the advertising of the survey, thus increasing participation rates. This could come in the form of further advertising the survey via Facebook (snowballing) and other Australian university health services. Future instrument designs may benefit from identifying and developing a data collection strategy that addresses the aforementioned limitations

FUTURE RESEARCH DIRECTIONS

Looking to the future, further research is needed around new initiatives that are underpinned by the Internet and provide opportunities for increased e-health knowledge management in the early 21st century. Findings from this study may help guide future research and policy and assist Australian university health services to develop the necessary e-health platforms for delivering effective health promotion. However, to date, there is little research indicating any substantial coordinated approach to addressing these recommendations (Australian Institute for Primary Care, 2008).

More importantly, the findings from this study indicate that future e-health initiatives (across all Australian universities) should include the development of e-health platforms that demonstrate practical e-healthcare delivery models for current and future Australian university students. The development and implementation of an e-health portal, designed to educate and reach Australian university students concerning the usage of reliable health websites for health care delivery and knowledge management would be one avenue. Given that young adults (primarily male) have been portrayed as reluctant to engage with traditional health services (Courtenay, 2000; White, 2006) this recommendation would seem plausible.

Comparable research, congruent with this study and its findings, has recognized that young people experience difficulties in accessing mainstream mental health services, particularly because of the stigma that remains associated with mental health problems (Horgan et al., 2010). One potential solution is to use the many interactive websites that are available and which offer information and support for mental health. Therefore, it seems conceivable that websites designed and managed by health services should have a predominant position among interventions which are specifically aimed at university students (Jimenez-Pernett and de Labry-Lima, 2010).

Furthermore, consideration should be directed towards newer forms of communication technology (i.e. SM – Web 2.0) which may present opportunities to engage with young adults pertaining to their health / medical issues. Social media (Web 2.0) technology allows its users to interact with other users or to change content, in contrast to non-interactive websites (i.e. the Internet - Web 1.0) where users are limited to the passive viewing of health information that is provided to them (Seeman, 2008). Young & Simon (2005) define social media technology as,

The literal fusion of multiple electronic, communications, computer, and media technologies. The art of listening, learning and sharing is being transformed through, for example, the development of social forums (Twitter, Facebook, Myspace), content sharing platforms (Wikis, Blogs, Diigo, Nigs, Google Docs) and high performance computing / advanced networking (Second Life, podcasts, instructional design, 3-D stereoscopic) (p. 14).

From such an identified research gap, further empirical data will be presented so as to highlight the shifting paradigms that have occurred over the past 5 years. This shift has been primarily caused by the increased technological advances when it comes to modern forms of communication technologies, namely wireless monitoring devices. Therefore, the forthcoming section will give specific reference to contemporary literature and research that goes to re-enforce and build on previous research in this field of investigation.

Web 2.0 or social media (SM) technology has become very popular among undergraduates, with usage rates upwards of 90% at most campuses (Lampe *et al.*, 2007; Stutzman, 2006). Specifically, there has been a great deal of recent research activity directed towards various aspects of Facebook use, such as the use of Facebook in academic settings (Hewitt & Forte, 2006). Steinfield *et al.*, (2008) suggest that more research on the role of social network sites among young adults is needed, since maintaining friendships through SNSs like Facebook may play an important role in psychological (emotional health) development. Social networking sites affordances help reduce barriers that lower self-esteem students might experience in forming the kinds of large, heterogeneous networks that are sources of bridging social capital (Steinfield *et al.*, 2008). Social capital is an elastic construct used to describe the benefits one receives from one's relationships with other people (Lin, 1999). Among young adults, relationships with peers are important both for generating offline benefits and for psychosocial development.

Moreover, Ellison et al., (2007) found evidence that self-esteem may operate as a moderator of the relationship between social network site use and social capital. That is, young people with lower self-esteem appeared to benefit more from their use of SNSs than those with higher self-esteem. As young adults are closely linked to social media as a way of communication (Seeman, 2008) and university students demonstrate higher mental health issues when compared to the general population (Stallman, 2011), further research that explores the use of Web 2.0 technologies for heightening e-health knowledge management and social capital would seem reasonable. Australian secondary schools have been seen more as a setting for promoting better mental health, but it hasn't occurred in the tertiary sector to the same degree (Higher Education, 2011).

Contemporary and future technologies (i.e. Web 2.0) which assist in generating, acquiring and disseminating health information will require new forms of literacy, to which this is another point of contention surrounding e-health knowledge management in the early 21st century (Usher, 2009). The concept of e-health literacy has been defined in terms of social action not just information processing as,

The ability to seek, find, understand and appraise health information from electronic sources and apply the knowledge gained to addressing or solving a health problem (Norman & Skinner, p., 57, 2006).

Social Media (Web 2.0) and University Students

O'Reilly (2007) identifies how the introduction of Web 2.0 technologies have created a new *'architecture of participation',* emphasising that there is a growing nexus which has emerged between such communication platforms as the Internet (Web 1.0) and SM (Web 2.0) technologies. This relationship has co-operatively changed the way providers of 21st century healthcare and consumers alike, deliver, access and implement health services and access health information. Since their introduction, Web 2.0 technologies (Facebook, Twitter, Instagram, MySpace and Flickr have attracted millions of international users', with many integrating these platforms into their daily health and communication practices (Boyd & Ellison, 2007, p 9). Boyd and Ellison (2007) comment:

While their key technological features are fairly consistent, the cultures that emerge around SNSs (Web 2.0) are varied. Most sites support the maintenance of pre-existing social networks, but others help

strangers connect based on shared interests, political views, or activities. Some sites cater to diverse audiences, while others attract people based on common language or shared racial, sexual, religious, or nationality-based identities. (p. 12).

What is more, Hackworth and Kunz (2011) identify that "Web 2.0 technologies provide the means for health care providers and marketers alike to provide actual content—not just marketing to the consumer, but providing the consumer with valuable information about health care topics, concerns, issues and controversies" (p. 3). Currently, Twitter, YouTube and Facebook are the most popular social media for hospitals, and the most effective in driving traffic to a web site (Cummins, 2010).

A framework, by Usher (2011), identifies four important health enabling qualities that Web 2.0 technologies collectively promote. These enabling aspects promote and allow for individuals to manage personal health conditions – by heightening the access and implementation of health information. The four (4) health enabling qualities are:

1. Multimodality;
2. Networkability;
3. Temporal flexibility; and
4. Message tailoring capabilities.

The 'overlapping' of these 4 qualities, brings about a number of *'Health Outcome Commonalities'*, being:

1. An increase in self-efficacy;
2. The ability to communicate and control information either synchronously or asynchronously;
3. The ability to manipulate text; and
4. The ability to narrow/segment information for a particular audience, target group or individual (Usher, 2011).

Simililarly, research by Ernst and Young (2012) reported that such enabling technologies, as above, potentially, offer and support for individuals to become increasingly more connected into any health-care ecosystem and can deliver actionable information, overcoming the barriers of multiple data silos across many platforms. Such attributes create unique opportunities to promote positive and sustainable behavioral changes amongst various populations.

Usher *et al.*, (2015) investigated how SM platforms create pathways for accessing widely available information; particularly those favored by the younger generations. The aim was to investigate the way university students use communication technologies in an attempt to access health information. The results ($n = 696$) indicated that communication technologies were used to extensively search for health information which ultimately resulted in positive health behavioural changes in participants' health patterns; however they perceived lack of reliability of the information as a pressing issue. The results suggested that appealing, persuasive and reliable SM can be used extensively to promote health amongst Australian youth.

Interestingly, Usher et al., (2015) further identified that the most preferred technology platforms were identified as being:

1. Smartphones, and
2. Facebook.

Similarly, Ernst and Young (2012) maintain that the transformation in health information access is being driven by modern technology's unique capacity for increased convenience, access to information, social connectedness and diversity. It is further understood that smartphones have become widespread and for most youth indispensable (World Economic Forum 2011). What is more, in this study, participants indicated that Instagram was used as the most likely technology for distributing and storing pictures on health information related to topics as: dietary intake, recipes and menu choices (Usher et al., 2015). Hochman *et al.* (2012: 6) explained such a trend:

Individuals are increasingly seeking ways to visualise, analyse and discover concealed socio-cultural characteristics and trends in an ever-growing flow of visual information.

Current and past research identifies the potential for utilising a variety of SM network for disseminating health information and for improving dietary habits, in a timely and accurate manner, and as such warrants further research regarding its effectiveness in achieving positive behaviour modification. Similar claims by Wong, Merchanta and Morenoc (2014), maintain that SM networks can provide prospects to heighten adolescents' and young adults' engagement in health care delivery. However, further study is required to outline a clear value proposition and develop evidence-based frameworks for measuring the impact of SM networks (such as Instagram) on young people's health. Of most significance, were results from this study (Usher *et al.*, 2015) which indicated that health related topics, such as exercise or diet, were the most frequently accessed types of health information. Ernst & Young (2012) also state that given the increasing trend of many CD are occurring at an older age, this information is important establishing preventive measures and delivering tailored and timely health related information. To minimise future CD epidemics, further research is necessary to explore how modern forms of communication technologies can be better harnessed to both equip and enable young adults as a means of preventing lifestyle diseases and that will sustain positive health behavioral changes.

Whilst positive behavioural changes were observed in this study, due to use of Web 1.0 (Internet) and Web 2.0 (social media), it is important to note that a small negative behaviour change, as a result of accessing mobile wireless devices (smartphones) and SM was also observed. It is possible that the inherent nature of modern technologies that exposes individuals to pervasive product marketing, powerful social norms and mass media, could account for the acquisition of various negative health behaviours evident in this research (Usher *et al.*, 2015).

SOLUTIONS AND RECOMMENDATIONS

Important to this chapter are specific recommendations for future practices and policies surrounding youth health (Cheung, Yip, Townsend and Scotch; 2008). Specifically, it is predicted that mental health issues among the student population are likely to escalate as Australian universities attract more young people from disadvantaged backgrounds (Higher Education, 2011). Similarly, Stallman (2011) further highlighted a need for Australian universities to take a broad and proactive approach to the mental health and wellbeing of students, in addition to targeting specific problems such as alcohol abuse.

Importantly, this study raises several questions that need to be addressed if e-health amongst Australian university students is to be successful. Firstly, what structural / environmental supports are needed to engage with university students from disadvantaged socio-economic groups? Secondly, what critical appraisal and e-literacy skills, do young adults attending universities, need to acquire to successfully access, comprehend and implement online health information? Lastly, what initiatives are required to ensure that gender resistance to e-health knowledge management is understood and subsequently minimized? However, firm conclusions, about the relationship between race, gender, and Internet use, are difficult to draw (Jones et al., 2009).

An initial start for Australian university health services could come in the form of adopting rigorous practices which maintain high ethical standards concerning e-health promotion and information dissemination. Discussions surrounding the importance of online practices and ethical guidelines are cause for further research (Risk & Dzenowagis, 2001). Notwithstanding, contemporary international literature and findings from this research, do provide guidelines that should be a consideration by current and future Australian University health services. In brief, these include the:

1. Establishment of third-party rating systems that enable students to filter harmful health information and to identify and select high-quality information ("downstream filtering") through health website content labels.
2. Creation of enforcement infrastructures.
3. Introduction educational modules which address reliability scales and seals associated with health websites.
4. The active encouragement of health information providers / services to conform to ethical codes of conduct.
5. Development of health information that is trustworthy and up-to-date.
6. Establishment of health information via providers who possess a high quality of service delivery through the application of meta tags and labeling technologies.
7. Implementation of a broad and proactive approach to the mental health and wellbeing of students – these to include e-health knowledge management initiatives.
8. Provision of on-line health services that follow Hi-Ethical principles.

As this is the first Australian study that has examined e-health knowledge management by Australian university students, further research should be undertaken to investigate possible avenues for the successful design and implementation of future university wide e-health initiatives. Therefore, again, it would be assumed that a larger cross-cultural study should be advocated for and undertaken. Primary prevention campaigns and strategies should be aimed to assist university students to reduce major risk factors associated with tobacco consumption, poor diet, insufficient physical activity, being overweight or obese, mental health, unsafe alcohol use, infectious diseases and exposure to ultraviolet radiation (AIHW, 2011). Moreover, results from this study, albeit drawn from a relatively small sample size, have been found to mirror many of the findings from similar international studies and literature. The results and recommendations presented throughout this paper are an opportunity for Australian university health services to develop and implement future effective health promoting strategies and campaigns.

CONCLUSION

This chapter has explored and presented how Web 1.0 (Internet), Web 2.0 (SM) and to a further extent mobile wireless devices (smartphones), are used by Australian university students for accessing personal health information, particularly for enhancing social connectedness, personal health care management, and the access and dissemination of health related information. It further presents, more contemporary and broader research and a theoretical basis of claim, which investigates the impact Web 2.0 and mobile wireless devices (smartphones) has had on youth and their health information access. The information and knowledge generated from this research has provided insights through which it could be determined how Australian university students use modern forms of communication technologies in an attempt to access and implement health information. What is clear, is that young Australians are turning to SM and similar devices / tools for accessing and implementing health related information. It is suggested that a possible way forward is to design effective electronic platforms that culminate the e-technologies so as to have the maximum health benefits for this generation. Future studies should be aimed at exploring how the health of young Australians could be enhanced by developing e-health platforms that mitigate a number of identified SM tools and devices that are frequently used by Australian youth (Usher *et al.,* 2015).

Lastly, futurists in the area of health care delivery, are looking to explore the possibilities of utilising, a third generation of Internet-based services – Web 3.0. It is envisaged that 'The Semantic Web' (Web 3.0) will simplify human–computer interfaces by enabling computers to 'understand' the actual/intended meanings of the content as they process it. When combined with such technologies as health apps (applications), smartphones, wireless devices and mobile technologies, an ecosystem will be created that will be useful to the medical and health related professionals because they are agile, handheld, easy to use and can be used on the move. A recommendation from this chapter is for further research and cross-cultural studies to be undertaken to investigate possible collaborative avenues which will explore how such a health ecosystem could better deliver health information to Australian youth. Lastly, such recommendations and predictions, as proposed in this chapter, offer opportunities rather than barriers and needs to be embraced with a degree of optimism for creating better health for all Australians.

REFERENCES

American College Health Association. (2007). National College Health Assessment Spring 2006 Reference Group data report. *Journal of Health.*, *55*, 195–206. PMID:17319325

Anderson, K. J. (2001). Internet use among college students: An exploratory study. *Journal of American College Health*, *50*(1), 21–26. doi:10.1080/07448480109595707 PMID:11534747

Arnett, J. J. (2000). Emerging adulthood: A theory of development from the late teens through the twenties. *The American Psychologist*, *55*(5), 469–480. doi:10.1037/0003-066X.55.5.469 PMID:10842426

Australian Bureau of Statistics (ABS). (2011). *Households using the Internet.* Retrieved September 12, 2012, from: http://www.abs.gov.au/ausstats/abs@.nsf/mf/8146.0

Australian Institute for Primary Care. (2008). *System reform and development for chronic disease management.* Australian Institute for Primary Care. Retrieved October 21, 2009, from: http://www.health.gov.au/internet/nhhrc/publishing.nsf/Content/038-aipclatrobe/$FILE/038%20Australian%20Institute%20for%20Primary%20Care,%20La%20Trobe%20University%20Attachment%20B.pdf

Australian Institute of Health and Welfare. (2011). *Authoritative information and statistics to promote better health and wellbeing*. Retrieved September 12, 2012, from: http://www.aihw.gov.au/cancer-control-health-priority-area/

Avendaño, C., Mata, A., Villanueva, A. M., Martínez, V. S., & Sarmiento, C. A. (2010). Laptop expositions affect motility and induce DNA fragmentation in human spermatozoa in vitro by a non-thermal effect: A preliminary report. *Journal of Fertility and Sterility*, *94*(4), 73. doi:10.1016/j.fertnstert.2010.07.284

Barker, E. T., & Galambos, N. L. (2007). Body dissatisfaction, living away from parents, and poor social adjustment predict binge eating symptoms in young women making the transition to University. *Journal of Youth and Adolescence*, *36*(7), 904–911. doi:10.1007/s10964-006-9134-6

Bernhardt, J., & Hubley, J. (2001). Health education and the Internet: The beginning of a revolution. *Health Education Research*, *16*(5), 643–645. doi:10.1093/her/16.6.643

Binkowska-Bury, M., & Januszewicz, P. (2010). Sense of coherence and health-related behaviour among University students--a questionnaire survey. *Journal of Public Health*, *18*(3), 145–150. PMID:21033609

Borzekowski, D. (2001). Adolescent cyber-surfing for health information: A new resource that crosses barriers. *Archives of Pediatrics & Adolescent Medicine*, *155*(7), 813–817. doi:10.1001/archpedi.155.7.813 PMID:11434849

Boyd, D. M., & Ellison, N. B. (2007). Social network sites: Definition, history, and scholarship. *Journal of Computer-Mediated Communication*, *13*(1), 210–230. doi:10.1111/j.1083-6101.2007.00393.x

Boyer, C., & Geissbuhler, A. (2006). Health and the Internet for all. *International Journal of Medical Informatics*, *75*(1), 1–3. doi:10.1016/j.ijmedinf.2005.07.039 PMID:16325462

Brodie, M., Flournoy, E., Altman, D., Blendon, R. J., Benson, J. M., & Rosenbaum, M. D. (2000). Health information, the Internet, and the digital divide. *Health Affairs*, *19*(6), 255–265. doi:10.1377/hlthaff.19.6.255 PMID:11192412

Cain, J., Brent, I., & Fox, P. (2009). Web 2.0 and pharmacy education. *American Journal of Pharmaceutical Education*, *73*(7), 1–11. doi:10.5688/aj7307120 PMID:19960079

Charles, S., Nicole, E., & Cliff, L. (2008). Social capital, self-esteem, and use of online social network sites: A longitudinal analysis. *Journal of Applied Developmental Psychology*, *29*(200), 434–445.

Cheung, K., Yip, K., Townsend, J., & Scotch, M. (2008). HCLS 2.0/3.0: Health care and life sciences data mashup using Web 2.0/3.0. *Journal of Biomedical Informatics*, *41*(5), 694–705. doi:10.1016/j.jbi.2008.04.001 PMID:18487092

Cormode, G., & Krishnamurthy, B. (2008). Key differences between Web 1.0 and Web 2.0. *First Monday*, *13*(6). doi:10.5210/fm.v13i6.2125

Courtenay, W. (2000). Construction of masculinity and their influence on men's well-being: A theory of gender and health. *Social Science & Medicine*, *50*(10), 1385–1401. doi:10.1016/S0277-9536(99)00390-1 PMID:10741575

Cummins, J. (2010). *Few hospitals use social media effectively, says study*. Health Leaders Media. Retrieved from October 13, 2011, from http://www.healthleadersmedia.com/content/TEC-245418/Few-Hospitals-Use-Social-Media-Effectively-Says-Study.html

Department of Health and Ageing. (2008). *Towards a National Primary Health Care Strategy: a discussion paper from the Australian Government*. Retrieved Feburary 6, 2009, from http://www.health.gov.au/primaryhealthstrategy

eBizMBA Rank. (2010). Retrieved March 13, 2010, from http://www.ebizmba.com/articles/health-websites

Ellison, N., Steinfield, C., & Lampe, C. (2007). The benefits of Facebook "friends:" Social capital and college students' use of online social network sites. *Journal of Computer-Mediated Communication, 12*, 1143–1168.

Ernst & Young. (2012). Mobile technology poised to enable a new era in health care. *EYGM Limited.* Retrieved April 5, 2013, from http://www.ey.com/Publication/vwLUAssets/mHealth_Report_January_2013/$FILE/mHealth%20Report_Final.pdf

Escoffery, C., Miner, K., Adame, D., Butler, S., McCormick, L., & Mendell, E. (2005). Internet use for health information among college students. *Journal of American College Health*, *53*(4), 183–188. doi:10.3200/JACH.53.4.183-188 PMID:15663067

Fox, S., & Jones, S. (2009). *The social life of health information*. Pew Internet and American Life Project. Retrieved March 13, 2010, from http://www.pewinternet.org/Reports/2009/8-The-Social-Life-of-Health-Information.aspx

Fox, S., & Rainie, L. (2006). The Online Health Care Revolution: How the Web Helps American Take better Care of Themselves. *ElectronicHealthcare*, *8*(5), 110–113.

Fox, S., Rainie, L., & Horrigan, J. (2000). The online health care revolution: How the web helps Americans take better care of themselves. *Pew Internet and American Life Project*, *91*, 235–245.

Gehl, R. W. (2011). The archive and the processor: The internal logic of Web 2.0. *New Media & Society*, *13*(8), 1228–1244. doi:10.1177/1461444811401735

Hackworth, B. A., & Kunz, M. B. (2011). Healthcare and social media: Building relationship via social networks. Morehead State University. *Academy of Health Care Management Journal*, *7*(2), 34–45.

Head, A., & Eisenberg, M. (2011). How college students use the Web to conduct everyday life research. *First Monday*, *16*(4), 2. doi:10.5210/fm.v16i4.3484

Hendricks, C., Murdaugh, C., & Pender, N. (2006). The Adolescent Lifestyle Profile: Development and psychometric characteristics. *Journal of National Black Nurses' Association*, *17*(2), 1–5. PMID:17410753

Hewitt, A., & Forte, A. (2006). *Crossing boundaries: Identity management and student/faculty relationships on the Facebook.* Poster presented at the ACM Special Interest Group on Computer-Supported Cooperative Work, Banff, Canada.

Higher Education. (2011). *Mental health issues among students to escalate*. Retrieved October 5, 2012, from http://www.theaustralian.com.au/higher-education/mental-health-issues-among-students-to-escalate/story-e6frgcjx-1226111953584

Hitlin, P., & Rainie, L. (2005). Teens, technology, and school. *Pew Internet & American Life Project, 93*, 124–201.

Hochman, N., & Schwartz, S. (2012). *Visualizing Instagram: Tracing Cultural Visual Rhythms AAAI Technical Report WS-12-03. Social Media Visualization.* Association for the Advancement of Artificial Intelligence. Retrieved June 11, 2012, from http://www.aaai.org/ocs/index.php/ICWSM/ICWSM12/paper/viewFile/4782/5091

Horgan, A., & Sweeney, J. (2010). Young students' use of the Internet for mental health information and support. *ElectronicHealthcare, 17*(2), 117–123. PMID:20465756

Huang, T. T., Harris, K. J., Lee, R. E., Nazir, N., Born, W., & Kaur, H. (2003). Assessing overweight, obesity, diet, and physical activity in college students. *Journal ofAmerican College Health, 52*(2), 83–86. doi:10.1080/07448480309595728 PMID:14765762

Jimenez-Pernett, J., & Olry de Labry-Lima, A. (2010). Use of the internet as a source of health information by Spanish adolescents. *BMC Medical Informatics and Decision Making, 10*(1), 6. doi:10.1186/1472-6947-10-6 PMID:20113486

Johnson-Yale, S., Millermaier, S., & Seoane Perez, F. (2009). Everyday life, online: U.S. college students' use of the Internet. *First Monday, 14*(10), 1.

Jones, S., Johnson-Yale, C., Millermaier, S., & Seoane Perez, F. (2009). Everyday life, online: U.S. college students' use of the Internet. *First Monday, 14*(10), 5. doi:10.5210/fm.v14i10.2649

Kamel Boulos, M. N., & Wheeler, S. (2007). The emerging Web 2.0 social software: An enabling suite of sociable technologies in health and health care education. *Health Information and Libraries Journal, 24*(1), 2–23. doi:10.1111/j.1471-1842.2007.00701.x PMID:17331140

Kenneth, B. (2005). *Internet Enhances Patient Education.* U.S Publications. Retrieved from http:www.uspharmacist.com/oldformat.asp

Korp, P. (2006). Health on the Internet: Implications for health promotion. *Health Education Research, 21*(1), 78–86. doi:10.1093/her/cyh043 PMID:15994845

Lampe, C., Ellison, N., & Steinfield, C. (2007). A familiar face(book): Profile elements as signals in an online social network.*Proceedings of the SIGCHI conference on human factors in computing systems* (pp. 435–444). New York: ACM. doi:10.1145/1240624.1240695

Landsberg, B., Plachta-Danielzik, S., Lange, D., Johannsen, M., Seiberl, J., & Müller, M. J. (2010). Clustering of lifestyle factors and association with overweight in adolescents of the Kiel Obesity Prevention Study. *Public Health Nutrition, 13*(10A), 1708–1715. doi:10.1017/S1368980010002260 PMID:20883570

Laska, M. N., Pasch, K. E., Lust, K., Story, M., & Ehlinger, E. (2009). Latent Class Analysis of Lifestyle Characteristics and Health Risk Behaviors among College Youth. *Preventative Science*, *5*, 12. PMID:19499339

Lin, N. (1999). Building a network theory of social capital. *Connections*, *22*, 28–51.

Lowery, R., Galuska, D. A., Fulton, J. E., Wechsler, H., Kann, L., & Collins, J. L. (2000). Physical activity, food choice, and weight management goals and practices among U.S. college students. *American Journal of Preventive Medicine*, *18*, 8–27. PMID:10736536

Madden, M., & Zickuhr, K. (2011). *65% of online adults use social networking sites*. Washington, DC: Pew Internet and American Life Project, Pew Research Centre. Retrieved March 8, 2012, from http://www.pewinternet.org/~/media//Files/Reports/2011/PIP-SNS-Update-2011.pdf

Mitra, A., Willyard, J., Platt, C., & Parson, M. (2005). Exploring Web usage and selection criteria among male and female students. *Journal of Computer-Mediated Communication*, *10*(3), 10.

Nielsen's Internet & Technology Report. (2010). Retrieved March 13, 2011, from http://www.emerchant.com.au/blog/nielsen%E2%80%99s-2010-internet-technology-report/

Norman, C., & Skinner, H. (2006). Ehealth Literacy: Essential skills for consumer health in a networked world. *Journal of Medical Internet Research*, *8*(2), 9. doi:10.2196/jmir.8.2.e9 PMID:16867972

Nöthlings, U., Ford, E., Kröger, J., & Boeing, H. (2010). Lifestyle factors and mortality among adults with diabetes: Findings from the European Prospective Investigation into Cancer and Nutrition–Potsdam study. *Journal of Diabetes*, *2*(2), 112–117. doi:10.1111/j.1753-0407.2010.00069.x PMID:20923493

O'Reilly, T. (2007). What is Web 2.0: Design patterns and business models for the next generation of software. *Communications & Stratégies*, *65*(1), 17.

Office of National Statistics. (2009). *National Omnibus Survey*. Retrieved April 23, 2012, from http://www.statistics.gov.uk/default.asp

Pew Internet & American Life Project. (2009). *Usage over time*. Retrieved April 4, 2012, from http://pewInternet.org//trends/UsageOverTime_Jan_2009.xls

Pullman, A. W., Masters, R. C., Zalot, L. C., Carde, L. E., Saraiva, M. M., & Dam, Y. Y. etal. (2009). Effect of the transition from high school to University on anthropometric and lifestyle variables in males. *Applied Physiology, Nutrition, and Metabolism*, *34*(2), 162–171. doi:10.1139/H09-007 PMID:19370046

Reddy, P., Rankins, D., Timoshanko, A., & Dunbar, J. (2011). Life! in Australia: Translating prevention research into a large-scale intervention. *Br J Diabetes Vasc Dis*, *11*(4), 193–197. doi:10.1177/1474651411410724

Risk, A., & Dzenowagis, J. (2001). Review Of Internet Health Information Quality Initiatives. *Journal of Medical Internet Research*, *3*(4), 8. doi:10.2196/jmir.3.4.e28 PMID:11772543

Seeman, N. (2008). Web 2.0 and chronic illness: New horizons, new opportunities. *ElectronicHealthcare*, *6*(3), 104–110. PMID:18326388

Stallman, H. (2011). *Mental illness running high among uni students*. The World Today. Retrieved from http://www.abc.net.au/news/2010-11-23/mental-illness-running-high-among-uni-students/2348772

Steptoe, A., Wardle, J., Cui, W., Bellisle, F., Zotti, A. M., Baranyai, R., & Sanderman, R. (2002). Trends in smoking, diet, physical exercise and attitudes toward health in European University students from 13 countries. *Preventive Medicine*, *35*(2), 97–104. doi:10.1006/pmed.2002.1048 PMID:12200093

Stutzman, F. (2006). *An evaluation of identity-sharing behavior in social network communities.Paper presented at the International Digital Media Arts*. Association and the Miami University Center for Interactive Media Studies CODE Conference, Oxford, OH.

Towards a National Primary Health Care Strategy: A discussion paper from the Australian Government. (2008). Department of Health and Ageing, Commonwealth of Australia. Retrieved October 6, 2011, from http://www.health.gov.au/primaryhealthstrategy

Uden-Kraan, C. F. (2009). Health-related Internet use by patients with somatic diseases: Frequency of use and characteristics of users. *Informatics for Health & Social Care*, *34*(1), 18–29. doi:10.1080/17538150902773272 PMID:19306196

Usher, W. (2009). Gold Coast general practitioners' understanding pertaining to reliability, interactive and usability components associated with health websites. *International Journal of Behaviour and Information Technology*, *28*(1), 39–44. doi:10.1080/01449290802187736

Usher, W. (2011). Types of social media (Web 2.0) usage by Australian Allied Health professionals' for early 21st century practice promotion and e-health care delivery. *Social Work in Health Care*, *50*(4), 305–329. doi:10.1080/00981389.2010.534317 PMID:21512953

Usher, W., Gudes, O., & Parekh, S. (2015). Exploring the use of technology pathways to access health information by Australian university students: A multi - dimensional approach. *Health Information Management Journal*, *4*, 1–12. PMID:26113541

White, A. (2006). Men's Health in the 21st Century. *International Journal of Men's Health*, *5*(1), 1–17. doi:10.3149/jmh.0501.1

Wong, C., Merchanta, R., & Morenoc, M. (2014). Using social media to engage adolescents and young adults with their health. *Health Care*, *31*(3), 56–58. PMID:25984444

Wood, G. (2004). Academic Original Sin: Plagiarism, the Internet, and Librarians. *Journal of Academic Librarianship*, *30*(3), 237–242. doi:10.1016/j.acalib.2004.02.011

World Economic Forum. (2011). *Personal Data: The Emergence of a New Asset Class*. Geneva, Switzerland: World Economic Forum.

World Health Organisation (WHO). (2010). *The social determinants of health*. WHO. Retrieved November 2, 2012, from http://www.who.int/social_determinants/en/

Yee, K. C., Miils, E., & Airey, C. (2008). Perfect match? Generation Y as change agents for information communication technology implementation in healthcare. *Studies in Health Technology and Informatics*, *136*, 496–501. PMID:18487780

Young, J., & Simon, W. (2005). iCon: Steve Jobs, the greatest second act in the history of business. *Studies in Health Technology and Informatics*, *23*, 45–50.

KEY TERMS AND DEFINITIONS

Web 1.0: An early stage of the conceptual evolution of the World Wide Web, where users could only view websites but could not contribute to the content of the website. Technically, Web 1.0 webpage's information is closed to external editing. Web 1.0 concentrated on presenting, not creating so that user-generated content was not available (Cormode & Krishnamurthy, 2008).

Web 2.0: Social media (SM), has been characterised as 'representing various forms of consumer-generated content such as blogs, virtual communities, wikis, social networks, collaborative tagging, and media files shared on sites like Facebook, Instagram, YouTube and Flickr' (Young & Simon, 2005).

Web 3.0: Viewed as the first-generation (convergence of the virtual and physical world) of web development layers that include TV-quality open video, 3D simulations, augmented reality, human-constructed semantic standards, and pervasive broadband, wireless, and sensors (Gehl, 2011).

Wireless Monitoring Devices: Technologies that allow an electronic device to exchange data wirelessly (using radio waves) over a computer network, including high-speed Internet connections (Avendaño et al., 2010). Examples include, activity monitoring arm brace, foot sensors and GPS positioning supported by Android phones / e-platforms and smartphones.

Chapter 4
Intelligent Medication Adherence Monitoring System

Athanasios Anastasiou
National Technical University of Athens, Greece

Georgia Koutsouri
National Technical University of Athens, Greece

Kostas Giokas
National Technical University of Athens, Greece

Dimitra Iliopoulou
National Technical University of Athens, Greece

ABSTRACT

This chapter presents the architecture and implementation of an automatic medication dispenser specifically for users who take medications without close professional supervision. By relieving the users from the error-prone tasks of interpreting medication directions and administrating medications accordingly, the device can improve the required level in compliance and prevent serious medication errors. By taking advantage of the scheduling flexibility provided by medication directions, the device makes the user's medication schedule easy to adhere and tolerant to tardiness whenever possible. This work is done collaboratively by the medication scheduler and dispenser controller in an action-oriented manner. An advantage of the action-oriented interface between the components is extensibility, as new functions can be added and existing ones removed with little or no need to modify the dispenser control structure. This chapter first describes the action-oriented design, major components and hardware structures of the smart device. It then provides an overview of the heuristic algorithms used by the medication scheduler and their relative merits. The different available user options will be presented depicting the user-specific operating modes of the device/service. The scope of this chapter is to describe the development of a smart electronic drug dispenser unit for the pharmaceutical adherence of patients.

INTRODUCTION

Thanks to years of advances in medical and pharmaceutical technologies, more and more drugs can cure or control, previously fatal diseases and help people live actively for decades longer. The benefits of the drugs would be even more wondrous were it not for the high rate of preventable medication errors (Veacez, 2006; Lisby et al., 2005; Law et al., 2003; Wertheimer, 2003). Medication errors are known to occur throughout the medication use process of ordering, transcription, dispensing, and administration.

DOI: 10.4018/978-1-5225-1724-5.ch004

They lead to many hundred thousands of serious adverse drug events, thousands of deaths and billions of Euros in hospital cost each year. These alarming statistics have motivated numerous efforts in research, development and deployment of information technology systems and tools for prevention of medication errors (Kuperman et al.,2007 ; Baron et al.,2005).

Medication adherence usually refers to whether patients take their medications as prescribed, as well as whether they continue to take a prescribed medication. Medication nonadherence is a growing concern to clinicians, healthcare systems, and other stakeholders because of mounting evidence that it is prevalent and associated with adverse outcomes and higher costs of care. To date, measurement of patient medication adherence and use of interventions to improve adherence are rare in routine clinical practice. The proposed solution aims to develop a medication adherence monitoring system, comprising of a portable medication dispenser with communication capabilities and a software platform allowing monitoring by medical personnel and/or carer. The patient data recorded by the dispenser (rate of medication intake) will be collected and will be transmitted in real-time to the hospital (via any Internet link), where it will be analyzed, and any alerts will be raised.

This will enable the doctors to:

- Monitor the progress of the patient and intervene in the case of an anomaly.
- Monitor treatment compliance of the patient.

On the other hand, it will also enable the carer to:

- Monitor the depletion of one or more medication.

Our system addresses the needs of patients with chronic illnesses that require encouragement and supervision with their medication. Monitoring is achieved through the use of a medication dispenser, which collects information about the patients' medication adherence. The dispenser will contain electronics that record automatically the time and date the dispenser is accessed. These data will be transmitted via an Internet connection to the clinical team base.

BACKGROUND

According to the International Society for Pharmacoeconomics and Outcome Research (ISPOR), adherence is "the extent to which a patient acts, in accordance with the prescribed interval, and a dose of a dosing regimen." Medication nonadherence can affect patient health adversely, negatively impact a patient's relationship with his/her care provider, skew results of therapy clinical trials, and increase health resource consumption. Medication nonadherence remains a common health care problem. Poor adherence causes approximately 33% to 69% of medication-related hospitalizations and accounts for $100 billion in annual health care costs. Irrespective of disease, medication complexity, or how adherence is measured, the average adherence rate to chronic medication therapy is approximately 50%. Adherence monitoring should be performed routinely to ensure therapeutic efficacy, avoid unnecessary dose and regimen changes, contain health care costs, and in certain cases, prevent resistance to therapy from emerging.

Medication adherence is a growing concern to clinicians, healthcare systems, and other stakeholders because of mounting evidence that nonadherence is prevalent and associated with adverse outcomes and higher costs of care. Medication nonadherence is likely to grow as the EU population ages and as patients take more medications to treat chronic conditions. Moreover, the rise of performance measures that reward quality based on the attainment of treatment targets such as blood pressure and low-density lipoprotein (LDL) levels or outcomes such as 1-year mortality after hospitalization for conditions like acute myocardial infarction reinforces the import of longitudinal medication adherence. Unlike other quality measures that are under the more direct control of care providers and healthcare systems (e.g., prescribing medications at discharge), the achievement of longer-term therapeutic and outcome goals requires a partnership with patients. To date, measurement of patient medication adherence and use of interventions to improve adherence are rare in routine clinical practice. (Cutler, D. et.al 2005).

Methods to measure adherence, including patient self-reports, pill counts, refill rates, biological monitoring, and electronic monitoring, have limitations and are only proxy measures. Patient self-reports rely on memory and are prone to inaccuracies and recall bias. Pill counts are unreliable if patients fail to return bottles or dump pills before the count. Biological monitoring (e.g., sampling blood, urine) is either impractical, invasive, or intrusive and does not measure adherence unless the time and dose administered before sampling are verified. Refill rates or electronic monitoring cannot determine whether patients actually take the medication. Although the process of cap removal does not necessarily reflect dose ingestion, medication electronic monitoring systems are useful for calculating adherence rates for dose taking and dose timing and often are viewed as the best method to measure adherence. Nonetheless, despite their limitations, all of these methods are adequate for documenting nonadherence, but in general, only self-report methods can distinguish among the various types of nonadherence described below. (Davis, 2005).

The cause of medication nonadherence varies among patients and is broadly categorized as unintentional or intentional. Unintentional nonadherence involves intending to take medication as instructed but failing to do so for some reason (e.g., forgetfulness, carelessness). Unintentional nonadherence is influenced by patient characteristics, treatment factors, and patient–provider issues. In contrast, intentional nonadherence involves making a reasoned decision not to take medication as instructed based on perceptions, feelings, or beliefs. Intentional nonadherence reflects a rational decision-making process by the patient whereby the benefits of treatment are weighed against any adverse effects of the treatment. Broadly characterizing nonadherence may oversimplify the complexities involved with nonadherence, but it is practical and illustrates that mitigating nonadherence requires different interventions.

Most medication adherence models are based on several social cognition models, including the health belief model, social cognitive theory, and theory of planned behavior. These models are similar, and all assume that beliefs developed by individuals shape how they interpret information and experiences and ultimately influence their behavior. Accordingly, health behavior (e.g., medication taking) results from rational decisions based on all available information.

Many methods to improve medication adherence have been studied. Most methods attempt to change patient behavior by using reminders, counseling, reinforcement, education, dosage simplification, or a combination of these methods. Generally, adherence interventions are categorized as behavioral, educational, or organizational based on modifying the patient's environment or incentives, providing more information, or lifting barriers associated with medication complexity and communication with care providers (Durso, 2001).

Most studies on improving adherence involve behavioral interventions (Yeh, H. et. al., 2006) Data suggest that patient education is one of the best methods for improving adherence, especially for those simultaneously managing more than six medications. Depending on the type of nonadherence and patient characteristics, using a combination of tailored interventions such as patient education, patient self-monitoring of specialized care, and stimuli to take medications have the greatest potential for improving adherence (Anastasiou, et.al., 2015).

MAIN FOCUS OF THE CHAPTER

Methodology

In order to acquire the most of our system, the proposed solution consists of four basic components:

1. **Medication Dispenser:** A dispenser that will provide the patient with the prescribed medication and will be able to record whether the drug has been taken. The patient's doctor or the pharmacist will provide the dispenser together with the right dosage of drugs needed by the patient. They will then insert the right amount of drugs dosage in each compartment of the dispenser according to the medication prescribed to each patient. The medication dispensers will be integrated with a communications device, which will transmit the patient's data to the clinic for monitoring. The data will be transmitted from the dispensers to the clinic for monitoring by the medical staff via cloud-based services. The dispenser will alarm the doctor, nurse or any other relatives of the patient that the patient has taken his drug and at which time of the day. The doctor will define the threshold values describing the patients' compliance to the treatment and when these values are reached, an alarm will be triggered letting the doctor know that the patients' compliance is not satisfactory (Tsai, P. et. al., 2008).
2. **Telematics Infrastructure:** The recordings from each medical dispenser will be transmitted to the clinic immediately. This will allow the clinic to monitor the patient in real-time and take action in the case of an anomaly. It is envisaged that the dispenser will transmit the patient's data (i.e. if he took a medicine and what dosage of medicine he received) to the server at the clinic. From this point of view, our system is non-obtrusive to the everyday life of the patient and his/her family, since it will not even use their telephone line. Concerning security issues, the system will incorporate 128-bit cryptography – a virtual private network will be set up during data transfer between the patient's home and the server at the clinic. Besides, the patient is only known by a code stored in our system. One would have to cross-check the code with the clinic's records, which are locally held at the clinic, in order to reveal the identity of the patient.
3. **Datastore with Patient Records:** This already exists in the electronic form in clinics around Europe. The proposed solution will develop a flexible interface for the integration of the system to the patient datastore.
4. **User Interface (UI) for the Medical Staff and Patients:** From the side of the clinic, the UI will enable complete control of the system by the operator, be that a doctor or a nurse. It is envisaged that different privileges will be given in order to access/write/modify the content of the system, according to the authority of the operator. From the side of the patient and, indeed, his family and carers, his record will be accessible via the Internet, using a password provided by the clinic. The patient/family/carer will also have access to an information library, which will assist them to assess the state of the patient and take action (i.e. call the doctor) if needed.

Clinicians will be able to connect to the System's web app. The web app will include the following data:

1. A list of personal details.
2. The current patient thresholds and alert types.
3. Each patient's medication prescription and historical data.
4. Medication dispensers' identification numbers.
5. Adherence events and alerts generated by the medication dispenser.

The hospital doctors will also be able to connect to the System's web app. This database will include the following elements:

- Personal information for the patient.
- The predetermined limits for the particular patient and various types of signals of danger
- The pharmaceutical education of patient.
- Unique code-number for the medical dispenser allocated to the specific patient.
- The compliance of the patient to the regime and the alerts that the dispenser has transmitted.

Among these systems, it is important that we use HL7 messages. Before discussing HL7, it is critical to understand that each healthcare establishment is radically different in terms of politics, business relationships, payment structures, data collected, database structures, and software systems. That means every hospital, clinical lab, imaging center, outpatient surgery center, podiatrist's office, and acupuncture center have unique requirements for interacting with data and patients (Smalling, J., et.al 2005).

If we multiply the uniqueness of each healthcare setting by the number of countries or political settings where care will be delivered we can expect the result to be an almost infinite number of unique requirements that like English, Spanish, and German are close in terms of their needs but not exactly the same.

It is in this hazardous arena where all care settings and users of clinical systems are different that HL7 attempts to establish a single, flexible, worldwide standard for the representation/movement of clinical data. Hospitals and other healthcare provider organizations typically have many different computer systems used for everything from billing records to patient tracking. All of these are based on the HL7 Reference Information Model (RIM) and the HL7 Version 3 Data Types. The CDA specifies that the content of the document consists of a mandatory textual part and optional structured parts. The structured part relies on coding systems (such as from SNOMED and LOINC) to represent concepts (Wan, D. 1999).

The service of our system begins when a supplier of medical services (e.g. a pharmacist or a nurse) programs the dispenser with the satisfactory doses for a determined period, which is bigger than the time interval that intervenes up to the visit for the next supply. As soon as the dispenser is provided with the medication, the electronic operations of the distributor as autonomous "sensor" will record various data with first and most important the time when the dispenser will open and close. All the above will shape the personal profile of the patient with regards to the continuous observation of his pharmaceutical adherence. The omissions of doses are characterized as alerts when they take place systematically for a time period and not as isolated incidents. Moreover, if one patient loses at least 50% of one week's doses an alert for the direct attention of the supplier responsible for the medical service is provided. Each time the patient will use each unique medical compartment, there will be a direct connection between his profile and his medical record according to the HL7 standards, and the latter will be updated thus letting know both sides if any changes are required.

The adoption of the HL7 standard is allowing for the creation of better tools with which to transfer critical information. This will make every aspect of healthcare more efficient and dynamic and will lessen the opportunity for mistakes (Kuperman, et al.. 2007).

These days, a patient's visit to a clinic or a doctor's office goes like this: A nurse measures a patient's weight, which is electronically populated into his or her medical record. The nurse then takes the patient's blood pressure, and the result is also electronically populated into the medical record. Next, the doctor selects criteria for a lab order, and the lab receives it electronically almost instantly. The lab performs the order and electronically populates the patient's medical record with the results (Governo, et.al. 2003).

HL7 certainly doesn't make these types of technological advancements happen, but the adoption and implementation of the HL7 message standard certainly help make them possible among different systems.

State of the Art

Our proposed platform is innovative both in the use of the technology (state of the art electro-mechanics, latest telecommunication standards, sophisticated interface features) but also in the business concept, as a medication adherence monitoring application. It is a truly innovative solution that reduces the cost of treatment and the hospitalization period while at the same time drastically improves the monitoring of the post-surgery or chronically ill patient enabling him to enjoy lower hospitalization costs and improved quality of life.

It introduces a ground-breaking communication channel between doctor and patient through a simple but intelligent device. The bi-directional communication offers the grounds for an effective reminder-compliance process. Also, through the series of features, the system possesses, critical, top-quality information is provided to the monitoring doctor at real-time. The device itself is highly sophisticated, with electromechanical features that provide highly efficient and secure medication management (compartment locking, intelligent medication allowance, remote dosage update, etc.). Also, being wireless and fully portable it offers ubiquitous service and ultimate efficiency. This device, coupled with the sophisticated supporting platform constitutes a pioneering application for widespread health home-monitoring.

The mechanical part of our system features an advanced design since it is able to accept changes in medication dosage and apply them in an ad-hoc manner. Likewise, it has the ability not only to increase or reduce (through doctors' specific online prescription) the dosage of a specific drug, but it can also implement an increase or a reduction in the time intervals between the dosages. It offers the ability to have different drugs at different times of day (as long as it is preloaded with these drugs). (Fulton, M. 2005).

If the dispenser is coupled with the innovative platform through the web interface, it becomes an innovative integrated solution for monitoring chronic patients.

SYSTEM ARCHITECTURE

In this section, the overall architecture of the proposed platform and how the various components will be connected to each other, are depicted. The main components of the system can be seen in Figure 1, and are described in the successive sections in greater detail.

Figure 1. System architecture

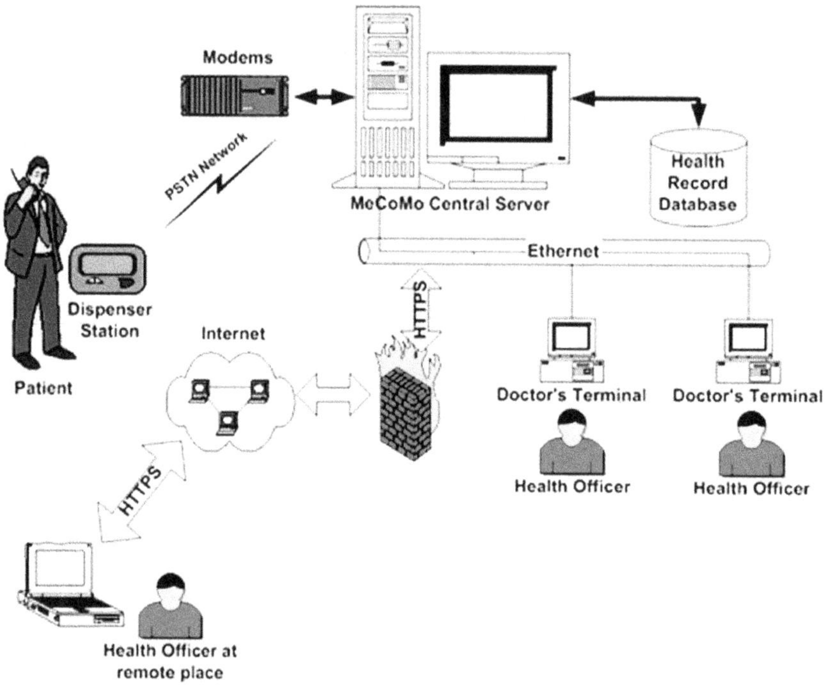

Health Record Database (HRD)

These databases already exist in numerous hospitals around Europe and contain patients' medical records that contain comprehensive information relating to the patient and his medical state. The proposed system will develop a flexible interface for the integration of the health record database (HRD) in order to acquire patient's information. This will enable the platform's server to query and enter/ retrieve information to/ from the hospital health record database.

Central Server

The central server is the heart of the system and is composed of several modules, responsible for the integrity as well as the performance of the system:

1. **Monitoring Module:** This is the main management system of the patient. The control functions on the server-side relate to continuous automatic monitoring of the dispenser's malfunctioning as well as patient's medication adherence. According to the specific medical scenario monitored, the dispenser will provide as input to the monitoring module a range of parameters, which will depend on the patient's case and the choices of the treating doctor.
2. **Presentation Module:** This module is responsible for producing adherence medication diagrams proving the medical staff with a brief and comprehensive view of the patient's medication adherence status. These diagrams will be customized according to doctor's preferences and patient parameters.

3. **Administration Module:** This module handles the requests for addition/removal/modification of patients, medical staff, and medication data. This module also audits user privilege and protects the system from any user errors.

Clinic User Interface (CUI)

At the side of the clinic, the CUI will enable complete control of the system by the operator, be that a doctor or a nurse. It is envisaged that different privileges will be given in order to access/write/modify the content of the system, according to the authority of the operator. All functions of the Control Module will be managed by the CUI. The CUI will be developed as a user-friendly Windows environment; it will be accessed through the clinic LAN and/or via a web server.

Medication Dispenser

As mentioned above, the medication dispenser will be a user-friendly device, capable of monitoring patient's medication adherence. The dispenser will provide the patient with the prescribed medication and record whether and when this has been taken. The doctor is able to program the medication dispenser according to medication prescription remotely. The medication dispenser records the timestamp of accessing a medication and conveys the recorded data to the hospital central server over a GPRS link. A detailed description of the medication dispenser's functionality and design requirements is given in the respective section.

Patient User Interface (PUI)

From the side of the patient and his family and carers, the patient record, including the system's readings, will be accessible via the Internet. The patient/ family/ carer will also have access to an information library, which will assist them to assess the state of the patient and take action (i.e. call the doctor) if needed.

HARDWARE COMPONENTS DESCRIPTION

Dispenser Components

The medication dispenser will be of the shape of a computer hard disk drive with a detachable rotating Carousel. It will enclose rechargeable batteries, the necessary GPRS modem, and respective antenna, an alarm bell, as well as the user interface for medication dispensing (LCD, buttons, etc).

The carousel will be doughnut-shaped, with a hole in the middle to couple with the base unit. It will contain a number of compartments, one for each dose. Considering that each dose usually does not exceed 4 pills, each compartment will be sized accordingly. It will have a single opening door, which should be locked when the carousel is not coupled so that the medication is not accessible by the patients or children. When coupled, the carousel door will open only when the patient chooses to take his medication (see Figure 2).

Figure 2. Medication dispenser (carousel)

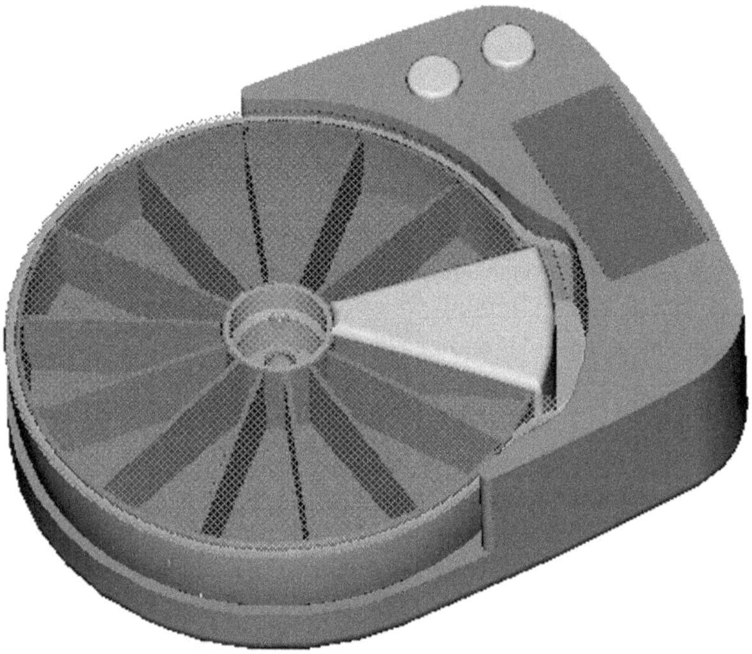

Dispenser Operation

The two modules (carousel and base unit) will couple together in an easy and fault tolerant way, with no need of external aid (e.g. keys). Attention will be given to make the door opening mechanism as tamperproof as possible. Medication will be provided only when requested by the patient and allowed by the logic, which will be programmable by the supervising doctor.

Specific Technical Requirements

The dispenser will be portable, and thus:

- **Wireless:** The only cable connection should be the power cable for recharging the battery. Normal operation will be with the dispenser being entirely wireless.
- **Ubiquitous:** This concerns the use of the GPRS networks for the communication purposes of the dispenser. Roaming will be supported for use in more than one country.
- **Of Limited Size and Weight:** The dispenser will be carried around by the patient, so it should even fit a pocket if possible.
- **Autonomous:** In terms of power consumption. It should have battery autonomy of at least two weeks of normal operation. Rechargeable batteries should be used.

After being filled with the right dosage of the drug, the dispenser will be locked so that the patient does not have direct access to more than the daily dosage. Following the above, the dispenser:

- Must be tamperproof– in terms of design and materials used in its manufacture. This means that it will not be possible for the patient to access its whole contents at once. Also, if it is opened by force, a notification must be sent to the monitoring server.
- An alarm, reminding the patient to take the prescribed dosage is also desirable. It will be activated according to the desire of the patient, and the programming will be done through the PC interface and data link. The patient will be able to deactivate the alarm.
- There will be an indicator warning for signal loss, low battery or system malfunction, showing blocking of the dispenser, errors in the logic circuit, etc.
- The dispenser will be robust, built so that it withstands being occasionally dropped. For this reason, high-quality materials shall be used. Furthermore, the design should be attractive and without sharp corners.
- The dispenser should be intuitive to use. Special skills will not be required for its use. Patients will be given a set of simple instructions for the use of the dispenser. This will include advice not to open the dispenser unless they plan to take their medication at that time, to remove the prescribed dose only when opening the dispenser and to close it immediately after removing the dose and should be sufficient for the complete understanding of the dispenser operation.
- The operation of the dispenser should not be intrusive to the patient's life. This means that the patient should not need to change any of his/her habits concerning the acquisition of medication.
- The dispenser will be childproof as it concerns access to the medication. To ensure that, coordinated action will be needed to access the dosage. This could be achieved by the use of a button that needs rotating before pushing or a door that opens only when a button is kept pressed, etc.

OPERATIONAL SCENARIO

This section describes the medication adherence monitoring procedure, focusing on points important for decisions to be made concerning the design of the system:

1. The doctor prescribes medication for a patient, who is then registered with the platform's service. The timing and frequency of taking medication are specified (the frequency of medication is estimated to be up to 4 times a day).
2. The patient is given a medication dispenser by the hospital pharmacist (or nurse). The dispenser contains the correct amount of medication that will be sufficient until the patient's medication is next reviewed by the doctor and a new prescription is issued (either a repeat or a change in medication). The system can handle any interval between medication reviews.
3. The pharmacist will program the dispenser on his PC terminal – the commands will be transmitted to the dispenser over the GPRS link (this task should be simplified as much as possible).
4. The dispenser should lock, i.e. in a single day, it should not allow the patient to take more medication than that prescribed on that specific day. This is a precaution against accidental access to medicine by children or other individuals and also a safeguard against accidental or deliberate overdose by the patient. Additionally, at any given dispensing time the patient has access only to the medication in the relevant compartment and not to the entire supply of medicines in the dispenser.
5. The patient uses the dispenser to take his/her medication. This should be made as simple as possible: e.g. by pressing just one button. Every time the patient accesses the dispenser for taking his

medication, the system's monitoring server should be notified by the dispenser automatically. It is, of course, impossible to know if the patient actually took his or her medication just based on a single recording (although one can infer this from the pattern of accessing over a period of a few days). However, the dispenser may "sense" whether the patient tipped it over to remove the tablet.

6. Medical Staff is interested in knowing how many times per day and the exact time the patient accesses his medications. Therefore timestamp recording of the access events is important – this will also be addressed in the presentation module.
7. The notification messages arriving at the central monitoring server are compared to the profile of the respective patients. If they indicate a wrongful medication pattern (e.g. omission of more than 50% of dosages for a week), an alert is generated and sent to two members of the medical staff responsible for the concerned patient. The alerts can be sent by the "preferred" means, as chosen by the receiver – this can be SMS, email, recorded telephone call, etc.
8. The nurse (or doctor) can review the patients' access to medication record from a terminal at the hospital or even online. They can generate a patient profile that they can discuss with the patient at regular medication reviews. Alternatively, the nurse or doctor can log on to the system after they have received specific alert messages regarding medication non-adherence. They should log on to the system's server via a terminal at the hospital (Internet access is also available), acknowledge the receipt of the alert and take any necessary action (phone call to the patient, schedule a visit at the patient's home, etc). Logging on to the system, the members of the medical staff will be able to edit/browse through the patients' details, log files showing messages arriving from the dispensers and edit the thresholds for the generation of alerts for each patient as well as the medication patterns that should be followed. The user interface of the system should be very user-friendly, minimizing the time spent on it.

RESULTS

Results are grouped according to five themes: Ease of Use, Reliability, Medication Management Assistance, Routine Task Performance, and Acceptability.

1. **Ease of Use**: On a scale of 1 to 5, where 1 indicated "very difficult" and 5 indicated "very easy", 94% (90 of 96) participants rated the medication dispenser as "very easy" to use and 2% (2 of 96) rated it "very difficult". In addition, 3% (3 of 96) of participants rated it a "4" and 1% (1 of 96) rated it a "3" on this same scale. Five participants commented on the need for the nurses' help if they were to continue to use the machine due to difficulty with pill set up.
2. **Reliability**: On a scale of 1 to 5, where 1 indicated "very reliable" and 5 indicated "very unreliable", 95% (91 of 96) participants rated the medication dispenser as "very reliable" and 1% (1 of 96) rated it "very unreliable". In addition, 3% (3 of 96) of participants rated it a "4" and 1% (1 of 96) rated it a "3" on this same scale.
3. **Medication Management Assistance**: Ninety-nine percent (95 of 96) of participants responded "yes" that the medication dispenser helped them manage their medications. According to one participant, the dispenser "does not let you forget".
4. **Routine Task Performance**: Ninety percent (86 of 96) of participants indicated that the dispenser did not affect their ability to do things for themselves. Ninety-two percent (88 of 96) of participants

indicated that the dispenser did not affect their ability to get around or leave the house. Ninety-eight percent (94 of 96) of participants indicated that the medication dispenser did not affect their ability to talk with or reach their nurse. Ninety-nine percent (95 of 96) of participants indicated that the dispenser did not interfere with their other activities.

5. **Acceptability**: Ninety-five percent (91 of 96) of participants responded positively that the dispenser gave them peace of mind. Eighty-four percent (81 of 96) of participants indicated that they would like to use the medication dispenser in the future.

The results show that nearly all participants perceived the medication dispensing device as very easy to use, very reliable and helpful in the management of their medications. In addition, nearly all participants reported that the machine did not interfere with other activities or the ability to reach their nurses. To a lesser degree, most participants reported that the device did not interfere with their independence or their ability to get around or leave the house. Many participants were initially not comfortable with the machine. However, as the study progressed, their comfort increased. For some participants, the machines became a key part of their home environment

CONCLUSION

Previous sections described the design and operations of a smart medication dispenser. Except for setting up operation and retrieval of individual doses from medication containers, the dispenser would be fully automatic. By monitoring the user's actions during set up, the dispenser prevents errors in medication identification. By automating the choices of dose sizes, the dispenser relieves the user from the burden of interpreting medication directions and special administration instructions and thus prevents the common errors due to misinterpretation.

By using algorithms that can take advantage of the scheduling flexibility provided by the sizable ranges of dosage parameters of modern medications, the scheduler can often adjust dose times of medications to keep compliance when the user is tardy. The bulk of the critical work in medication administration is done collaboratively by the dispenser controller and medication scheduler.

The medication dispensing device was designed to simplify the complex task of medication management with the aim of reducing medication errors and improving communication with providers. Medication error reduction and better communication are important to reach the larger goals of improved outcomes in older adult health status, rates of hospitalization, rates of nursing home admission, total costs of care and costs per quality-adjusted life year.

Older adults in this study accepted the medication dispensing device as reliable, easy to use and useful in coordinating personal medication management. These results indicate that technology-enhanced medication dispensers can be acceptable tools for older adults to help manage their care in collaboration with home care nurses. These results are encouraging because acceptance of technology-enhanced medication management is a requirement for improved monitoring of unpredictable responses to drug therapy in older adults.

The design is an iterative process, and implementations in a real-world context often reveal opportunities for better design. With older adults, it is particularly important to match personal abilities to device controls for medication management activities.

Future research should include:

1. Design studies for medication management devices
2. Research into new cost models that enable better access to medication management devices
3. Comparison of medication management devices with and without home services and
4. Integration studies of medication management interventions and data bundled with other informatics interventions for holistic support of older adults.

Last but not least, a challenge would be how to dispense the correct dose size of each medication given that medications can come in arbitrary shapes and forms. Our system answers the need for cost-effectiveness, fast-response, ubiquitous patient monitoring, focusing on the adherence medication area. Offering such an innovative solution, it brings itself ahead of the competition, setting the pace of the fast-moving healthcare technology area.

REFERENCES

Anastasiou, A., Giokas, K., Koutsouris, D. (2015). Monitoring of compliance on an individual treatment through mobile innovations. *EMBC*, 7320-7323.

Baron, R. J., Fabens, E. L., Schiffman, M., & Wolf, E. (2005). Electronic health records: Just around the corner? Or over the cliff? *Annals of Internal Medicine*, *143*(3), 222–226. doi:10.7326/0003-4819-143-3-200508020-00008 PMID:16061920

Cutler, D. M., Feldman, N. E., & Horwitz, J. R. (2005). U. S. Adoption of Computerized Physician Order Entry Systems. *Health Affairs*, *24*(6), 1654–1663. doi:10.1377/hlthaff.24.6.1654 PMID:16284040

Davis, R. L. (2005). Computerized Physician Order Entry Systems: The Coming of Age for Outpatient Medicine. *PLoS Medicine*, *2*(9), e290. doi:10.1371/journal.pmed.0020290 PMID:16173835

Durso, S. C. (2001). Technological advances for improving medication adherence in the elderly. *Annals of Long Term Care: Clinical Care and Aging*, *9*, 43–48.

Fulton, M. M., & Riley Allen, E. (2005). Polypharmacy in the elderly: A literature review. *Journal of the American Academy of Nurse Practitioners*, *17*(4), 123–132. doi:10.1111/j.1041-2972.2005.0020.x PMID:15819637

Governo, M., Riva, V., Fiorini, P., & Nugent, P. P. (2003). *MEDICATE Teleassistance System*. The 11th International Conference on Advance Robotics.

Kuperman, G. J., Bobb, A., Payne, T. H., Avery, A. J., Gandhi, T. K., Burns, G., & Bates, D. W. et al. (2007). Medication related clinical decision support in computerized provider order entry systems: A Review. *Journal of the American Medical Informatics Association*, *14*(1), 29–40. doi:10.1197/jamia.M2170 PMID:17068355

Law, A. V., Ray, M. D., Knapp, K. K., & Balesh, K. K. (2003). Unmet needs in medication use process: Perceptions of physician, pharmacists, and patients. *Journal of the American Pharmaceutical Association*, *43*(3), 394–402. doi:10.1331/154434503321831111 PMID:12836790

Lisby, M., Nielsen, L. P., & Mainz, J. (2005). Errors in the medication process: Frequency, type, and potential clinical consequences. *International Journal for Quality in Health Care*, *17*(1), 15–22. doi:10.1093/intqhc/mzi015 PMID:15668306

Smaling, J., & Holt, M. A. (2005, April). Integration and automation transform medication administration safety. *Health Care Management Technology*.

Tsai, P. H., Shih, C. S., & Yu, C. Y. (2008). *Smart Medication Dispenser Design, Architecture and Implementation* (Technical Report TR-IIS-08-010). Institute of Information Science, Academia Sinica.

Veacez, P. J. (2006). An individual based framework for a study on medical error. *International Journal for Quality in Health Care*, *18*(4), 314–319. doi:10.1093/intqhc/mzl011 PMID:16672255

Wan, D. (1999). Magic Medicaine Cabinet: A situated portal for consumer healthcare. *Proceedings of First International Symposium on Handheld and Ubiquitous Computing (HUC '99)*. doi:10.1007/3-540-48157-5_44

Wertheimer, A. I., & Santella, T. M. (2003). Medication compliance research. *Journal of Applied Research in Clinical and Experimental Therapeutics*, *3*(3), 254–261.

Yeh, H. C., Hsiu, P. C. C., Shih, S., Tsai, P. H., & Liu, J. W. S. (2006). APAMAT: A Prescription Algebra for Medication Authoring Tool. *Proceedings of IEEE International Conference on Systems, Man and Cybernetics*. doi:10.1109/ICSMC.2006.384807

KEY TERMS AND DEFINITIONS

Compliance: Compliance describes the degree to which a patient correctly follows medical advice.

Hardware Design: Allows hardware designers to understand how their components fit into system architecture and provides to software component designers important information needed for software development and integration.

Medical Dispensers: Are Items which release medication at specified times. Their purpose is to help senior citizens and other people who may suffer from impaired ability to adhere to their prescribed medication regime.

M-Health: is A general term for the use of mobile phones and other wireless technology in medical care.

Software Design: Is The process of implementing *software* solutions to one or more sets of problems.

Chapter 5 Robotics in Surgical Techniques Robotics in Surgical Techniques: Present and Future Trends

Vassilia Costarides
National Technical University of Athens, Greece

Kostas Giokas
National Technical University of Athens, Greece

Apollon Zygomalas
University of Patras, Greece

Dimitris Koutsouris
National Technical University of Athens, Greece

ABSTRACT

Healthcare robotic applications are a growing trend due to rapid demographic changes that affect healthcare systems, professionals and quality of life indicators, for the elderly, the injured and the disabled. Current technological advances in robotic systems offer an exciting field for medical research, as the interdisciplinary approach of robotics in healthcare and specifically in surgery is continuously gaining ground. This chapter features a review of current applications, from external large scale robotic devices to nanoscale swarm robots programmed to interact on a cellular level.

INTRODUCTION

Since the beginning of human history, surgical operations even in their primitive form have been on the frontier of medicine, due to the lack of non-invasive diagnostic techniques and the traumatic nature of the majority of health issues resulting from centuries of wars and battles. Surgeon, a term introduced in the 14th century means 'a person who heals by manual operation on the patient and has its roots in the Latin world chirurgiae from Greek *cheirourgiki (χειρουργική) and* more specifically their – hand and ergon – work. Surgery, the physical manipulation of the body aimed at the diagnosis, prevention and eventually treatment of diseases and traumas and from early on, the most critical factors that had to be dealt with, were bleeding, pain and infections.

DOI: 10.4018/978-1-5225-1724-5.ch005

Among the first surgical operations were laceration suturing, amputations, cauterization of wounds and trepanation with evidence such as prehistoric remains in cave paintings and ancient Greek writers' descriptions. In ancient Egypt engravings of surgical tools and papyri with recipes and pharmacopeia for the treatment of numerous diseases have been discovered and in China, physicians performed surgery with the aid of anesthesia, 1600 years before it was adopted in Europe. The evolution and incorporation of anatomy in medical education in the middle ages and Renaissance provided the basis for the systematic research that established the discipline of modern scientific surgery, as a common and safe practice.

Nowadays challenges such as pain management and infections are addressed with the latest technological advances in anesthesia, antisepsis, and novel diagnostic procedures. In our never ending quest for lower mortality rates, less pain and quality services, current economic and social trends guide surgical advances to less invasive techniques that eventually lead to lower hospitalization and recovery times, thus ensuring profit and quality of life to all relevant stakeholders and patients relatively.

BACKGROUND

In the delicate balance between minimally invasive surgery and high-cost state of the art technology, lies robot-assisted surgery, a field rapidly evolving in conjunction with other disciplines, such as micro and nano machines, wireless communications, bioengineering and information technology.

Minimally invasive procedures refer to techniques that target at limiting the incision site, so that wound healing times, pain and infection risk are controlled and minimized. It is widely used by interventional radiologists, employing imaging techniques and catheters, used as interventional instruments directed at the targeted vessel or organ, but also by general surgeons with laparoscopic procedures.

There are several techniques that surgeons use to perform minimally invasive surgery with the patient under general or local anesthesia, depending on the procedure. Usually, laparoscopic instruments either have a telescopic rod lens system that is connected to a camera, or the laparoscope is digital and the charged – couple device is placed at the end of it (Swanstrom, 2013).

The demand of robots in healthcare and specifically in surgery comes from the finite human capability to perform certain actions with adequate efficiency. As described above, latest trends in healthcare align towards automatization, robot – assisted surgery and minimization and therefore efficiency must be maximized along with patient safety, security and sensitivity. The manipulation of robotic instruments via a console, directly or indirectly that translate the surgeon movements to precision actions, was first introduced in 1983 with the Arthrobot (Paul, 1992), a bone mountable hip arthroplasty surgery robot and in 1985 the PUMA 560 (Piltan, 2012) was introduced, for a needle brain biopsy, under CT guidance. In 1988 it was used to perform a transurethral resection and a year earlier for the first laparoscopic cholecystectomy. In 1992 the Robodoc was introduced to mill out precise fittings in the femur for hip replacement (Schulz, 2007).

IDENTIFIED NEEDS

Robot-assisted surgery originally developed to overcome certain limitations of minimally invasive procedures. Based on the analysis of sensor information, healthcare robots use systems capable of doing mechatronic actions to provide healthcare services, such as diagnosis, interventions, treatment, support rehabilitation and prevention (Bogue, 2011). Patients, healthcare professionals and relevant stakeholders such as public institutions, insurance companies, and researchers, are setting the clear lines around the needs and challenges regarding technological evolution and turning points in robot-assisted surgery.

Safety is the most important requirement from patient's point of view and at the same time, professionals like doctors and nurses must maintain safety because of their obligation due to the nature of their profession. Therefore, procedures performed by robotic systems or with their assistance must ensure safety to both patient and healthcare professionals. In general, robots offer newer, better and safer treatments compared to the traditional approaches in many procedures (Finkelstein, 2010).

Even though quality improvements in diagnosis and treatment are crucial and recognized as a need, this must never outweigh safety issues as well as accuracy and consistency in delivering stable, reproducible and predictable results. Surgical accuracy and efficiency, as well as quick recovery times, are important factors, as they are directly affecting indicators of overall efficiency of health systems, and consequently improving the quality of life for patients and working conditions for healthcare professionals.

A specific need that initially triggered the development of telemedicine is medical care in remote areas on earth or even in space missions and even disaster scenarios, where medical facilities as we know them may not be available (Zygomalas, 2015). It is important therefore to develop and evolve flexible and portable, autonomous or remotely controlled semi-autonomous robotic surgical systems that can function in the above cases. From macro-world to micro and macro again, robotic-assisted surgery offers the possibility to access otherwise inaccessible human body areas, without major incisions and perform delicate operations, even on a cellular level in the future.

In the era of big data and information technology, robot-assisted surgical interventions have the possibility to provide detailed information about each case, which can be analyzed and contribute to further research. Furthermore, extended documentation of the procedures provides traceability, improved surgical and recovery time, and consequently lower costs which make health care accessible to all social classes in a long-term perspective.

CLASSIFICATION OF SURGICAL ROBOTS

Several classification systems have been suggested for robotic systems in healthcare in general (Kim, 2016), most distinguishing between imaging, rehabilitation, simulation, prostheses and surgical assistance technologies. The hypothesis behind classification lies on pillars such as potential benefits, technological challenges, and configuration. Factors such as accuracy, space constrictions, compatibility and extension issues, user experience and interface, application specific functionalities, size, sterilization and imaging (CT, C-Arm, MRI) compatibility, sensing and haptic technological challenges, degree of autonomy (passive, active, teleoperative and interactive systems) are also taken into consideration, allowing for future clinical and technological advances to be explored.

Two major categories of surgical robots for general abdominal surgery can be identified, distinguishing in relation to the positioning of the main robotic system and the effective arms with the medical instruments in relation to the human body and the targeted surgical field (Zygomalas, 2015); A) External robotic systems, and B) Internal robotic systems.

The external surgical robots have their basic operating mechanism outside of the surgical field, yet instrumentation is inside the abdomen (or the target area), regardless of the incision approach, which can either be through multiple incisions, one incision (Laparo-Endoscopic Single-Site), or through the body's natural orifices (Natural Orifice Transluminar Endoscopic Surgery) (Rosen, 2011). The external workstations are usually large installations that have to be situated inside the operating room. External endoscopic workstations, specifically oriented towards NOTES surgical techniques have been developed, as well as flexible endoscopic systems (Bardaro, 2006) that allow navigation and surgery in tight workspaces. As it is mentioned above, current trends in surgery are incision minimization with quality improvement and external robotic systems, have been under interdisciplinary research, in terms of miniaturization, in research activities and implementation, offering a new area for development with miniaturized external robots (Sanchez, 2013).

Regarding internal robotic systems, miniaturized laparoscopic systems, that are located entirely inside the human body, have been described and developed (Lehman, 2007; Oleynikov, 2005) that are introduced into the abdominal cavity via various methods and once positioned, function completely inside the abdomen. For applications in NOTES techniques, internal endoscopic miniature systems, that can be swallowed and self- assembled have been proposed (Assembling Reconfigurable Endoluminal Surgical system, 2014).

In addition to mini-robotic devices, endoscopic swallowable capsules have been developed that allow for imaging, telemetry, and even histology if provided with appropriate biopsy tools (Saurin, 2016). Finally, the evolution of nanotechnology contributes positively to surgical technologies, with the introduction of swarm intelligence robotics, interacting on a cellular and intra-cellular level (Mavroidis, 2013).

External Laparoscopic Robotic Systems

Laparoscopic surgery in which operations are performed through small incisions (usually 0.5–1.5 cm) reduces patient trauma and diminishes recovery times but at the same time limits surgeon's dexterity and vision because of the degrees of freedom that are lost due to the entry incisions, the rigidity of the laparoscopic instruments and the two-dimensional visual feedback.

The best known robotic system today is the da Vinci® Surgical System (Intuitive Surgical (2002) which incorporates a magnified vision system with a 3D high-definition view of the area and robotic technology that allows surgeons' hands movements to be translated into smaller, precise movements of its tiny wristed instruments inside the patient's body. Currently, there are several surgical systems under development that are marketed as daVinci's rivals, such as the SportTM Surgical System (Titanic Medical, 2016), the Telelap AlF-X (TransEnterix, 2016), the Raven Surgical robot (Kehoe, 2014) and the Araknes project (Sanchez, 2013) among others.

The daVinci surgical system is a proprietary technology, consisting of the surgeon's console, a patient-side cart, a vision system and instruments. The surgeon operates from the console, viewing the 3D image of the surgical field. It seamlessly translates the surgeon's movements in real time into precise, movements of the surgical instruments. More specifically, the 3D image featured in the console, provides HD vision and natural colors, up to 10x magnification, and the patented instruments have 7 degrees of freedom and a range of motion, greater than the human hand. The surgeon's hand tremors are minimized, and the console features built-in microphone in order to facilitate operating room communication.

The laparoscopic robot arm is equipped with a 3D camera and a light at the end. The camera sends the images from the abdominal cavity to the video monitor in the operation room and the surgeon console. The surgeon is at all times 100% in control of the system. Since its operation it has brought minimally invasive surgery to more than 3 million patients, covering various medical specialties such as cardiac, colorectal, general, gynecologic, head & neck, thoracic, and urologic surgery.

The SPORT™ Surgical System, which is yet under development comprises a robotic platform, surgeon – control for a single incision that incorporates a 3D HD vision system and multi articulating instruments for minimally invasive surgery. There is also a surgeon workstation that provides surgeons with an interface for controlling the instruments as well as the 3D view during the minimally invasive procedures. It is a surgical system, designed to provide the multi-articulating instruments and the 3D vision system for insertion into the patient's body cavity through a single incision of approximately 25mm with the surgeon being able to control it from the workstation. The instruments are designed to be coupled with sterile single use tools so that quality is ensured. The robotic platform is also designed to include a mast, a boom and wheels for optimal configurability for a variety of surgical indications and the ability to be maneuvered around the operating room and surgical centers where applicable.

The Telelap ALF-X surgical system, acquired by Transenterix Inc., is granted a CE mark, intended to be used for laparoscopic surgery in the abdomen and pelvis (Stark, 2015). It features haptic feedback, which leads to improved safety and allows for certain maneuvers to be performed with greater confidence. The system also tracks the surgeon's eye movements, positioning the camera, so the field of view is centered where the eyes are looking. The system is highly adjustable for an optimal ergonomic experience.

The SurgiBot System, by TransEnterix as well is designed to be a minimally invasive surgical platform that allows multiple instruments to be introduced and deployed through a single incision. The flexible instruments may be controlled directly by the surgeon from inside the sterile field, with robotic assistance. Its arm stabilizes the camera and alleviates the need for a dedicated person to hold it, and the instruments were developed to minimize incisions.

The Raven Surgical Robotic System was developed by the universities of Berkeley, Davis, and Santa Cruz mainly. It is a state-of-the-art open architecture (software & hardware) surgical robotic system and a prototype system including four arms which is currently available at the Bionics Lab (UCSC), while several other identical systems are to be distributed among leading groups across the US (Harvard, Hopkins, U. Nebraska, UCLA, UCB, UCSC, UW). The system uses a new statistical approach, Apprenticeship learning in terms of robot learning, targeted at allowing at robotic surgical assistants a higher level of autonomy, by being able to execute specific subtasks with performance exceeding human potential in regards to speed and smoothness. The latest version of the Raven Surgical System is IV, which was developed at the University of California – Santa Cruz and it includes two cameras and four robotic arms, and it facilitates a collaborative effort of two surgeons interacting with the surgical site in teleportation. The surgical arms are based on a spherical mechanism with a remote center located at the point of entry of the tool into the human body. Two surgeons in different remote locations can be connected via UDP protocol, as it is designed in the system architecture, with the use of a proprietary client interface and thus remotely operate the robots in the master/slave standard configuration. In experiments, several fundamental laparoscopic surgeries were completed while using a sampling rate of 1kHz.

Miniature External Robotic Systems

The Araknes Project, under the Large-scale integrating project (IP), FP7-ICT-Challenge 3: Components, systems and engineering/Micro/nanosystems funding scheme (Sanchez, 2013), is targeted at engaging micro and nanotechnologies from on-bench applications to in vivo surgical scenarios in endoluminal surgical approaches, thus further reducing operative trauma and enhancing therapeutic outcome of minimally invasive procedures. The system is based on an array of micro robotic instrumentation with components that include a flexible oro-pharyngo-esophageal access port and an umbilical access port, assistive and operative micro-robots allowing a bi-manual operation, an imaging system consisting of an endoscopic camera for global vision and a stereoscopic camera for visualizing the operative area, biosensors for tissue analysis (normally not available during laparoscopy) and an operating console incorporating the image of the operative field.

The developed robot under the project - ARAKNES SPRINT, Single-Port Laparoscopy bimanual robot - is yet a single incision master-slave robotic platform in terms of configuration, which consists of two high dexterity anthropomorphic manipulators, a stereoscopic camera and a master console for the robot control by the surgeon.

Even though external surgical robots have been an established reality in the medical community, there are still facing many challenges, mostly of technological and financial nature that must be addressed in the years to come, with an interdisciplinary approach and methodology (Vitiello, 2013; Marcus, 2013). In order for such an expensive technology to be incorporated in the services of health care systems, extensive cost- benefit analyses and needs assessments must be performed in mentioned environments, so that potential benefits can be substantiated.

At all times, the pre-operative diagnostic data must be matched in the surgical field so that localization of pathology is accurate. Furthermore, the tissue deformation that occurs by the manipulation of the tissue with either tools or physiological processes must be modeled and characterized in real time so that pathology may be identified in real time and deformations predicted. Haptic environments and tools may offer significant benefit together with visual technologies that will improve the restricted vision provided from current cameras.

Above all, as surgical robots are designed for all case scenarios, there is the size factor, that dictates new systems to be light-weight (versus current bulky systems) and with flexible access platforms (Noonan, 2011) that incorporate actuators and sensors.

Internal Laparoscopic Robotic Systems

Internal surgical laparoscopic robots aim at overcoming the obstacles of the classic and even the robotic laparoscopic surgery by including systems that augment vision and improve dexterity, using externally controlling robots that are completely located inside a body cavity. In vivo miniature robots, with either fixed-base or mobile platform, that fit entirely inside the peritoneal cavity, are now a novel technology offering a different approach (Rentschen, 2004; Zygomalas, 2015).

When it comes to fixed based laparoscopic robots, the main purpose is to provide an enhanced view of the surgical field, by augmenting vision and depth perception. Robots are placed with classical laparoscopic tools and are possible to be moved throughout the procedure, without the need to change the sterile field and make a new incision. Miniature PT (pan tilt) cameras have been developed as initial work allowing for panning of 360o and tilting of 45o, rotating two independent axes and with the use of LED lights (Oleynikov, 2004). Such robots were inserted within the standard laparoscopic port into the peritoneal cavity and had provided additional views of the cavity.

Laparoscopic robots, which feature a movable platform, remotely controlled, consist of systems that provide forward, reverse and turning motion (Rentschen, 2006). There is usually a mechanism that allows for counter rotation prevention and wheels are incorporated so that it is possible to maneuver on organs, like liver, spleen and bowels without causing damage. Similar robotic mobile laparoscopic systems have been developed (Rentschen, 2006) that feature adjustable focus cameras to improve depth perception within the peritoneal cavity, thus eliminating the need for camera port incisions eventually.

Biopsy instrumentation in addition to vision assistance has been added in several systems for one-port laparoscopic biopsy. Forceps providing adequate biopsy samples in porcine subjects have demonstrated promising results, with the onboard camera used to locate the biopsy site as the robot traverses the peritoneal cavity (Rentschen, 2007).

Apart from fixed base camera and wheeled robots, magnetic drive robots for biopsy, vision, and task assistance has been developed (Lehman, 2007), and tested in vivo. These robots assisted surgeons in laparoscopic surgery by providing manipulators with a dexterity not limited by the entry incision, alongside with an enhanced view.

Internal Endoscopic Robotic Systems

In advancing minimally invasive surgery an evolving field that initiated interest in the medical community since 2005 is Natural Orifice Transluminal Endoscopic Surgery. NOTES features operations where scar-less abdominal operations are performed with the use of endoscopic systems or miniaturized robots that are passed through the natural orifices of the human body and then through internal incisions, therefore avoiding external incisions and scars. NOTES is the integration of laparoscopic surgical techniques with endoscopic instrumentations and the current technological focus of the development of flexible or autonomous wireless platforms that incorporate robotic technology, thus using micro or nanoscale robotic devices providing capabilities such as imaging, retraction, tissue and organ manipulation, and precise maneuverability in the abdominal cavity. NOTES can be classified according to primary routes of access as transvaginal, transrectal and trans gastric (Kaloo, 2004; Marescaux, 2007).

The transvaginal entrance has already been established as a beneficial technique, as it is performed under direct visualization and through 2010 in 64% of the cases, rigid endoscopes were used in hybrid procedures (Auyang, 2011). Transrectal procedures are less common (Bulian, 2014) and trona gastric access has been less frequently used, as it had the technical challenge of gaining peritoneal access and a challenging gastrostomy closure.

Swallowable microsystems, which can be reassembled in the stomach cavity are proposed and developed, with potential to change their configuration according to location and task assigned, while monitored by navigation systems and controlled via wireless communication consoles operated by surgeons or healthcare professionals (Nagy, 2009). Within the ARES project (Assembling Reconfigurable Endoluminal Surgical system, 2014) such a system was developed, that can be disassembled after the operation, into individual models or reconfigured for a consequent intervention, eventually reassembled into a snake type structure. The modular nature of the proposed system can incorporate various extra modules, even during operations or dispose of unnecessary modules that can be discarded or replaced, with the use of magnets as the driving mechanism of self-assembly. Magnets can provide a reversible connection – disconnection platform due to the nature of the phenomenon per se and can enhance re-configuration options. Modular mini robots for possible use in NOTES or laparoendoscopic single site (LESS) surgery, have also been investigated in-silico using professional robotics simulation software with promising results (Zygomalas, 2011, 2012, 2014).

Magnetic anchoring and guidance systems (MAGS), that usually consist of an external magnet and an intracorporeal device with a camera or surgical instrumentation, have been proposed to be used for NOTES. The idea features insertion of the internal part through either an incision or a natural orifice and coupling via magnetic fields, across the skin tissue layer. The use of cameras with LED-wrapped trocars (Park, 2007) and the insertion of cautery and retractors modules have been tested in experimental models (Zeltser, 2007).

Endoluminar miniaturized robots are a much promising technological field for minimally invasive surgery, even though for the time being, implementation in real practice is limited mainly due to size constraints (Zygomalas, 2015).

ROBOTIC CAPSULES

In addition to miniaturized robotic devices that are endoscopically inserted into the abdominal cavity, capsule endoscopy, is a trend that has been an uprising in current medical research and it has started from imaging and telemetry capsules, used for diagnostic issues. A robotic system for capsule endoscopy has modules for power, vision, telemetry, localization and diagnosis and/or manipulation. Robotic capsules are now incorporating locomotion capabilities and are evolving into devices able to perform interventional tasks. One of the most critical issues is the development of an adequate propulsion system that will be delicate enough not to damage tissues, yet powerful enough to advance in complex tissue structures and perform surgical tasks with accuracy, safety and efficiency. The propulsion system is part of the overall design of the capsule that has a critical role in the successful deployment of the device. It can either be internal, external or hybrid where more than one propulsion mechanisms are used. Various methods have been proposed according to the geometry of the target area, like leg or paddle like mechanisms, activated by micro motors, magnetic actuators, or wall-to-wall motion with the aid of micro-propellers.

When it comes to internal propulsion mechanisms, the robotic system is more autonomous, having better control of its mobility. Legged propulsion systems have already been developed (Gorini, 2006), extending from 3 to 12 legged as nature is providing inspiration with bio-mimetic (bio – inspired) systems, that can vary from earthworm/inchworm-like that are based on piezo actuators or shape memory alloy springs (Kim, 2004, 2005, 2009). In such nature-inspired propulsion systems, the modules are to be swallowed and then reassembled inside the gastrointestinal track, using magnetic or wireless communication systems (Kim, 2013; Fang, 2015).

Cilia and flagella, cell organelles, similar in structure but with different functions, provide different motions, with the motion of flagella undulating and wave-like, whereas cilia motion is more complicated, 3D and with a power and recovery stroke. Both have been suggested and used as the basis for propulsion mechanisms of robotic endovascular systems (Li, 2006; Feng, 2007; Kosa, 2007) while other systems have been created with paddling based propulsion robots, that mimic canoeist paddling (Park, 2006, 2007). These feature linear actuators with dual cylinders that perform a cyclic motion, which helps the robot to advance in cycles.

Apart from external mechanisms, it is possible to use the electrical stimuli produced by the natural contractions of the intestinal smooth muscles that can be applied via electrodes to the robot (Woo, 2009, 2011). The peristalsis that occurs (the natural movement of the bowels) creates a force that allows potentially for a robot to move opposite to the contraction end of the lumen and it can be bidirectional depending on which electrode is activated.

Vibratory propulsion is a concept where the robot has an eccentric rotating motor that generates a (Carta, 2011; Zabulis, 2008) centripetal force thus allowing for the horizontal component of the force to propel the robot.

In the principle of internal reaction propulsion, the robot moves by the reaction force caused by the movement of an internal mass, without legs or wheels as in other systems (Liu, 2008), exploiting the piezoelectric phenomenon, incorporating a linearly-moving mass generate the reaction force. The most common mechanism for external propulsion, which bypasses the issue of internal actuators, releasing space for other instrumentation, is external propulsion by means of an external magnetic field interacting with internal magnetic components. It can be either guided by an MRI device, with its magnetic field interacting with potential coils incorporated in the robot or by an external permanent magnet that can be operated by a healthcare professional or even a robotic navigation system (Lien, 2012).

In order to combine advantages of internal and external propulsion systems and reduce risks and disadvantages mentioned above, hybrid systems have been developed that combine magnetic and motor mechanisms (Menciassi, 2009) with motion achieved by external magnetic fields and orientation by internal mechanisms. Other hybrid systems, bring together legged actuators with external magnetic dragging (Simi, 2010).

With the microelectromechanical systems advances, it is possible to integrate into miniature robotic capsules several tools like sensors for pH measurements, pressure and temperature sensors and blood detection platforms. Integration of interventional tools, is still under development. However interventions such as biopsy, suturing, clipping and drug delivery, have already been tested in vitro or in vivo in porcine models (Iddan, 2000).

NANOTECHNOLOGY AND SURGICAL ROBOTS

Since the miniaturization of electromechanical systems (MEMS) and their incorporation in general surgery (Rebelo, 2004), the next goal set by science was to advance further on the nanoscale, thus manipulation of the matter on an atomic, molecular, and supramolecular scale, with at least one dimension sized from 1 to 100 nanometers. Nanotechnology in medical applications and more specifically in surgery has been part of research, from drug delivery systems to diagnostics and interventions. Nanorobots, controllable electromechanical systems, are capable of actuation, sensing, communication, propulsion, signal and information processing and interaction with tissue. They can also manifest swam behavior and have a unique potential in delivering clinical results of high quality and accuracy (Mavroidis, 2013).

Apart from diagnosis and treatment of diseases with nanoscale delivery systems (Lenaghan, 2013; Dadkhah, 2013), monitoring and treatment of chronic diseases (Cavalcanti, 2008) or even incisionless surgery is the next potential application. In order for the nanorobots to be functional, several conditions must be met. Initially, the swarm intelligence (Bonabeau, 1999), which is the collective behavior of nanorobots that can self-organize them, should be accompanied by appropriate propulsion so that movement and navigation inside the human body can be realized. For sensors and actuators, communications, control, and decision-making functions, it is important to incorporate a power supply system, capable of supporting the described functions for the estimated time of the surgical intervention.

Nanorobots will be scaled to fit inside a drop of saline and then can be programmed to move to specific locations, to areas of interest and interact with cells directly, instead of manipulating tissue in a macro scale. This interaction on a cellular level means that cells can be guided to either die or regenerate with simple commands, inspired by computer programming. The input taken from cells will serve as logical input that can train and enhance logical function and cognitive behavior of the nanorobots, sustaining and advancing their autonomous intelligence.

Apart from collecting information and interacting with living cells, nanorobots can be integrated or even compiled of compatible biomaterials and serve as scaffolds in surgical interventions that require bone or soft tissue reconstruction.

CONCLUSION

As the world marches towards a new era of intelligent technologies, interacting autonomously within an environment of shared information and big data, it is but certain that self-aware cognitive robotic systems will be incorporated into everyday medical practice. Minimally invasive surgeries, performed with micro and nano-robots, will be ensuring minimal tissue damage, high accuracy, and quality, as technological advances will be incorporated into the discipline, along with accumulated experience. New capabilities and procedures will be developed, and it is likely that human horizon and possibilities will expand including thought controlled devices and what once was science fiction, will become mundane reality.

REFERENCES

Assembling Reconfigurable Endoluminal Surgical System. (2014). CORDIS. Retrieved June 8, 2016, from http://cordis.europa.eu/publication/rcn/10899_en.html

Auyang, E. D., Santos, B. F., Enter, D. H., Hungness, E. S., & Soper, N. J. (2011). Natural orifice translumenal endoscopic surgery (NOTES®): A technical review. *Surgical Endoscopy*, *25*(10), 3135–3148. doi:10.1007/s00464-011-1718-x PMID:21553172

Bardaro, S. J., & Swanström, L. (2006). Development of advanced endoscopes for natural orifice transluminal endoscopic surgery (NOTES). *Minimally Invasive Therapy & Allied Technologies*, *15*(6), 378–383. doi:10.1080/13645700601038069 PMID:17190663

Bogue, R. (2011). Robots in healthcare. *Industrial Robot: An International Journal*, *38*(3), 218–223. doi:10.1108/01439911111122699

Bonabeau, E., Dorigo, M., & Theraulaz, G. (1999). *Swarm intelligence: from natural to artificial systems (No. 1)*. Oxford University Press.

Bulian, D. R., Runkel, N., Burghardt, J., Lamade, W., Butters, M., Utech, M., & Lehmann, K. S. et al. (2014). Natural Orifice Transluminal Endoscopic Surgery (NOTES) for colon resections—analysis of the first 139 patients of the German NOTES Registry (GNR). *International Journal of Colorectal Disease*, *29*(7), 853–861. doi:10.1007/s00384-014-1883-1 PMID:24798629

Carta, R., Sfakiotakis, M., Pateromichelakis, N., Thoné, J., Tsakiris, D. P., & Puers, R. (2011). A multi-coil inductive powering system for an endoscopic capsule with vibratory actuation. *Sensors and Actuators. A, Physical*, *172*(1), 253–258. doi:10.1016/j.sna.2011.03.036

Cavalcanti, A., Shirinzadeh, B., & Kretly, L. C. (2008). Medical nanorobotics for diabetes control. *Nanomedicine; Nanotechnology, Biology, and Medicine*, *4*(2), 127–138. doi:10.1016/j.nano.2008.03.001 PMID:18455965

Dadkhah, M., Kumar, N., & Yoon, J. (2013). Design and simulation of a 3D actuation system for magnetic nano-particles delivery system. In *Intelligent Robotics and Applications* (pp. 177–187). Springer Berlin Heidelberg. doi:10.1007/978-3-642-40852-6_20

Fang, H., Wang, C., Li, S., Wang, K. W., & Xu, J. (2015). A comprehensive study on the locomotion characteristics of a metameric earthworm-like robot. *Multibody System Dynamics*, *35*(2), 153–177. doi:10.1007/s11044-014-9428-5

Feng, Y., Li, W., Li, M., & Sun, L. (2007, December). Structure optimization of the endoscopic robot ciliary leg based on dimensional analysis. In *Robotics and Biomimetics, 2007. ROBIO 2007. IEEE International Conference on* (pp. 109-114). IEEE.

Finkelstein, J., Eckersberger, E., Sadri, H., Taneja, S. S., Lepor, H., & Djavan, B. (2010). Open Versus Laparoscopic Versus Robot-Assisted Laparoscopic Prostatectomy: The European and US Experience. *Reviews in Urology*, *12*(1), 35–43. PMID:20428292

Gorini, S., Quirini, M., Menciassi, A., Pernorio, G., Stefanini, C., & Dario, P. (2006, February). A novel SMA-based actuator for a legged endoscopic capsule. In *Biomedical Robotics and Biomechatronics, 2006. BioRob 2006. The First IEEE/RAS-EMBS International Conference on* (pp. 443-449). IEEE. doi:10.1109/BIOROB.2006.1639128

Iddan, G., Meron, G., Glukhovsky, A., & Swain, P. (2000). Wireless capsule endoscopy. *Nature*, *405*(6785), 417. doi:10.1038/35013140 PMID:10839527

Intuitive Surgical. (2002). *The da Vinci Surgical System*. Retrieved June 8, 2016, from http://www.intuitivesurgical.com/

Kalloo, A. N., Singh, V. K., Jagannath, S. B., Niiyama, H., Hill, S. L., Vaughn, C. A., & Kantsevoy, S. V. et al. (2004). Flexible transgastric peritoneoscopy: A novel approach to diagnostic and therapeutic interventions in the peritoneal cavity. *Gastrointestinal Endoscopy*, *60*(1), 114–117. doi:10.1016/S0016-5107(04)01309-4 PMID:15229442

Kehoe, B., Kahn, G., Mahler, J., Kim, J. H., Lee, A., Nakagawa, K., . . . Goldberg, K. (2014, May). Autonomous multilateral debridement with the raven surgical robot. In *Robotics and Automation (ICRA), 2014 IEEE International Conference on* (pp. 1432-1439). IEEE. doi:10.1109/ICRA.2014.6907040

Kim, B., Lee, S., Park, J. H., & Park, J. O. (2004, August). Inchworm-like microrobot for capsule endoscope. In *Robotics and Biomimetics, 2004. ROBIO 2004. IEEE International Conference on* (pp. 458-463). IEEE.

Kim, B., Lee, S., Park, J. H., & Park, J. O. (2005). Design and fabrication of a locomotive mechanism for capsule-type endoscopes using shape memory alloys (SMAs). *Mechatronics, IEEE/ASME Transactions on, 10*(1), 77-86.

Kim, B., Park, S., Jee, C. Y., & Yoon, S. J. (2005, August). An earthworm-like locomotive mechanism for capsule endoscopes. In *Intelligent Robots and Systems, 2005. (IROS 2005). 2005 IEEE/RSJ International Conference on* (pp. 2997-3002). IEEE.

Kim, B., Park, S., & Park, J. O. (2009, July). Microrobots for a capsule endoscope. In *Advanced Intelligent Mechatronics, 2009. AIM 2009. IEEE/ASME International Conference on* (pp. 729-734). IEEE. doi:10.1109/AIM.2009.5229926

Kim, J., Gu, G. M., & Heo, P. (2016). Robotics for Healthcare. In Biomedical Engineering: Frontier Research and Converging Technologies (pp. 489-509). Springer International Publishing. doi:10.1007/978-3-319-21813-7_21

Kim, L., Tang, S. C., & Yoo, S. S. (2013, October). Prototype modular capsule robots for capsule endoscopies. In *Control, Automation and Systems (ICCAS), 2013 13th International Conference on* (pp. 350-354). IEEE. doi:10.1109/ICCAS.2013.6703922

Kósa, G., Jakab, P., Hata, N., Jólesz, F., Neubach, Z., Shoham, M., . . . Székely, G. (2008, October). Flagellar swimming for medical micro robots: theory, experiments and application. In *Biomedical Robotics and Biomechatronics, 2008. BioRob 2008. 2nd IEEE RAS & EMBS International Conference on* (pp. 258-263). IEEE. doi:10.1109/BIOROB.2008.4762812

Kósa, G., Shoham, M., & Zaaroor, M. (2007). Propulsion method for swimming microrobots. *Robotics. IEEE Transactions on*, *23*(1), 137–150.

Lehman, A. C., Rentschler, M. E., Farritor, S. M., & Oleynikov, D. (2007). The current state of miniature in vivo laparoscopic robotics. *Journal of Robotic Surgery*, *1*(1), 45–49. doi:10.1007/s11701-007-0019-9 PMID:25484938

Lenaghan, S. C., Wang, Y., Xi, N., Fukuda, T., Tarn, T., Hamel, W. R., & Zhang, M. (2013). Grand challenges in bioengineered nanorobotics for cancer therapy. *Biomedical Engineering. IEEE Transactions on*, *60*(3), 667–673.

Li, W., Guo, W., Li, M., & Zhu, Y. (2006, June). A novel locomotion principle for endoscopic robot. In *Mechatronics and Automation,Proceedings of the 2006 IEEE International Conference on* (pp. 1658-1662). IEEE. doi:10.1109/ICMA.2006.257445

Lien, G. S., Liu, C. W., Jiang, J. A., Chuang, C. L., & Teng, M. T. (2012). Magnetic control system targeted for capsule endoscopic operations in the stomach—design, fabrication, and in vitro and ex vivo evaluations. *Biomedical Engineering. IEEE Transactions*, *59*(7), 2068–2079.

Liu, Y., Yu, H., & Yang, T. C. (2008). Analysis and Control of a Capsubot. *City*, *10*, 2.

Marcus, H., Nandi, D., Darzi, A., & Yang, G. Z. (2013). Surgical robotics through a keyhole: From today's translational barriers to tomorrow's "disappearing" robots. *Biomedical Engineering. IEEE Transactions on*, *60*(3), 674–681.

Marescaux, J., Dallemagne, B., Perretta, S., Wattiez, A., Mutter, D., & Coumaros, D. (2007). Surgery without scars: Report of transluminal cholecystectomy in a human being. *Archives of Surgery (Chicago, Ill.)*, *142*(9), 823–826. doi:10.1001/archsurg.142.9.823 PMID:17875836

Mavroidis, C., & Ferreira, A. (Eds.). (2013). *Nanorobotics: current approaches and techniques*. Springer Science & Business Media. doi:10.1007/978-1-4614-2119-1

Menciassi, A., Valdastri, P., Quaglia, C., Buselli, E., & Dario, P. (2009, September). Wireless steering mechanism with magnetic actuation for an endoscopic capsule. In *Engineering in Medicine and Biology Society, 2009. EMBC 2009. Annual International Conference of the IEEE* (pp. 1204-1207). IEEE. doi:10.1109/IEMBS.2009.5332426

Nagy, Z., Fluckiger, M., Oung, R., Kaliakatsos, I. K., Hawkes, E. W., Nelson, B. J., & Abbott, J. J. et al. (2009). Assembling reconfigurable endoluminal surgical systems: Opportunities and challenges. *International Journal of Biomechatronics and Biomedical Robotics*, *1*(1), 3–16. doi:10.1504/IJBBR.2009.030054

Noonan, D. P., Vitiello, V., Shang, J., Payne, C. J., & Yang, G. Z. (2011, September). A modular, mechatronic joint design for a flexible access platform for MIS. In *Intelligent Robots and Systems (IROS), 2011 IEEE/RSJ International Conference on* (pp. 949-954). IEEE. doi:10.1109/IROS.2011.6094907

Oleynikov, D., Rentschler, M., Hadzialic, A., Dumpert, J., Platt, S. R., & Farritor, S. (2005). Miniature robots can assist in laparoscopic cholecystectomy. *Surgical Endoscopy And Other Interventional Techniques*, *19*(4), 473–476. doi:10.1007/s00464-004-8918-6 PMID:15742124

Park, H., Park, S., Yoon, E., Kim, B., Park, J., & Park, S. (2007, April). Paddling based microrobot for capsule endoscopes. In *Robotics and Automation, 2007 IEEE International Conference on* (pp. 3377-3382). IEEE. doi:10.1109/ROBOT.2007.363994

Park, S., Bergs, R. A., Eberhart, R., Baker, L., Fernandez, R., & Cadeddu, J. A. (2007). Trocar-less instrumentation for laparoscopy: Magnetic positioning of intra-abdominal camera and retractor. *Annals of Surgery*, *245*(3), 379–384. doi:10.1097/01.sla.0000232518.01447.c7 PMID:17435544

Park, S., Park, H., Park, S., & Kim, B. (2006). A paddling based locomotive mechanism for capsule endoscopes. *Journal of Mechanical Science and Technology, 20*(7), 1012-1018.

Paul, H. A., Bargar, W. L., Mittlestadt, B., Musits, B., Taylor, R. H., Kazanzides, P., & Hosainpour, A. et al. (2012). PUMA-560 Robot Manipulator Position Computed Torque Control Methods Using MATLAB/SIMULINK and Their Integration into Graduate Nonlinear Control and MATLAB Courses. *International Journal of Robotics and Automation*, *3*(3), 167–191.

Rebello, K. J. (2004). Applications of MEMS in surgery. *Proceedings of the IEEE, 92*(1), 43–55. doi:10.1109/JPROC.2003.820536

Rentschler, M., Hadzialic, A., & Dumpert, J. (2004). In vivo robots for laparoscopic surgery. *Studies in Health Technology and Informatics*, *98*, 316–322. PMID:15544298

Rentschler, M. E., Dumpert, J., Platt, S. R., Ahmed, S. I., Farritor, S. M., & Oleynikov, D. (2006). Mobile in vivo camera robots provide sole visual feedback for abdominal exploration and cholecystectomy. *Surgical Endoscopy And Other Interventional Techniques*, *20*(1), 135–138. doi:10.1007/s00464-005-0205-7 PMID:16333551

Rentschler, M. E., Dumpert, J., Platt, S. R., Iagnemma, K., Oleynikov, D., & Farritor, S. M. (2006). Modeling, analysis, and experimental study of in vivo wheeled robotic mobility. Mechanical Engineering Faculty Publications.

Rentschler, M. E., Dumpert, J., Platt, S. R., Iagnemma, K., Oleynikov, D., & Farritor, S. M. (2007). An in vivo mobile robot for surgical vision and task assistance. *Journal of Medical Devices*, *1*(1), 23–29. doi:10.1115/1.2355686

Sanchez, L. A., Le, M. Q., Rabenorosoa, K., Liu, C., Zemiti, N., Poignet, P., & Dario, P. (2013). A case study of safety in the design of surgical robots: The ARAKNES platform. In *Intelligent Autonomous Systems 12* (pp. 121–130). Springer Berlin Heidelberg. doi:10.1007/978-3-642-33932-5_12

Saurin, J. C., Beneche, N., Chambon, C., & Pioche, M. (2016). Challenges and Future of Wireless Capsule Endoscopy. *Clinical Endoscopy, 49*(1), 26.

Schulz, A. P., Seide, K., Queitsch, C., von Haugwitz, A., Meiners, J., Kienast, B., & Jürgens, C. (2007). Results of total hip replacement using the Robodoc surgical assistant system: Clinical outcome and evaluation of complications for 97 procedures. *International Journal of Medical Robotics and Computer Assisted Surgery*, *3*(4), 301–306. doi:10.1002/rcs.161 PMID:18000945

Simi, M., Valdastri, P., Quaglia, C., Menciassi, A., & Dario, P. (2010). Design, fabrication, and testing of a capsule with hybrid locomotion for gastrointestinal tract exploration. *Mechatronics. IEEE/ASME Transactions on Mechatronics*, *15*(2), 170–180. doi:10.1109/TMECH.2010.2041244

Stark, M., Pomati, S., D'Ambrosio, A., Giraudi, F., & Gidaro, S. (2015). A new telesurgical platform–preliminary clinical results. *Minimally Invasive Therapy & Allied Technologies*, *24*(1), 31–36. doi:10.3109/13645706.2014.1003945 PMID:25627435

Swanstrom, L. L., & Soper, N. J. (2013). *Mastery of endoscopic and laparoscopic surgery*. Lippincott Williams & Wilkins.

Titanic Medical. (2016). *The SPORT Surgical System*. Retrieved June 8, 2016, from http://www.titanmedicalinc.com/product/

Transenterix. (2016). *The Telelap ALF-X Surgical Robotic System*. Retrieved June 8, 2016, from http://www.alf-x.com/en/

Vitiello, V., Lee, S. L., Cundy, T. P., & Yang, G. Z. (2013). Emerging robotic platforms for minimally invasive surgery. *Biomedical Engineering. IEEE Reviews in*, *6*, 111–126.

Woo, S. H., Kim, T. W., Lee, J. H., Kim, P. U., Won, C. H., & Cho, J. H. (2009). Implemented edge shape of an electrical stimulus capsule. *International Journal of Medical Robotics and Computer Assisted Surgery*, *5*(1), 59–65. doi:10.1002/rcs.235 PMID:19170130

Woo, S. H., Kim, T. W., Mohy-Ud-Din, Z., Park, I. Y., & Cho, J. H. (2011). Small intestinal model for electrically propelled capsule endoscopy. *Biomedical Engineering Online*, *10*(1), 108. doi:10.1186/1475-925X-10-108 PMID:22177218

Zabulis, X., Sfakiotakis, M., & Tsakiris, D. P. (2008, August). Effects of vibratory actuation on endoscopic capsule vision. In *Engineering in Medicine and Biology Society, 2008. EMBS 2008. 30th Annual International Conference of the IEEE* (pp. 5901-5904). IEEE. doi:10.1109/IEMBS.2008.4650557

Zeltser, I. S., Bergs, R., Fernandez, R., Baker, L., Eberhart, R., & Cadeddu, J. A. (2007). Single trocar laparoscopic nephrectomy using magnetic anchoring and guidance system in the porcine model. *The Journal of Urology*, *178*(1), 288–291. doi:10.1016/j.juro.2007.03.001 PMID:17499803

Zygomalas, A., Giokas, K., & Koutsouris, D. (2012). Modular assembly micro-robots for natural orifice transluminal endoscopic surgery, the future of minimal invasive surgery. *International Journal of Reliable and Quality E-Healthcare*, *1*(4), 43–55. doi:10.4018/ijrqeh.2012100104

Zygomalas, A., Giokas, K., & Koutsouris, D. (2014). In Silico Investigation of a Surgical Interface for Remote Control of Modular Miniature Robots in Minimally Invasive Surgery. *Minimally Invasive Surgery*, *2014*, 307641. doi:10.1155/2014/307641 PMID:25295187

Zygomalas, A., Gkiokas, K., & Koutsouris, D. D. (2011). In silico development and simulation of a modular reconfigurable assembly micro-robot for use in natural orifice transluminal endoscopic surgery. *Hellenic Journal of Surgery*, *83*(4), 190–196. doi:10.1007/s13126-011-0037-y

Zygomalas, A., Kehagias, I., Giokas, K., & Koutsouris, D. (2015). Miniature surgical robots in the era of NOTES and LESS: Dream or reality? *Surgical Innovation*, *22*(1), 97–107. doi:10.1177/1553350614532549 PMID:24828382

KEY TERMS AND DEFINITIONS

Laparoscopy: A type of surgical procedure, in which the incisions are small and through which instruments and a viewing tube are inserted.

Micro – Electro – Mechanical Systems: Mechanical and electromechanical structures and devices that are made with microfabrication techniques and with dimensions that vary from below one micron to several millimeters.

Modular Microrobots: Robotic Systems that consist of diverse several subunits that could be assembled in order to construct a functional miniature robot.

Natural Orifice Transluminal Endoscopic Surgery: A novel surgical technique that uses the natural orifices of the human body in order to approach the peritoneal cavity.

Robotic Surgery: Surgical procedures that incorporate as aid, the latest technological developments in robotic systems.

Chapter 6
Ob/Gyn EMR Software:
A Solution for Obstetricians and Gynecologists

Konstantinos Bougoulias
National Technical University of Athens, Greece

Marios Prasinos
National Technical University of Athens, Greece

Ioannis Kouris
National Technical University of Athens, Greece

Kostas Giokas
National Technical University of Athens, Greece

Dimitris Koutsouris
National Technical University of Athens, Greece

ABSTRACT

In this chapter, the collection and the analysis for the development of an Ob/Gyn EMR software for small Obstetrics and Gynecology organizations is analyzed. The necessary gynecological information was gathered via research concerning the needs of the practice and was organized and categorized according to its importance to the clinicians. The user interface of the developed software provides access to obstetrics, gynecological, surgical, sterilization and PAP test data, along with video and image file storage capabilities. An integrated appointment scheduling module, as well as an expected labor day prediction module, are also part of the application. The developed software is self-contained so that it can be installed on the clinician's computer or accessed within the clinic.

INTRODUCTION

The increase in computer usage and the cooperation between Medicine and Informatics has a lead over the past 40 years to the development of important research and educational activity as well as high-quality infrastructure in the field of Biomedicine. Concentrating on Health Information Management (HIM) and Health Information Exchange (HIE) systems, Electronic Health Record (EHR) and Electronic Medical Record (EMR) software is being developed, in order to provide efficiency in Health Care and improve patient – doctor relationship. Various sizes of Health Care Organizations and unique needs of each Medical specialty have created the need for a wide range of software.

DOI: 10.4018/978-1-5225-1724-5.ch006

Information Technology has rapidly become over the past years one of the most important concepts in almost all daily activities and has expanded its influence over Health Care as well. Health Informatics combines Information Science, Computer Science and Health Care possibilities. A new level of cooperation and coordination is provided in managing and organizing data and Health Care services, for both research and knowledge application purposes. Health Informatics optimizes the acquisition, storage, retrieval and usage of information in Health and Biomedicine through the resources, devices and methods that Information and Computer Science can provide. Health Informatics tools are not limited to computers, but also include medical devices and information and communication systems, as well as clinical guidelines and clinical data management software. The cooperation of Health Informatics tools opens up new ways of practicing medicine and contributes highly to improving the quality of health care services.

The interdisciplinary nature of Health Informatics allows the simplification of every Health Care concerning activity. It is applied to various areas of Health Care including direct medical services for any specialty, pharmacy, public health analysis, therapy, and research. Efforts in improving Health Informatics systems have transformed Health Care by optimizing information and communication systems, enhancing provided services (in the level of analysis, therapy coordination methods, results evaluation techniques, etc.), improving patient care and clinician – patient relationship. This cooperation has been essential in developing and designing the necessary tools to implement health care with improved safety, efficiency, accuracy and making it more patient-centered.

Considering the continuously rising importance of Health Informatics and analyzing its benefits and applications in international Health Care systems we concentrate on designing an EMR Software that can be applied in Greek Obstetrics and Gynecology Health Organizations. Our software was designed by evaluating the usage and efficiency of similar software used in more highly advanced Health Care systems of other countries and adjusting the results of the analysis to the Greek Health Care system and the needs of the specialty in Greece. The analysis concentrated in the Health Informatics solutions mainly available in the US and the UK and the modern technologies used to implement Information Technology tools in Medicine. In addition, local factors such as specific methods of testing, therapy, and data management were taken into consideration and implemented in the software in order for it to better fit the exact needs of Obstetricians and Gynecologists.

BACKGROUND

Worldwide use of Information Technology in Health Care began in the early 1950's with the rapid increase of computers usage. In 1949 Gustav Wager established the first professional organization of informatics in Germany. During the 1960's various specialized university departments were established in France, Germany, Belgium, Holland developing Informatics educational programs, while Health Informatics research facilities began during the next decade in Poland and the US. Since then the development of high-quality research, education, and facilities of Health Informatics was the prime goal in the USA and the European Union (Hovenga, 2010).

In its beginning, Health Informatics was not referred to using one specific term and was usually known as medical computing, medical computer science, computer medicine, medical electronic data processing, medical automatic data processing, medical information processing, medical information science, medical software engineering, and medical computer technology.

Health Informatics community is still growing and is not as highly organized and well-structured as other technological communities. However, the work of the UK Council of Health Informatics Professions has led to the proposal of eight main areas of interest in an attempt to extend it more rapidly. Specifically it was proposed that advancements in domain - information management, knowledge management, portfolio/program/project management, ICT, education and research, clinical informatics, health records (service and business-related), health informatics service management are expected to lead to assisting not only health care professionals but also academics and would contribute to the development of commercial applications and the improvement of health care services in general. Since 1970 this effort's most prominent international coordination association has been the International Medical Informatics Association (IMIA) (Haux, 2010).

Health Informatics in the USA

Although the idea of using computers in Medicine was considered innovative even since early 20th century, it had not even widely applied in the USA before the 1950's (Hovenga, 2010). The first use of computers in Medicine was when for dental activities during this decade, at the National Bureau of Standards, Robert Ledley used them for his projects (Sittig, Ash, & Ledley, 2006). The next step was in mid-1950's when MYCIN and Internist-I were designed. In 1965 the National Library of Medicine started using MEDLINE and MEDLARS. At about the same time Neil Pappalardo, Curtis Marble, and Robert Greens designed MUMPS (Massachusetts General Hospital Utility Multi-Programming System) in Octo Barnett's Laboratory of Computer Science, at Massachusetts General Hospital in Boston (Reilly, 2003). For the next two decades, this has been the most commonly used programming language for clinical applications. As of 2004, a descendant of this system is used in the United States Veterans Affairs hospital system, which covers the electronic medical record needs of over 1000 health organizations. After the 1970's a vast number of commercial applications of electronic medical records management became available.

Health Informatics in the United Kingdom

The history of Health Informatics was summed up in the book "UK Health Computing: Recollections and reflections, Hayes G, Barnett D (Eds.), BCS (May 2008)". As of 1960, the application of Informatics in Medicine became a reality for several specialties, including pathology (1960), radiotherapy (1962), immunization (1963) and prime care (1968). Most of the applications used up until the next decade were designed by specialists to fulfill their needs. The Health Informatics community has played a key role internationally. The first ever Health Informatics conference in Europe was held in Cambridge. After all, it was in the UK where the IMIA was founded and originally named International Federation of Information Processing in 1969, before getting its current name in 1979.

Health Informatics Law

While Health Informatics research was being conducted and was applied in software and information systems designed, the ethical and operational limits of Health Informatics were established. Health Informatics Law is usually complicated in most of the cases, since all the advancements made in the field have always to be taking into account issues like personal medical data security, ethical issues in using the newfound medical tools in general, as well as the way information and methods of Health Care are used in practice. Of course, Health Informatics Law also applies to using Information Technology in Medicine, the interaction of information with the Health Care system and the circumstances under which medical data and records are available to other fields that support or enhance Health Care services. For example, in the US, Privacy Act of 1974 regulates information collected by the federal government and its agencies, allowing citizens to know what information is collected about them, assure the veracity of that data and obtain copies of the information. In Greece, Health Informatics Law is moving towards the harmonization with the European Directive 2011/24/EU for the application of patients' rights in cross-border healthcare (Buzek & Gyori, 2011).

HIM / HIE: THE BASIS OF ELECTRONIC HEALTH SYSTEMS

Two of the most important concepts amongst the Health Informatics community are HIM and HIE. These two concepts are nowadays the foundation of every Health Care system since they play a key role in organizing, managing and transmitting medical information, some of the most important fields of interest as proposed by the UK Council of Health Informatics Professions. The current goal of Health Informatics is the efficient utilization of information technology in enhancing HIE and HIM systems. Health Information Management is the practice of maintaining and organizing medical records, either in the traditional printed form or electronically, in hospitals, clinics, Health Care centers, insurance companies or any other organization that provides Health Care services or maintains medical records. The widespread computerization of medical records and other medical data sources has led to a wide utilization of information technology in Health Care data management.

HIM specialists design information systems, develop Health Care strategies and recognize the current or future medical information collecting and managing needs. They also apply computer science in collecting, storing, using and transmitting of medical data according to the legal, professional, ethical and administrative requirements of health records management and Health Care services. Specifically, they handled clinical, epidemiological, demographical, financial, reference and coded Health Care data. It has been indicated that the appropriate collection, storage, and use of data in Health Care Systems "will determine the system's effectiveness in detecting health problems, defining priorities, identifying innovative solutions and allocating resources to improve health outcomes" (Stansfield, 2005). For example, health information administrators have been described to "play a critical role in the delivery of healthcare in the United States through their focus on the collection, maintenance and use of quality data to support the information-intensive and information-reliant healthcare system" (LaTour & Eichenwald, 2006). As the field grows, and Information Technology becomes vital in Medicine, HIM moves away from traditional record keeping, approaching an era of more efficient electronic management, using for example Electronic Health Records (EHR). The main goal is still the same; analyzing, organizing and evaluating Health Care information, while Health Care organizations are provided the opportunity to access this information whenever it is necessary (LaTour & Eichenwald, 2006).

Latest developments in HIM field are concentrated mainly in three goals. Electronic Health Records (EHRs), educational applications and online availability. Electronic Health Records are the evolution in maintaining medical records. Due to the fact that they are kept electronically, EHRs must follow specific privacy and security rules to ensure that the confidential information will not be compromised. To ensure those rules, national and international standards have been developed to protect the medical records, such as the HIPAA Privacy Rule in the US (Herold & Beaver, 2004) and the EC Data Protection Directive 95/46/EC and in Directive 2002/58/EC on privacy and electronic communications in the European Union (Directive, 1995).

Health Information Exchange (HIE) is the mobilization of Health Care information electronically across organizations within a region, community or a hospital system. It provides the capability of transferring clinical information to remote Health Care information systems while maintaining the integrity and the quality of the information transferred. The main goal is simplifying access to and retrieval of clinical data that could provide efficient resource management, speed, and security in Health Care services. It is also extremely useful to public health authorities since it contributes greatly to analyzing population health levels. HIE systems help clinicians provide high-level Health Care services to patients by participating electronically to the patient's continuity of care with different providers, while the installation of HIE systems leads to economic profit for an organization, due to a reduction in the repetition of laboratory tests. Furthermore, patient care time is reduced due to the fast access to the necessary information, while paper and ink usage (note taking), physical mailing and phone expenses (referrals, verification of test results, etc) are lowered (Hillestad et al., 2005).

Medical Records Computerization

Electronic Health Records is the evolution in data processing for Health Care organizations, simplifying data processing and the development of efficient HIM and HIE systems. Computerization of vast amount of medical information implements computer science capabilities to Medicine, and it is rapidly becoming the most reliable way of managing and organizing medical data. EHR and EMR are usually thought to be the same, though there are discrete differences. An EMR is a computerized Health Care record created by a Health Care organization (hospital, clinic) and is usually part of a local Health Care system that allows storing, retrieval and editing of medical data. So, in a way, it is the data source for an EHR which includes much more information (demographics, public health data, etc.) that can be used even by users of a remote system. It is clear that an EHR is a far more complex system and contains additional information that an EMR would in general not.

An EHR is a systematic collection of electronic health information about an individual patient or populations (Gunter & Terry, 2005). It is a digital record that can theoretically move across various health organizations. In some cases, this exchange can occur via network-connected information systems or other information networks. EHRs may include a wide range of information, demographic, medical history, pharmaceutical treatment and allergies, immunization, lab tests findings, radiology images, vital signs, personal information, or even billing information.

An EMR is a digital medical record that is created within a Health Care organization. It is usually part of an autonomous, local information system that allows data are storing, retrieval and editing. Paper-printed records are still the most common method used by doctors for data managing purposes. Most of the doctors find it hard to let go of how easy it is to store data using paper. However, as easy as it might be to write down all the necessary information, paper-based records require increased storing room in comparison to digital records. In addition to that, health records need to be stored for a significant amount of time making paper-based records storage costs increase even more. Additionally, it is obviously far easier to move the information whenever necessary when it is digitalized. A study has estimated that EMR systems improve a Health Care organization's productivity by around 6%, while EMR monthly cost is less than what a doctor could save by not repeating a few unnecessary tests (Evans, Nichol, & Perlin, 2006).

In comparison with traditional paper-based methods, EMR/EHR systems can offer long term profits for Health Care organizations, while improving Health Care services, by avoiding medical mistakes, duplicate tests and by providing decision-making support. They also offer storing and transmission advantages because of the digital nature of data, increasing productivity and remote access to the data. On the other hand, those who are favored to paper-based records, argue about the time needed to digitize already obtained data, and the data security issued related to the electronic records. The time spent to digitize the medical records is spent only in the initial phase of transferring from paper-based to digital records, while regarding security issues, role access and multiple stage verification access, along with data encryption can ensure the safekeeping of the data (Gostin et al., 1993; Li, Yu, Zheng, Ren, & Lou, 2013; Win, Susilo, & Mu, 2006).

HEALTHCARE SOFTWARE

There are differences between software that is used in large health organizations, like hospitals, and software used in smaller organizations like a private clinic, or a doctor's office. In that sense, the requirements for each implementation are different. In a hospital system that can maintain many different types of data is required, to cover the requirements of clinicians from different specialties and departments. In that sense, it is necessary for each hospital with an HIE system to be able to exchange medical information with other external services (hospitals, clinics, government services). All hospital information systems should be designed using a client-server architecture to provide networking and data processing flexibility. Such solutions are developed as modular systems, to cover a number of hospital information subsystems, such as Laboratory Information System (LIS), Radiology Information System (RIS), Picture Archiving and Communication System (PACS), pharmacy, billing, and management.

The requirements of a smaller size health organization are different. Those systems focus on providing to the doctor the ability to store and manage medical information suited to their exact needs, rather than providing a holistic solution. Clinicians are usually working alone, or in small groups (private clinics), so they require a less complex system, adjusted to the exact nature of their everyday professional activities. Instead of storing general type of data, for these organizations, it is vital that the information maintained and provided are organized in a manner that is as close as possible to the clinicians way of working and thinking. The software solutions must be highly adjusted to the exact needs of each clinicians' specialty, in order to urge them to prefer electronic rather than paper-based record keeping. It is vital that these systems do not offer more than what the clinicians need, to maintain a high quality of information stored and data organizing methods. The client-server architecture is usually less important for such organizations, given the fact that information exchange needs are significantly decreased in comparison to larger health organizations. Of course, this does not mean that HIE systems for these organizations are unnecessary, just that their structure and functionality would be quite simpler than systems used in a large hospital.

Developing the Software

In Greece, Obstetrics and Gynecology related software availability is quite low. The data management needs of Obstetricians and Gynecologists are fulfilled mostly by more general software that is not adjusted to their specific needs, but is designed to cover all fields of Medicine. This usually leads to either lack of required data specialization of the software to Ob/Gyn needs, or to usage of software that cannot provide all the necessary information managing possibilities, to lower functionality due to the fact that the information needed is not organized in a well-structured manner for Gynecologists and seems lost among the vast amount of fields that are of no interest to them. This causes doctors of the specialty to favor the traditional paper-based record keeping method, feeling that it better suits their needs.

Before developing our solution, research on the functionalities of large scale Ob/Gyn EMR software was conducted, to identify the required features. In that sense, a series of software solutions were examined (both desktop and web-based). The key features that were common in all the solutions were:

1. Recording of the pregnancy history;
2. Storage of ultrasound images;
3. Creation of ultrasound flow sheets;
4. Recording of prenatal tests and results;
5. Obs/Gyn physical exam findings;
6. Calculation of expected delivery date;
7. Billing module; and
8. Appointment module.

Analyzing that Obstetrics and Gynecology health organization software needs and requirements, our software addressed to smaller Ob/Gyn clinics and offices was developed. The main goal was to provide software of high user interface familiarity that would offer improved functionality for these health organizations. Design-wise we attempted to include as few schemas as possible while including all specialty necessary quality information storing and processing capabilities, in order to enhance system efficiency and data accessibility while using the software. Of course, this occurs while providing all useful information management functions, making the software less complex and organizing information structure in a way that user interaction is as efficient as possible.

Information structure and software design are such that allows management of a wide variety of specialty related information without the additional burden of specialty unnecessary information. Considering that even among doctors of the same specialty there are different data processing needs to fulfill, a general set of gynecological fields were originally chosen and were implemented by some more detailed sets of data in order to achieve as high coverage of specialty related information management needs as possible. Through this process, a full medical information management system is provided while ensuring that there is no loss of quality information among unnecessary or useless fields. Furthermore in order to manage even information that might not have been predicted to be as important as it really is, there are fields that provide free, non-predefined type of input that allow the user to store any additional information.

Time scheduling features are also included, as every modern health organization of any level can benefit highly from such workflow management modules. Specifically, these features include setting and revising a daily, weekly or even monthly work schedule, having a fast preview of a patient's past or future appointments and predicting expected labor days for each patient. This combination of information can provide users with the chance to have full supervision of their work with as less time spent as possible.

The software itself is not designed in client-server architecture. The goal was not offering the capability of medical information exchange with other information networks or systems, but rather maintaining a full medical record that would allow the retrieval and analysis of patient information in an efficient manner. Therefore, there are no e-prescribing features that would unavoidably require some type of online information transmission. However, lack of connectivity to remote information systems features a feeling of security to the patients who would not question the safety of their private medical information since their doctors are the only ones that have physical and digital access to their data.

There is no billing and data statistical analysis features in the software solution. The financial part of the organizations this software is addressed to was omitted to emphasize on the pure medical information and the users interaction. Although, statistical analysis is of great importance in Health Care, and would enhance most of health organizations' service provision, it is mostly efficient for the larger ones. Statistical analysis is a whole different part of a software solution that would require exquisitely detailed work. moreover, as previously mentioned, the main goal in the development of this software is the improvement of theefficiency of the medical data organization and management.

Information is categorized in a clear manner and in a way that specific type of information is concentrated in separate parts of the software for smoother accessibility. Furthermore, all data are stored in one database that can be accessed through different local machines in the same workgroup. In order for the software to become efficient in larger health organizations, though, it should be implemented with storage, pharmacy, billing, e-prescribing, automatic analysis of laboratory findings and formatted input features. Another field that improved was the patient-doctor interaction. Image visualization of laboratory findings and images/videos, benefit the doctors while offering the opportunity to doctor to describe a patient's medical condition more efficiently and effectively.

METHODOLOGY

For a more efficient information structure, originally the specific needs of Obstetricians and Gynecologists were researched in general. This was the source of the main information structure design schedule. In addition to that, we contacted professionals occupied in the field to get further details on the subject, in order to better organize and categorize all the information gathered, and to implement our set of data with additional information that we might not have predicted to be useful. The knowledge base constructed this way was used to finally categorize our data depending on the type of patient-doctor interaction during each appointment, so that each time data is stored or retrieved, only the necessary fields are viewed by doctors.

The whole project was utilized in a way that the keyboard and the computer screen are as familiar to users-doctors as pen and paper, only providing more efficiency while processing data. Anonymous paper-based records that were collected during our meetings with various doctors were similar in many ways. These similarities significantly defined the software design and structure and the way information is categorized and organized in the database. The database was developed taking all those factors under consideration. User-software interaction was defined to provide ease of access and fulfill doctors' needs. The database was developed using the patterns that applied to the user interface, separating each set of data according to the doctor's interest, while securing each piece of information amongst the different users of the application.

Points of Interest

The software is practically focused on managing Ob/Gyn related information. For this purpose, it provides several different schemas to categorize the necessary information, including sterilization, gynecological, obstetrics, operational, PAP test, laboratory findings imaging and multimedia schemas. Maintaining and managing health information data is implemented with time scheduling and expected labor-day prediction features.

Seven different schemas cover the storing and processing needs of obstetric and gynecological interest. A full medical record is maintained containing data about individual patient medical history, family medical history, laboratory findings, doctor observations, guidelines and treatment suggestions, schematic visualization of test results, as well as image and video records of various operations like a colposcopy, laparoscopy or ultrasound tests. Various types of tests are categorized depending on their interest for the doctor and in this way, related data is requested to be filled in the database or is viewed after retrieval from it. Schematic imaging of test results offers a fast evaluation of a patient's condition. Video and image files collected during examination can be linked to the patient's medical record and viewed by the doctor either for analysis purposes or for presenting the results to the patients themselves. Multimedia files collected during various exams are observed through the software at the format they were captured, so no editing or format conversion is required.

The time-scheduling module is a simple and efficient date setting feature. Users-doctors are provided with the possibility to set upcoming dates with any patient at any specific date, or review past dates with specific patients or of specific days. In addition to that, this module automatically interacts with each patient's medical record, and the doctor can have full access to all previous and future date scheduling information concerning the patient at all times just by reviewing the patient's record. It is a simple, efficient, time-scheduling system that simplifies everyday workflow management. Additionally, expected labor days are predicted using a set algorithm that automatically utilizes data provided by the doctor and processes, providing predictions for up to the next nine months, further enhancing the software's time-scheduling features and the clinic's management.

Design Process Resume

Our software is mainly focused on medical information and the way medical data are processed and organized in a simple, offline method so that small health organizations can benefit from the computerization of their records. The features that were included are selected according to what is most needed in small clinics or doctors' offices, in order to make every-day workflow more efficient, offer a simple user interface to users-doctors and improve the patient-doctor relationship. The software aims to gain the trust of Ob/Gyn specialists through its simple structure and high efficiency and fully replace traditional paper-based record keeping methods of health organizations it is addressed to.

CONCLUSION

During the research leading to the development of this software, and throughout almost all sources reached, it was clear that Health Informatics is a constantly evolving field of Science. Health Informatics communities across the world, International Informatics companies, the constantly increasing number of software related to Health Informatics, innovative design schemas and evolving Health Informatics Legislation are only a few factors proving that Health Informatics is one of the fastest growing fields of Science today. EMR software has become an important Health Informatics tool and is the first step towards the development of medical applications. Therefore, EMRs are the foundation of digitalized health records and Health Informatics evolution is greatly going to be influenced by how fast EMRs can replace traditional record keeping methods.

The EMR software that was developed was adjusted to fulfill the needs of small health organizations. It attempts to utilize the benefits of Information Technology and apply them to Health Care organizations aiming to improve services provided, health care efficiency and patient-doctor relationship and replace previous record keeping methods. It is a solid suggestion that could instantly be applied to any health organization it is addressed to and fulfill its data computerization needs, taking into consideration the benefits of replacing paper-based records with digitalized ones. We can safely conclude that EMR software similar to the one we developed can be used as an efficient data computerization solution for small Health Care organizations.

REFERENCES

Buzek, J., & Gyori, E. (2011). Directive 2011/24/EU of the European parliament and of the council. Official Journal of the European Union, 45-65.

Directive, E. (1995). 95/46/EC of the European Parliament and of the Council of 24 October 1995 on the protection of individuals with regard to the processing of personal data and on the free movement of such data. *Official Journal of the EC, 23*(6).

Evans, D. C., Nichol, W. P., & Perlin, J. B. (2006). Effect of the implementation of an enterprise-wide Electronic Health Record on productivity in the Veterans Health Administration. *Health Economics, Policy, and Law*, *1*(2), 163. doi:10.1017/S1744133105001210 PMID:18634688

Gostin, L. O., Turek-Brezina, J., Powers, M., Kozloff, R., Faden, R., & Steinauer, D. D. (1993). Privacy and security of personal information in a new health care system. *Journal of the American Medical Association*, *270*(20), 2487–2493. doi:10.1001/jama.1993.03510200093038 PMID:8192748

Gunter, T. D., & Terry, N. P. (2005). The emergence of national electronic health record architectures in the United States and Australia: Models, costs, and questions. *Journal of Medical Internet Research*, *7*(1), e3. doi:10.2196/jmir.7.1.e3 PMID:15829475

Haux, R. (2010). Medical informatics: Past, present, future. *International Journal of Medical Informatics*, *79*(9), 599–610. doi:10.1016/j.ijmedinf.2010.06.003 PMID:20615752

Herold, R., & Beaver, K. (2004). *The practical guide to HIPAA privacy and security compliance*. CRC Press.

Hillestad, R., Bigelow, J., Bower, A., Girosi, F., Meili, R., Scoville, R., & Taylor, R. (2005). Can electronic medical record systems transform health care? Potential health benefits, savings, and costs. *Health Affairs*, *24*(5), 1103–1117. doi:10.1377/hlthaff.24.5.1103 PMID:16162551

Hovenga, E. J. (2010). *Health informatics: an overview* (Vol. 151). IOS Press.

LaTour, K. M., & Eichenwald, S. (2006). *Health information management: Concepts, principles, and practice*. Ahima.

Li, M., Yu, S., Zheng, Y., Ren, K., & Lou, W. (2013). Scalable and secure sharing of personal health records in cloud computing using attribute-based encryption. Parallel and Distributed Systems. *IEEE Transactions on Parallel and Distributed Systems*, *24*(1), 131–143. doi:10.1109/TPDS.2012.97

Reilly, E. D. (2003). *Milestones in computer science and information technology*. Greenwood Publishing Group.

Sittig, D. F., Ash, J. S., & Ledley, R. S. (2006). The story behind the development of the first whole-body computerized tomography scanner as told by Robert S. Ledley. *Journal of the American Medical Informatics Association*, *13*(5), 465–469. doi:10.1197/jamia.M2127 PMID:16799115

Stansfield, S. (2005). Structuring information and incentives to improve health. *Bulletin of the World Health Organization*, *83*(8), 562–562. PMID:16184268

Win, K. T., Susilo, W., & Mu, Y. (2006). Personal health record systems and their security protection. *Journal of Medical Systems*, *30*(4), 309–315. doi:10.1007/s10916-006-9019-y PMID:16978011

KEY TERMS AND DEFINITIONS

Data Processing: The collection and manipulation of items of data to produce meaningful information.

Electronic Health / Medical Record: A systematized collection of patient and population electronically-stored health information in a digital format.

Gynecology: The medical practice dealing with the health of the female reproductive systems (vagina, uterus and ovaries) and the breasts.

Health Informatics: The study of resources and methods for the management of health information.

Health Information Management: Information management applied to health and health care. It is the practice of acquiring, analyzing and protecting digital and traditional medical information vital to providing quality patient care.

Medical Software: Any software item or system used within a medical context, such as: (1) Software embedded in a medical device (often referred to as "medical device software"); (2) Software that acts as an accessory to a medical device; (3) Software that drives a medical device or determines how it is used; (4) Software that provides quality control management of a medical device; (5) Software used in the design, production, and testing of a medical device; or (6) Standalone software used for diagnostic or therapeutic purposes.

Chapter 7
Early Detection of Electroencephalogram Temporal Events in Alzheimer's Disease

Pedro Miguel Rodrigues
University of Porto, Portugal

João Paulo Teixeira
Polythecnic Institute of Bragança, Portugal

Diamantino Freitas
University of Porto, Portugal

Dílio Alves
Hospital de São João – Porto, Portugal

Carolina Garrett
Hospital de São João – Porto, Portugal

ABSTRACT

Alzheimer's Disease (AD) is considered one of the most debilitating illness in modern societies and the leading cause of dementia. This study is a new approach to detect early AD Electroencephalogram (EEG) temporal events in order to improve early AD diagnosis. For that, Self-Organized Maps (SOM) were used, and it was found that there are sequences of EEG energy variation, characteristic of AD, that appear with high incidence in Mild Cognitive Impairment (MCI) patients. Those AD events are related to the first cognitive changes in patients that interfered with the normal EEG signal pattern. Moreover, there are significant differences concerning the propagation time of those events between the study groups($p=0.0082<0.05$), meaning that, as AD progresses the brain dynamics are progressively affected, what is expected because AD causes brain atrophy.

INTRODUCTION

In the last decades, deep changes related to world population age structure happened with a progressive decrease of young people and a progressive increase of elderly people (Ballard, et al., 2011). The decrease of mortality and the simultaneous decrease of fertility levels have contributed to the phenomenon called overall aging of the population. The aging population has become a fact of scientific interest because

DOI: 10.4018/978-1-5225-1724-5.ch007

the elderly are most vulnerable to the onset of certain degenerative diseases (Jonker, Launer, Hooijer, & Lindeboom, 1996). Alzheimer's disease (AD) is a degenerative, chronic, progressive and irreversible illness and is the most common cause of dementia. In 2001 AD reached more than 24.3 million affected people around the world and it has the propensity to rise significantly in the coming years (Ballard, et al., 2011). AD also represents 60% of elderly diseases and has an unknown cause. As it is a cortical and progressive brain disorder, gradually, over time, most parts of the brain will suffer damage and AD symptoms will severely increase (Blennow, Leon, & Zetterberg, 2006). The first symptoms of AD are memory loss, particularly difficulty remembering newly learned information and concentration problems (Gwyther, 2001). As the disease progresses patients manifest general cognitive problems, confusion, personality / behavioral changes and also disorientation (Bird, 2001). Finally, there is a global brain atrophy and patients acquire a complete inability (Cummings, 2004). So, permanent aids of family members or caregivers are increasingly requested (Jeong, 2004).

AD progression is gradual and usually categorized into four stages. Each one presents typical symptoms of the disease progression. The pre-dementia stage is known as Mild Cognitive Impairment (MCI). At this stage subjects present subtle symptoms, daily life activities are preserved, and cognitive impairment is restricted to memory (Nestor, Scheltens, & Hodges, 2004). MCI confers a higher risk of developing AD but only between 6% and 25% of people affected with MCI actually develops AD (Shimokawa, et al., 2001). Mild and Moderate AD are the next two stages characterized by a significant increase of cognitive impairment and a marked loss of independence (Gwyther, 2001). The last stage is Severe AD where a complete deterioration of personality occurs; patients are unable to perform any tasks and caregiving becomes fully indispensable (Mesulam, 2000).

Researchers do not know yet why the brain cells deteriorate. Senile plaques and neurofibrillary tangles in the medial temporal lobe and cortical areas are two pathological hallmarks of brains destroyed by AD (Blennow, 2005; Mattson, 2004). These two abnormal structures are responsible for damaging and killing the nerve cells (Cummings, 2004). Parts of the brain start to shrink because the brain's nerve cells die. In AD the last stage, the damage is generalized, and the brain tissue volume decreases very significantly (Blennow, 2005; Blennow & Zetterberg, 2010).

Several factors are often associated with a higher risk of developing AD. Ageing is considered the main risk factor; after the age of 65, the risk of developing the disease doubles every five years. Another factor is family history; people who have a close relative who developed Alzheimer's disease have a slightly higher risk of eventually developing the disease themselves (Blennow, 2005). Gender is considered another factor; a higher percentage of women develop AD than men do. Heart diseases (namely: high cholesterol, hypertension or poorly controlled diabetes) are considered risk factors for developing AD. Many other factors, including stress, obesity, smoking, lower educational qualifications, Down's syndrome and head injuries are associated with a possible risk of developing AD (Blennow, Leon, & Zetterberg, 2006; Lahiri, Farlow, Greig, & Sambamurti, 2002).

Despite the progress in better understanding AD stages, there remains no prospect of cure at least shortly. Therapies currently available only soften and slow the symptoms progression, that is why new treatments must be developed to alter the disease process itself and not just to reduce some of the common symptoms (Ballard, et al., 2011). AD has been researched for years, but researchers have not yet discovered a good treatment for this complex and stressful disease and neither have discovered a reliable method to make an accurate AD diagnosis (Ballard, et al., 2011).

AD leads to death approximately seven years after being diagnosed (Mölsä, 1986). An early and accurate diagnosis is necessary to help intervention in order to reduce the brain damage. It is often difficult to diagnose AD, and the diagnosis is made by excluding other possible causes of dementia symptoms (Porth & Matfin, 2009). Besides, a definitive AD diagnosis can only be made by necropsy (Blennow, 2005). The development of methods that can assist in AD diagnosis may lead to reducing costs associated with this illness because AD is considered a modern epidemic with a large impact on the Health Care Systems (Lahiri, Farlow, Greig, & Sambamurti, 2002; Ferri, et al., 2005). AD is a public health problem and represents a challenge to the scientific community in order to find solutions to minimize its socio-economic effects (Machado, 2002).

The Electroencephalogram (EEG) has been used for several decades as a diagnostic tool for dementia. Therefore, it can be a useful tool in AD diagnosis. The EEG is a physiological technique that records the brain electrical activity originated by the neurons with high resolution (Sanei & Chambers, 2007). It is also a non-invasive and a cost-effective technique that presents no side effects and it is widely extended in clinical settings (Jeong, 2004; Stam, 2005). Nowadays, there are equipments with up to 32 channels of EEG with electrodes connected to the scalp to conduct the electro-cortical potentials to the amplification device. This device provides quite accurate readings, and the analysis is reliable enough (Sanei & Chambers, 2007). A system consists of EEG electrodes, connecting cables, amplifiers and a microcontroller to communicate with the main computer in order to visualize the brain signals (Sanei & Chambers, 2007). The recorded EEG signals have very complex shapes, which depend on the locations of the electrodes, given a large number of interconnections that the neurons have, as well as, the fact that the brain does not have a uniform structure (Sanei & Chambers, 2007). EEG is typically divided into several frequency bands, such as delta (1-4 Hz, δ), theta (4-8 Hz, θ), alpha (8-13Hz, α), beta (13-30 Hz, β) and gamma (30-40 Hz, γ). AD seems to affect the power in those different bands. Many studies have shown that AD causes "slow down" on EEG signals (Jeong, 2004; Stam, 2005). AD is associated with an increase of power in low frequencies (delta and theta band) and a decrease of power in higher frequencies (alpha and beta) (Jeong, 2004). This phenomenon also called "shift-to-the-left" appears in advanced and intermediate states of AD and it can be seen notably in the peak occurring in the alpha range (Jeong, 2004). These changes are related to the destruction of cholinergic synapses in the Meynert nucleus where transferase is produced, responsible for the synthesis of acetylcholine (Gawel, Szmidt-Salkowska, & Kowalski, 2009). A lack of acetylcholine is, in turn, responsible for disorders of the synchronization of synaptic potentials, and then, pathological activity reveals itself in the form of EEG slower waves (Gawel, Szmidt-Salkowska, & Kowalski, 2009).

STUDY OBJECTIVE AND CHAPTER ORGANIZATION

In this study, the authors want to create a methodology to better understand AD behavior during its progression. For that propose, as it is difficult to get an accurate AD diagnoses in early stages, in this study an unsupervised learning tool (Self-Organized Maps (SOM)) was used in order to search characteristic AD events in MCI patients by using EEG signals. The Wavelet Transform (*WT*) was applied to extract several EEG features, and genetics algorithms were used to search the best feature combinations. The features selection process was important in order to have the best accurate EEG information to search AD temporal events with better precision by an unsupervised learning tool. The paper is organized as follows: In the section Materials and Methods - the Materials are introduced together with the EEG analysis and the unsupervised tool that leads to the development of the proposed methodology and its fundamentals; In the section Methodology - the methodology is described; section Future Research

Directions indicates the future research lines of this work; and finally, in the section Discussion and Conclusions - the results are discussed and it concludes the paper emphasizing its main contributions.

MATERIALS AND METHODS

Selection of Study Participants and EEG Recording

A set of 24 subjects participated in this study (8 as Controls (C), 8 with MCI, 8 with AD). EEGs were recorded from the 19 scalp loci of the international 10-20 configuration using a digital electroencephalograph in "Hospital de São João - Porto", Portugal. The sampling frequency was 256 Hz and all recordings were digitally filtered with a band-pass filter with cut-off frequencies at 1-40Hz. In Table 1, additional information is provided regarding the participants in each group including the average age and Mini Mental State Examination (MMSE) average. All EEG were organized in segments of 5s (1280 epochs) and recorded with the eyes closed. All participants gave their informed consent prior for their participation in this study, and the study protocol was approved by the local Ethics Committee.

EEG Time-Frequency Representations

The EEG signals, in general, tend to have rapid oscillations in short intervals or slow variations in long intervals (Sanei & Chambers, 2007). The Fast Fourier Transform (FFT) was introduced in 1965 and it remains the spectral EEG signal processing most commonly used until today (Rodrigues & Teixeira, 2013). However, FFT is not able to provide information both in the time and frequency of signal characteristics. The spectral components do not reflect changes over time, what is a problem to analyze non-stationary signals, like the EEG (Haykin & Veen, 2003). As a result, it is convenient to use a transformation that provides a variable resolution time-frequency plane. This is the case of the *WT*, which provides a good time resolution for the high frequencies and good frequency resolution for low frequencies (Kaiser, 1994; Rioul & Vetterli, 1992). The EEG discrete signal is represented as $x[n] = x(n \cdot T_s)$, $n = 0,..,N-1$, sampled to F_s samples/s ($F_s = 1/T_s$) with N samples. The *WT* is an optimal tool for data analysis when time and frequency resolution are critical (Schiff & Milton, 1993). The Equation 1 represents the calculation of *WT* per scale, sometimes called child *WT* ($\psi(t)_{\tau,a}$) (Kaiser, 1994; Rioul & Vetterli, 1992)

$$\psi\left(t\right)_{\{\tau,a\}} = \frac{1}{\sqrt{\{\left| a \right|\}}} \cdot \psi\left(\frac{t-\tau}{a}\right), \tag{1}$$

Table 1. The dataset

Dataset			
	Control Subjects	**MCI Patients**	**AD Patients**
#	8	8	8
Age average	75	80	78
MMSE average	28,77	26,29	20,97

where τ is the translational parameter, t represents the bins in the time domain, $\psi(t)$ is the Wavelet Mother and a represents the basis functions range that acts as an enlargement factor if $a > 1$ or as a compression factor if $a < 1$.

The Discrete Wavelet Transform (*DWT*) uses a multiresolution analysis that consists in obtaining increasingly smaller signal resolution versions by successive filtering. The *DWT* uses one set of two functions: a scale function ($\varphi[n]$) and a Wavelet function ($\psi[n]$).

$$\varphi[n] = \sum_k h[k] \cdot \phi[2 \cdot n - k] \tag{2}$$

$$\psi[n] = \sum_k g[k] \cdot \phi[2 \cdot n - k] \tag{3}$$

where k is the discrete translation parameter and $h[k]$ and $g[k]$ respectively are the impulse responses of the low-pass and high-pass filters used in the *WT* analysis. The signal decomposition in different frequency bands is achieved by successive low-pass filters and high-pass filters in time, followed by subsampling by a factor of two until the maximum level of decomposition ($log_2(N)$) as is illustrated in the following equations 4 and 5.

$$DWT_A^{\varphi}[j,k] = \sum_{n=0}^{\frac{N}{2^{(j-1)}}} DWT_A^{\varphi}[j-1,n] \cdot h[2 \cdot k - n] \tag{4}$$

$$DWT_D^{\psi}[j,k] = \sum_{n=0}^{\frac{N}{2^{(j-1)}}} DWT_A^{\psi}[j-1,n] \cdot g[2 \cdot k - n] \tag{5}$$

where, $k = 0, ..., N/2j$; $j = 0, ..., log_2(N)$; A represents the *DWT* approximated coefficients; D the *DWT* detail coefficients and N the signal length. The Power Spectral Density (*PSD*) functions showed the variations strength of Power as a function of frequency. The Wavelet Packet Transform (*WPT*) spectrum was obtained by extracting the *WPT* coefficients corresponding to the terminal nodes. The *WPT* function was defined as (Rodrigues & Teixeira, 2011; Rodrigues & Teixeira, 2013):

$$X_{\varphi,\psi}[j,m,k] = \sum_{n=0}^{\frac{N}{2^j-1}} WP^{\varphi,\psi}[j,m,n] \cdot w_{j,m,k}[n],$$

$$w_{j,m,k}\left[n\right] = 2^{-\frac{j}{2}} \cdot w_m\left[2^{-j} \cdot n - k\right],$$

$$j = 1,\dots,J; m = 0,1,\dots,2^j - 1; k = 1,\dots,2^{J-j} \quad (6)$$

where $J=log_2(n)$, j represented the level of *WPT*. To estimate the *PSD* of *WT*, we used the *WPT* periodogram based on the observations of length $N=2^j$-1.

$$S_{x,\varphi,\psi}\left[m,k\right] = \left[\sum_{j=1}^{J} X_{\varphi,\psi}\left[m,k\right]\right]^2 ; m = 0,1,\dots,2^j - 1; k = 1,\dots,2^{J-j}; \quad (7)$$

To obtain the frequency spacing of *PSD* of *WT* of each level of decomposition we used the range,

$$\left[\frac{F_s}{2^{j+1}}, \frac{F_s}{2^{j+1-1}}\right], \quad j = 1,\dots,log_2(N) \ , \quad (8)$$

Summarizing, the absolute value of the coefficients was taken, and the Wavelet coefficients were ordered by frequency. The *PSD* was normalized (PSD_n) as below (Rodrigues & Teixeira, 2013):

$$PSD_n\left[m,k\right] = \frac{S_{x,\varphi,\psi}[n]}{\sum_{n=k_1}^{k_2} S_{x,\varphi,\psi}[n]}, \qquad m = 0,\dots,2^j - 1 \quad (9)$$

Feature Extraction

Several features were extracted in each frequency bands (δ, θ, α, β and γ) of the EEG signal. This feature characterized the waveform in terms of faster or slower and of greater or smaller variability as it is required to observe the "shift-to-the-left" phenomenon. It can be described by the values of maxima (*NMax*) and minima (*NMin*), the zero-crossing (*Zcr*) rate, the mean derivative value at a point (*Mdif*), the Relative Power (*RP*) and the spectrum energy deceleration represented by the spectral ratios (*r*). The extracted features were:

- ***NMax*** and ***NMin***: Accounting and calculation of all signal maxima and minima, respectively, by the variation of the signal waveform derivative (view Figure 1).
- ***Zcr***: The zero-crossing rate was calculated as (Chen, 1988):

$$Zcr_i = \frac{1}{N-1}\sum_{n=1}^{N-1}\mathbb{I}\left\{s_i\left(n\right)s_i\left(n-1\right) < 0\right\}, \quad (10)$$

Figure 1. Signal, maxima and minima, example

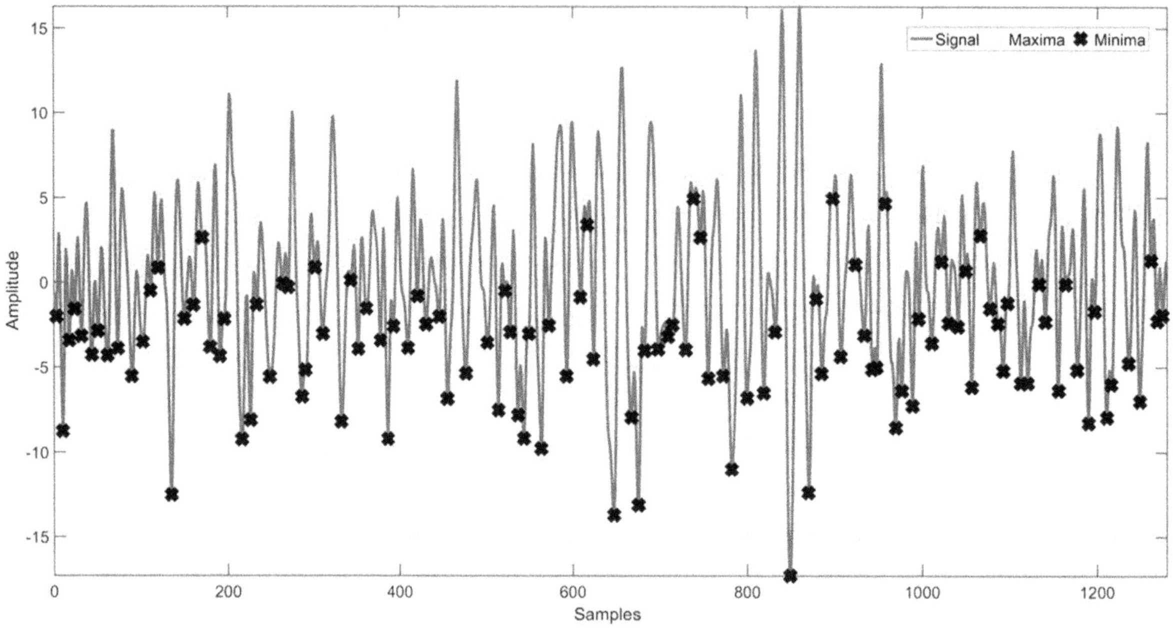

where $i = \{\delta,\theta,\alpha,\beta,\gamma\}$, s is a *DWT* coefficient signal of length N and $\mathbb{I}$ the indicator function. If the $\mathbb{I}$ value, in a certain position, is equal to 1 a signal zero crossing is found.

- ***Mdif***: The mean derivative value at a point was obtained by the equation 11 (Apostol, 1988),

$$Mdif_i = \frac{1}{N-6} \cdot \sum_{n=1}^{N-6} \left(s_i(n) - \sum_{b=n}^{n+5} s_i(b) \right), \tag{11}$$

where $i = \{\delta,\theta,\alpha,\beta,\gamma\}$.

- ***RP***: It was calculated as the sum of the components of the PSD_n in the conventional frequency bands: delta (1-4 Hz), theta (4-8 Hz), alpha (8-13Hz), beta1 (13-19Hz, *β1*), beta2 (19-30 Hz, *β2*) and gamma (30-40 Hz):

$$RP(\delta) = \sum_{f=1Hz}^{4Hz} PSD_n(f); \tag{12}$$

$$RP(\theta) = \sum_{f=4Hz}^{8Hz} PSD_n(f); \tag{13}$$

$$RP(\alpha) = \sum_{f=8Hz}^{13Hz} PSD_n(f); \tag{14}$$

$$RP(\beta 1) = \sum_{f=13Hz}^{19Hz} PSD_n(f); \tag{15}$$

$$RP(\beta 2) = \sum_{f=19Hz}^{30Hz} PSD_n(f); \tag{16}$$

$$RP(\gamma) = \sum_{f=30Hz}^{40Hz} PSD_n(f); \tag{17}$$

- ***r*:** Four spectral ratios were used to summarize the deceleration of the EEG spectrum of AD patients. r_1 is a spectral ratio that enabled us to detect changes when a slight slowdown in the EEG spectrum appears. The r_2 index summarizes the EEG globally slowing down. r_3 computes the relationship between high-frequency bands ($\beta 1$ and $\beta 2$) and the lowest frequency band (δ). r_4 is similar to r_3, but with a narrower high-frequency band (only $\beta 2$). (Rodrigues & Teixeira, 2013).

$$r_1 = \frac{RP(\alpha)}{RP(\theta)}, \tag{18}$$

$$r_2 = \frac{RP(\alpha) + RP(\beta 1) + RP(\beta 2) + RP(\gamma)}{RP(\delta) + RP(\theta)}, \tag{19}$$

$$r_3 = \frac{RP(\beta 1) + RP(\beta 2)}{RP(\delta)}; \tag{20}$$

$$r_4 = \frac{RP(\beta 2)}{RP(\delta)}; \tag{21}$$

Unsupervised Classification: Self-Organized Maps

Self-Organized Maps is one example of an unsupervised neural network that reduces the dimensionality of the input data, on a map of neurons (Kohonen, 2001). It is based on competitive learning where the output neurons compete with each other, and only one is activated. This activated neuron is called the winner neuron. The winner neuron will be the one whose weights in the input connections are closer to the input pattern in terms of Euclidean distance. Such competition can be induced by a negative feedback system between neurons. Finally, neurons are forced to organize themselves into groups enabling a good ability to form clusters (Kohonen, 2001). The phases of SOM algorithm are:

1. **Initialization:** Randomly initialize the vectors of weight w_j.
2. **Sampling:** Build an input vector from the training set.
3. **Correspondence:** Find the winner neuron $I(x)$ witch has a weight vector most similar to the input vector.
4. **Update:** Update the weights by the function:

$$\Delta w_{ji} = \eta(t) \cdot T_{j,I(x)}(t)(x_j - w_{ji}) \tag{22}$$

where Δw_{ji} represents the value of updating weights, $\eta(t)$ is the learning rate parameter, $T_{j,I(x)}(t)$ is the neighborhood function centered around the winner neuron and w_{ji} is the current weight value.

5. **Continued:** Back to step 2 until the map of "clustering" stops changing (Haykin, 1998).

Statistical Analysis and Features Selection

Each 5 seconds (1280 epochs) of EEG signal epoch has undergone an average process per electrode and per subject in order to make a statistical analysis of the extracted features (see example of EEG signal average in Figure 2).

In order to extract some information from the EEG signals of AD patients, MCI patients, and Control subjects, each signal resulting from the average process was decomposed to the level 5 by the Wavelet Biorthogonal (Bior) 3.5 *DWT.* Additionally the EEG signals were processed by Bior 3.5 *PSD* of *WT* technique to the level 8 of decomposition. These decomposition levels for both techniques provided the correct level of EEG signal decomposition to reach the conventional frequency bands of EEG (δ, θ, α, β and γ bands). In the case of the *PSD* of *WT* technique, the level 8 of decomposition allowed obtaining a *PSD* which ranges between 1Hz and 128Hz. Thus containing the frequency range of conventional EEG bands (1-40Hz) and in this way, the *PSD* of *WT* can be restricted to this range of frequencies. In the case of *DWT,* the level 5 of decomposition gives the detail coefficients *D*2 that corresponds to the Gamma band, *D*3 to the beta band, *D*4 to the alpha band, *D*5 to the theta band and the approximated coefficients *A*5 to the delta band. The *PSD* of *WT* and *DWT* were computed by Bior 3.5 because it proved to be a good choice in EEG previous studies (Rodrigues & Teixeira, 2011; Rodrigues & Teixeira, 2013). After this, the previously defined features were extracted from the averaged signals.

Figure 2. Example of signal averaging per electrode and per subject

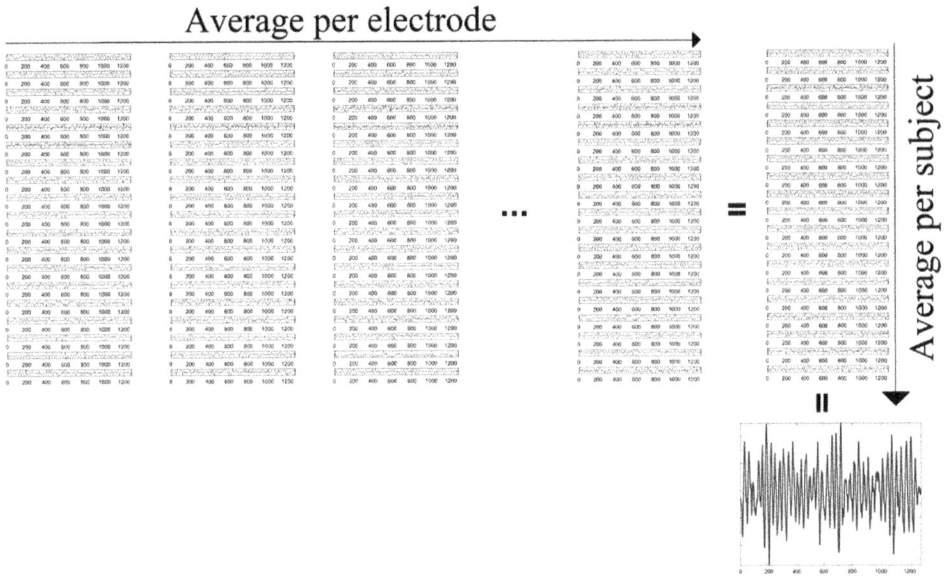

A linear classifier with a leave-one-out cross-validation procedure was performed to assess the features combination that reached the best classification performance. The classifier is intended to have the ability to discriminate AD patients from Control subjects and MCI patients. It was evaluated by using ROC curves (Williams, Lee, Fisher, & Dickerman, 1999). The ROC curve is a graphical representation of the trade-off between sensitivity and specificity. Sensitivity (Sens) measures the proportion of positives that are correctly identified, specificity (Spec) is the proportion of negatives that are correctly identified (Accu) is the percentage of the study participants correctly recognized. The Area Under the ROC Curve (AUC) is a single number that summarizes the diagnostic robustness of the parameter (Williams, Lee, Fisher, & Dickerman, 1999). The best features combinations were obtained by using genetic algorithms. After the process, the 19 features combination that achieved the best classification indexes were: r_1, $r_{2,}RP(\alpha)$, $Mdif_\delta$, $r_{4,}NMax_\gamma$, $NMin_\gamma$, $RP(\gamma)$, $NMax_\alpha$, $NMin_\alpha$, Zcr_β, Zcr_α, $RP(\theta)$, Zcr_α, $NMin_\theta$, $NMax_\theta$, r_3, $NMax_\beta$ and $NMin_\beta$.

METHODOLOGY

Each 5 seconds/1280 epochs of EEG signal epoch per electrode selected from this 24 subjects that participate in this study were split into twenty threads (each thread has 64 samples). After that, in each thread, the best-combined features that provided the best classification results for all dataset (24 subjects) it has been extracted. For that a linear classifier with leave-one-out cross-validation procedure was used, see previous section.

The EEG features extracted consisted in the set of 19 previous selected features: r_1, $r_{2,}RP(\alpha)$, $Mdif_\delta$, $r_{4,}NMax_\gamma$, $NMin_\gamma$, $RP(\gamma)$, $NMax_\alpha$, $NMin_\alpha$, Zcr_β, Zcr_α, $RP(\theta)$, Zcr_α, $NMin_\theta$, $NMax_\theta$, r_3, $NMax_\beta$ and $NMin_\beta$. In next step, as shown in Figure 3, the SOM was used to classify randomly in five groups all the twenty

Figure 3. Scatter plot example of the classification made with the values of two extracted features

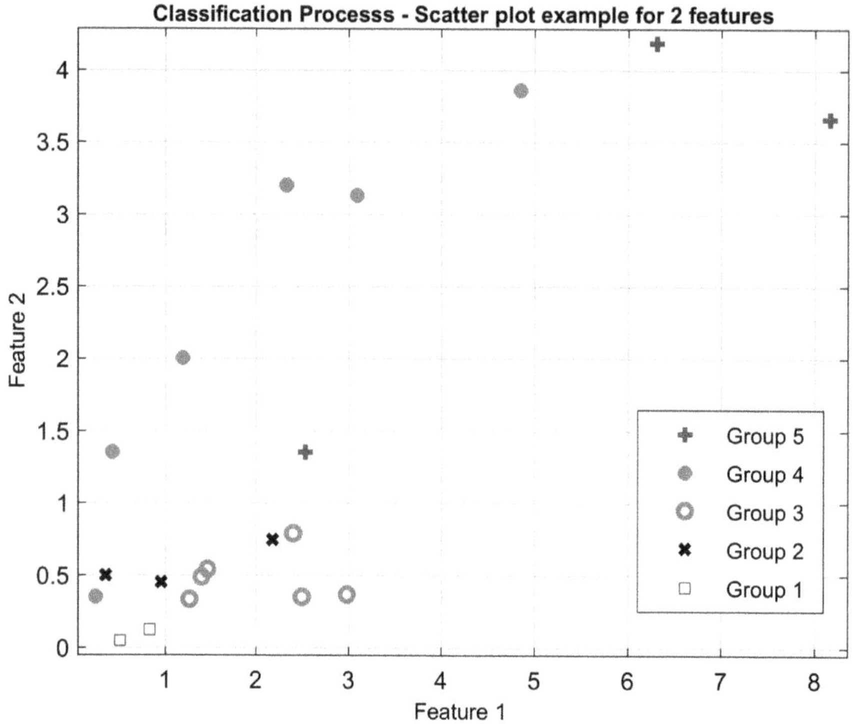

threads. SOM was forced to perform a logical classification in order to obtained groups. For all classifications, of twenty threads from a segment of 5 seconds length, the labels have been reordered in order to obtain a homogeneous classification (groups composed of characteristics with similar trends of values over all the classification process).

The Figure 4 represents sequentially, the SOM classification in the temporal domain, for a segment of 1280 epochs length. Depending on the threads classification, the segment threads were represented in Figure 4 with different colors. It can be observed a decrease of AD incidence degree from Group 1 to Group 5. AD patients tendentially present lower distributions of values from feature 1 and feature 2 than the healthy Controls and MCI patients. This was also observed in previous works for AD (Rodrigues P. M., 2011; Rodrigues & Teixeira, 2013; Rodrigues, Freitas, & Teixeira, 2013).

By observing the scatter plot of Figure 3 it can be seen that from the Group 1 to the Group 5 the median values of feature 1 and features 2 in each group increases progressively. Consequently, the incidence degree of AD in EEG will decrease along the classifying groups.

After performing SOM classification for the dataset, all four combinations of five groups (SOM classification groups) were verified for AD patients, MCI patients and for Control group in any temporal SOM classification of 5s segments - 1280 epochs (see, Figure 4). In order to analyze the results, two tables were made (Tables 2 and 3). Table 2 provided the difference ($Diff_{ADvsC}$) between the number of temporal sequences found at AD group (Seq_{AD}) and at Control group (Seq_C),

$$Diff_{ADvsC} = Seq_{AD} - Seq_C. \tag{23}$$

Figure 4. Example of the classification process in the temporal domain, for an EEG segment of 5s

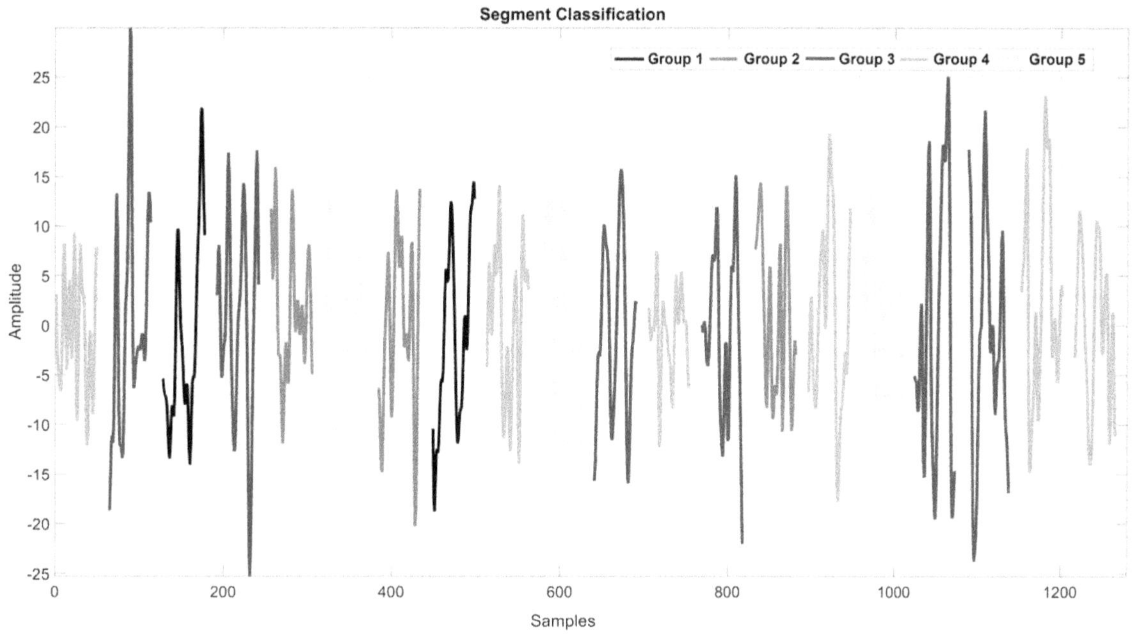

Table 2. The difference between the number of temporal sequences found at AD group and Control group

Seq	Diff	Seq	Diff	Seq	Diff	Seq	Diff	Seq	Diff	Seq	Diff	Seq12	Diff	Seq	Diff	Seq1	Diff	Seq1	Diff
1111	**41**	1333	33	**2111**	**29**	**2333**	**36**	3111	12	3333	3	**4111**	**31**	4333	18	5111	13	5333	-7
1112	**27**	1334	0	2112	12	2334	-16	**3112**	**46**	3334	-47	4112	8	4334	-4	5112	14	5334	-63
1113	25	1335	15	**2113**	**32**	2335	20	**3113**	**29**	3335	-3	4113	19	4335	-6	5113	9	5335	18
1114	15	1341	15	2114	9	**2341**	**30**	3114	16	3341	11	4114	20	**4341**	**31**	5114	-12	5341	17
1115	**39**	1342	6	**2115**	**47**	2342	-2	**3115**	**31**	3342	-2	4115	8	4342	-36	5115	19	5342	3
1121	22	1343	2	2121	1	**2343**	**35**	3121	18	3343	-12	4121	12	4343	-41	5121	0	5343	-23
1122	29	1344	10	**2122**	**32**	2344	-10	3122	-2	3344	26	4122	22	4344	-30	5122	23	5344	-14
1123	21	1345	11	2123	11	2345	2	**3123**	**26**	3345	-2	4123	25	4345	0	5123	20	5345	5
1124	11	1351	20	2124	14	**2351**	**33**	3124	11	3351	-12	4124	20	4351	4	5124	-1	5351	-22
1125	14	1352	-2	2125	3	2352	-3	3125	4	3352	-77	4125	12	4352	20	5125	11	5352	-32
1131	12	1353	0	**2131**	**28**	2353	1	3131	0	3353	-15	**4131**	**39**	4353	-6	5131	23	5353	7
1132	23	1354	-13	**2132**	**27**	2354	6	3132	3	3354	-15	4132	-13	4354	-17	5132	12	5354	-46
1133	**47**	1355	-24	2133	-1	2355	25	**3133**	**27**	3355	14	4133	-9	**4355**	**28**	5133	12	5355	9
1134	22	1411	22	2134	0	2411	19	3134	-12	3411	13	4134	-15	4411	-1	5134	-1	5411	16
1135	1	**1412**	**42**	2135	18	2412	6	3135	15	3412	12	**4135**	**38**	4412	7	5135	-7	5412	-4
1141	**34**	1413	-13	2141	9	**2413**	**47**	3141	3	3413	-9	4141	18	4413	14	5141	-3	5413	-3
1142	9	**1414**	**43**	2142	21	2414	0	3142	24	**3414**	**27**	**4142**	**39**	4414	36	5142	-10	5414	-23
1143	25	1415	7	**2143**	**34**	2415	6	3143	-3	3415	17	4143	-9	4415	21	5143	7	5415	11
1144	**27**	1421	14	2144	8	2421	10	3144	14	3421	27	**4144**	**29**	4421	-27	5144	2	**5421**	**35**
1145	-4	1422	11	2145	14	**2422**	**26**	3145	8	3422	-1	4145	13	4422	12	5145	1	5422	21
1151	3	1423	-3	2151	-2	2423	-22	3151	14	**3423**	**31**	4151	20	4423	-27	5151	-4	5423	-12

continued on following page

Table 2. Continued

Seq	Diff	Seq	Diff	Seq	Diff	Seq	Diff	Seq	Diff	Seq	Diff	Seq12	Diff	Seq	Diff	Seq1	Diff	Seq1	Diff
1152	22	1424	-10	**2152**	**28**	2424	7	3152	-15	3424	17	4152	7	4424	-36	5152	-1	5424	-29
1153	18	1425	4	2153	17	2425	14	3153	3	3425	3	4153	-4	4425	24	5153	-15	5425	-11
1154	11	1431	14	2154	8	2431	14	3154	25	3431	0	4154	8	4431	10	5154	-25	5431	17
1155	2	**1432**	**32**	2155	21	**2432**	**34**	**3155**	**41**	3432	27	4155	6	4432	17	5155	4	5432	-13
1211	**40**	**1433**	**46**	**2211**	**47**	2433	4	3211	14	3433	-41	4211	9	4433	-3	5211	9	5433	-34
1212	34	1434	9	2212	5	2434	15	3212	13	3434	-18	4212	-5	4434	9	**5212**	**42**	5434	-21
1213	22	1435	-4	2213	24	2435	12	3213	18	3435	11	**4213**	**32**	4435	25	5213	3	5435	-8
1214	12	**1441**	**55**	2214	19	2441	22	**3214**	**27**	3441	1	4214	23	4441	-63	5214	-19	5441	5
1215	25	1442	0	**2215**	**33**	**2442**	**32**	3215	24	3442	-1	**4215**	**30**	4442	-13	5215	17	5442	24
1221	13	1443	14	2221	-109	2443	-21	3221	8	3443	-32	4221	-4	4443	-49	5221	-47	5443	-42
1222	25	1444	2	2222	5	2444	-4	**3222**	**41**	3444	-18	4222	10	4444	-71	5222	14	5444	-4
1223	22	1445	-4	2223	-6	2445	17	3223	12	3445	14	4223	17	4445	2	5223	14	5445	-10
1224	**33**	1451	0	2224	-42	2451	23	3224	13	3451	12	4224	-9	4451	-10	5224	-13	5451	-41
1225	-34	1452	8	2225	25	2452	9	3225	24	3452	-25	4225	25	4452	-3	5225	8	5452	-14
1231	20	1453	13	**2231**	**36**	2453	-33	3231	-19	3453	-10	4231	2	4453	-40	5231	4	5453	-57
1232	11	1454	-12	2232	-2	2454	3	3232	-34	3454	-11	4232	11	4454	-31	5232	-7	5454	-88
1233	12	**1455**	**30**	**2233**	**34**	2455	8	3233	9	3455	0	4233	17	4455	-1	5233	2	5455	27
1234	**29**	1511	11	2234	-7	2511	2	3234	22	3511	-5	4234	9	4511	13	5234	-11	5511	20
1235	18	**1512**	**26**	2235	25	**2512**	**27**	3235	-1	**3512**	**30**	**4235**	**39**	4512	-7	5235	5	5512	14
1241	**33**	1513	1	2241	-13	2513	19	3241	25	3513	-7	4241	-24	4513	0	5241	-2	5513	-26
1242	25	1514	2	2242	-2	2514	6	3242	18	3514	-9	4242	9	4514	-8	5242	1	5514	-22
1243	**30**	1515	-14	**2243**	**55**	2515	14	3243	-17	3515	2	4243	-26	4515	11	5243	-20	5515	-8
1244	**30**	1521	23	2244	14	2521	-4	3244	-2	3521	7	4244	-22	**4521**	**29**	**5244**	**29**	5521	-41
1245	-8	1522	-2	2245	16	2522	-5	3245	15	3522	-16	4245	12	4522	-9	5245	5	5522	-23
1251	11	1523	22	2251	-41	2523	-41	**3251**	**54**	**3523**	**35**	4251	-24	4523	-18	5251	-47	5523	17
1252	4	1524	19	2252	8	2524	-16	3252	5	3524	-10	4252	15	4524	-30	5252	-14	5524	-46
1253	13	1525	-2	2253	-20	**2525**	**34**	3253	-5	3525	6	4253	-27	4525	10	5253	1	5525	1
1254	7	1531	-4	2254	-37	2531	-8	3254	-25	3531	-11	4254	-8	4531	24	5254	-29	5531	-12
1255	11	1532	8	**2255**	**29**	2532	20	**3255**	**40**	3532	-55	4255	-1	4532	-20	**5255**	**30**	5532	-34
1311	**42**	1533	16	2311	2	2533	1	3311	19	3533	8	4311	18	4533	-18	5311	24	5533	-3
1312	19	1534	13	2312	18	2534	-15	3312	6	3534	-43	4312	4	4534	-9	5312	13	5534	-39
1313	9	1535	5	**2313**	**30**	2535	-1	3313	11	3535	15	4313	5	4535	0	5313	3	5535	-20
1314	-9	1541	9	**2314**	**26**	2541	-23	3314	12	3541	15	4314	-3	4541	-1	5314	-5	5541	14
1315	2	1542	17	2315	17	2542	18	3315	15	3542	-29	**4315**	**33**	4542	-25	5315	18	5542	-15
1321	**29**	1543	-14	**2321**	**31**	2543	6	3321	4	3543	10	**4321**	**38**	4543	-47	5321	-6	5543	0
1322	**28**	1544	9	2322	-13	2544	-38	3322	2	3544	-21	4322	-12	4544	-73	5322	9	5544	-7
1323	13	1545	-6	2323	-12	2545	15	3323	-3	3545	4	4323	-4	4545	3	5323	9	5545	-63
1324	-7	1551	20	2324	22	2551	-26	3324	22	3551	-26	4324	-1	4551	-23	5324	-23	5551	18
1325	**33**	1552	9	2325	-4	2552	-5	3325	20	3552	-26	**4325**	**44**	4552	-29	5325	13	5552	17
1331	**29**	**1553**	**27**	2331	-9	2553	-5	3331	13	3553	-6	4331	17	4553	-21	5331	10	5553	3
1332	6	1554	3	2332	-39	2554	-71	3332	-50	3554	-51	4332	26	4554	-40	5332	-45	5554	-23
		1555	-28			**2555**	**34**			3555	12			**4555**	**30**			5555	-14

Table 3. The difference between the number of temporal sequences found at MCI group and Control group

Seq	Diff	Seq	Diff	Seq	Diff	Seq	Diff	Seq	Diff	Seq	Diff	Seq12	Diff	Seq	Diff	Seq1	Diff	Seq1	Diff
1111	-10	1333	-2	2111	-1	2333	9	3111	-1	3333	-43	4111	0	4333	-8	5111	4	5333	-30
1112	3	1334	-7	2112	7	2334	-20	**3112**	**29**	3334	-20	4112	4	4334	-19	5112	12	5334	-52
1113	19	1335	0	2113	16	2335	8	3113	15	3335	-23	4113	-1	4335	-9	5113	-6	5335	1
1114	14	1341	14	2114	10	2341	1	3114	10	3341	-27	4114	-6	4341	-9	5114	-12	5341	-25
1115	3	1342	7	2115	14	2342	7	3115	-11	3342	-26	4115	18	4342	-28	5115	21	5342	-9
1121	0	1343	-31	2121	-1	2343	-12	3121	-11	3343	-9	4121	-23	4343	-28	5121	-15	5343	-44
1122	-8	1344	2	2122	17	2344	-27	3122	-8	3344	-10	4122	-12	4344	-33	5122	-6	5344	-37
1123	10	1345	-18	2123	12	2345	-1	3123	12	3345	8	4123	-16	4345	-9	5123	-9	5345	8
1124	4	1351	-9	2124	-14	2351	-14	3124	-38	3351	-16	4124	3	4351	2	5124	-22	5351	-8
1125	0	1352	-7	2125	-2	2352	-24	3125	-12	3352	-30	4125	8	4352	10	5125	-6	5352	-50
1131	20	1353	-2	2131	-6	2353	4	3131	6	3353	-40	4131	25	4353	-10	5131	9	5353	0
1132	8	1354	-13	2132	1	2354	-18	3132	8	3354	-33	4132	-31	4354	-22	5132	-4	5354	-11
1133	**27**	1355	-22	2133	-18	2355	-8	3133	13	3355	-12	4133	-22	4355	-9	5133	6	5355	0
1134	7	1411	17	2134	-4	2411	-3	3134	-39	3411	-11	4134	-8	4411	-17	5134	-10	5411	-8
1135	12	1412	10	2135	16	2412	-3	3135	11	3412	-3	4135	4	4412	-7	5135	2	5412	-5
1141	8	1413	-3	2141	4	2413	3	3141	-13	3413	12	4141	9	4413	-6	5141	-16	5413	-6
1142	-3	1414	10	2142	-4	2414	-23	3142	14	3414	14	4142	0	4414	-9	5142	-24	5414	-19
1143	16	1415	14	2143	7	2415	-8	3143	-20	3415	-19	4143	-25	4415	14	5143	-8	5415	-12
1144	24	1421	-5	2144	6	2421	-9	3144	20	3421	-19	4144	25	4421	-46	5144	-7	5421	-11
1145	-20	1422	-10	2145	0	2422	13	3145	-8	3422	-14	4145	-22	4422	13	5145	7	5422	-12
1151	-12	1423	2	2151	3	2423	-25	3151	9	3423	-5	4151	20	4423	-57	5151	0	5423	-10
1152	16	1424	-20	2152	12	2424	-31	3152	-26	3424	15	4152	-7	4424	-19	5152	-34	5424	-34
1153	12	1425	8	2153	23	2425	-14	3153	-24	3425	-12	4153	-15	4425	3	5153	-28	5425	-16
1154	3	1431	12	2154	-1	2431	-8	3154	12	3431	2	4154	-1	4431	1	5154	-22	5431	-24
1155	-17	1432	8	2155	7	2432	22	3155	23	3432	-17	4155	0	4432	-30	5155	-14	5432	-32
1211	13	1433	-8	2211	20	2433	15	3211	7	3433	-46	4211	3	4433	-9	5211	-2	5433	-29
1212	12	1434	-12	2212	-18	2434	-11	3212	-8	3434	-20	4212	-25	4434	-26	5212	21	5434	3
1213	3	1435	6	**2213**	**26**	2435	-5	3213	9	3435	4	4213	0	4435	-21	5213	1	5435	-17
1214	6	1441	-8	2214	7	2441	-11	**3214**	**26**	3441	-23	4214	5	4441	-48	5214	1	5441	1
1215	2	1442	-7	2215	0	2442	-23	3215	21	3442	-24	4215	-5	4442	-12	5215	-5	5442	0
1221	**30**	1443	11	2221	-73	2443	-28	3221	4	3443	-16	4221	-40	4443	-105	5221	-31	5443	-54
1222	-24	1444	0	2222	-17	2444	-34	3222	17	3444	-25	4222	-38	4444	-62	5222	-21	5444	-26
1223	-8	1445	-19	2223	-39	2445	0	3223	-22	3445	-10	4223	-3	4445	-17	5223	10	5445	-20
1224	7	1451	-4	2224	-28	2451	0	3224	-36	3451	-8	4224	-11	4451	-27	5224	-15	5451	-54
1225	-50	1452	14	2225	-13	2452	-4	3225	18	3452	-41	4225	11	4452	-30	5225	-18	5452	-20
1231	3	1453	4	2231	-4	2453	-26	3231	-21	3453	-30	4231	-6	4453	-43	5231	24	5453	-45
1232	9	1454	-18	2232	-23	2454	-28	3232	3	3454	-21	4232	9	4454	-35	5232	-22	5454	-65
1233	1	1455	6	2233	10	2455	-4	3233	1	3455	-3	4233	12	4455	-6	5233	-30	5455	19
1234	-1	1511	3	2234	-41	2511	-14	3234	19	3511	5	4234	-21	4511	-23	5234	-4	5511	-5
1235	-14	1512	0	2235	7	2512	4	3235	1	3512	6	4235	-14	4512	-15	5235	-12	5512	4
1241	6	1513	-7	2241	-38	2513	-21	3241	-5	3513	-15	4241	-14	4513	-12	5241	-12	5513	4
1242	-5	1514	-17	2242	-19	2514	-6	3242	-5	3514	-6	4242	-19	4514	-10	5242	7	5514	-28

continued on following page

Table 3. Continued

Seq	Diff	Seq	Diff	Seq	Diff	Seq	Diff	Seq	Diff	Seq	Diff	Seq12	Diff	Seq	Diff	Seq1	Diff	Seq1	Diff
1243	17	1515	-30	2243	4	2515	6	3243	-30	3515	-7	4243	-33	4515	-2	5243	-48	5515	-16
1244	2	1521	19	2244	-10	2521	-2	3244	-15	3521	3	4244	-24	4521	-3	5244	14	5521	-42
1245	-7	1522	-12	2245	-24	2522	-6	3245	-5	3522	-13	4245	-7	4522	-26	5245	4	5522	-35
1251	-7	**1523**	**30**	2251	-45	2523	-43	3251	9	3523	1	4251	-16	4523	-29	5251	-17	5523	10
1252	2	1524	23	2252	-8	2524	-15	3252	-37	3524	-15	4252	-9	4524	-16	5252	-43	5524	-31
1253	-22	1525	-10	2253	2	2525	10	3253	-10	3525	3	4253	-16	4525	-24	5253	-14	5525	-8
1254	-12	1531	-1	2254	-60	2531	-23	3254	-24	3531	-42	4254	-7	4531	21	5254	-17	5531	-2
1255	-29	1532	-21	**2255**	**31**	2532	-11	3255	-18	3532	-38	4255	7	4532	-49	5255	14	5532	-23
1311	**34**	1533	-17	2311	-34	2533	-42	3311	10	3533	-19	4311	-17	4533	-26	5311	0	5533	-25
1312	-8	1534	-8	2312	-22	2534	-35	3312	-9	3534	4	4312	-8	4534	-14	5312	22	5534	0
1313	-5	1535	-11	2313	11	2535	1	3313	20	3535	3	4313	2	4535	0	5313	-21	5535	-43
1314	-6	1541	11	2314	14	2541	-52	3314	2	3541	-12	4314	-24	4541	-9	5314	-25	5541	-21
1315	-5	1542	0	2315	1	2542	2	3315	2	3542	1	**4315**	**28**	4542	-45	5315	7	5542	-20
1321	23	1543	-29	2321	-6	2543	12	3321	7	3543	-5	4321	0	4543	-39	5321	-27	5543	-47
1322	15	1544	-2	2322	16	2544	1	3322	-1	3544	-35	4322	-19	4544	-67	5322	0	5544	-76
1323	13	1545	-24	2323	-31	2545	-8	3323	-9	3545	-9	4323	-9	4545	-9	5323	-5	5545	-3
1324	-14	1551	16	**2324**	**27**	2551	-11	3324	-27	3551	-26	4324	-12	4551	-32	5324	-34	5551	-38
1325	10	1552	-9	2325	-15	2552	-18	3325	17	3552	-20	4325	-15	4552	-24	5325	13	5552	-37
1331	2	1553	25	2331	-6	2553	-35	3331	-11	3553	-34	4331	13	4553	-31	5331	-12	5553	-30
1332	-1	1554	-21	2332	-12	2554	-63	3332	-98	3554	-28	4332	-19	4554	-40	5332	-45	5554	-52
		1555	-46			**2555**	**28**			3555	-2			4555	14			5555	1

and Table 3 provided the difference ($Diff_{MCIvsC}$) between the number of temporal sequences found at MCI group (Seq_{MCI}) and at Control group (Seq_C),

$$Diff_{MCIvsC} = Seq_{MCI} - Seq_C. \tag{24}$$

1,2,3,4 and 5 represented the SOM classification in five groups. *Seq* represented the temporal sequences. The temporal sequences that have higher probability to appear in the EEG of AD patients and its respectively *Diff* score are shown at bold in Table 2 and Table 3.

The authors compared the sequences of four threads that appeared in Table 2 and Table 3 with a high incidence and concluded that the sequences 1133, 1311, 2255, 2555, 3112, 3214 and 4315 are the first sequences of AD that appear in early stages of the disease and constituted the denominated "AD early EEG Events". Based on the previous Events detection results, an analysis of the propagation of those events was performed. The propagation time is the time interval between the onset of the "AD early event" until its appearance/spread at other cerebral scalp zone, in another electrode, or until its demise. In Figure 5. It can be seen a boxplot; that shows that the average propagation time of the events detected in AD (approximately 850ms) is higher than in Control subjects (approximately 680 ms) and then in MCI patients (approximately 790ms), proving that the brain dynamism gets lower as the disease

Figure 5. Time events propagation differences between Alzheimer's, MCI's and controls groups

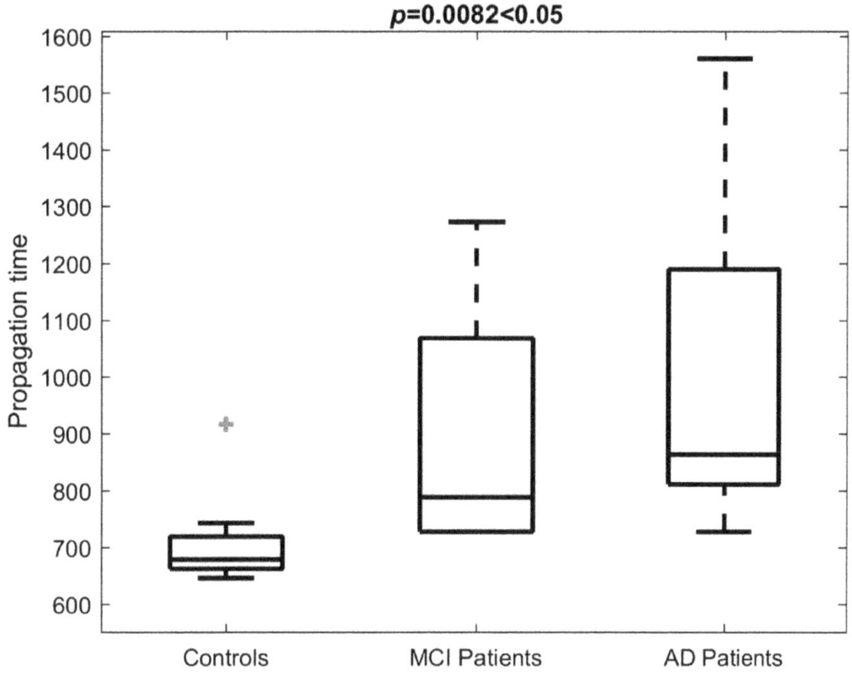

progresses. The statistical difference between those group relatively to the events propagation time is $p=0.0082<0.05$. The "AD early EEG events" detected in Control subjects results from a different kind of sources and have a different nature than the events found in AD and MCI patients, despite the EEG segments representative of those events being energetically similar to those found in AD and MCI patients.

FUTURE RESEARCH DIRECTIONS

The future lines of research that emerged from the work carried out include:

1. Modify the event detection methodology to get events with a longer time (250ms and 500ms);
2. Verify the possibility that an event appears and does not propagate by using magnetic resonance images; and
3. Results should be extended to a larger population to ensure generalization.

DISCUSSION AND CONCLUSION

The future holds challenges to mankind and one of them is AD. Despite all the technological advances and decades of research, the mankind has not yet discovered the origin and the cure of AD. However, the increasing incidence of this disease is a fact more and more frequent in developed countries where the aging population has significantly raised in recent decades, and the number of AD cases grew exponentially because the probability of developing AD increases with age. It is, therefore, urgent to find new ways to early diagnose and care for the disease in the near future. Therefore, this study represents a further contribution to the search for new techniques of AD early detection based on the EEG. Most of the literature focuses primarily on the frequency analysis of the EEG signal. However, the temporal analysis should also be considered for a better diagnosis of this disease, since the episodes that show the AD in the EEG can be sporadic and not permanent. In the present study, the approach of more temporal detail was based on the good results obtained in the classification of EEG segments depending on the distribution of Power Densities in time / scale analysis provided by *WT* in previous studies (Rodrigues P. M., 2011; Rodrigues & Teixeira, 2013; Rodrigues & Teixeira, 2011).

In short, the authors of this study extracted a set of preselected features with WT tool from threads of 64 epochs obtained from a segment of 5s length for both study groups and classified them in 5 clusters by SOM. After that, the clusters that represented a thread, respectively, were evaluated in sequences of 4 over time, and a diff score was performed between AD patients/Control subjects and MCI patients/ Control subjects (Tables 2 and 3). After the analysis of Table 2 and Table 3, it can be concluded that there were sequences of threads that appeared with a high incidence in both Tables (Table 2 and 3), such as, 1133, 1311, 2255, 2555, 3112, 3214 and 4315 with a high positive *Diff* scores, it means that these sequences were found in MCI patients and AD patients with a higher incidence. The sequences formed by two or more threads classified in Group 1 and Group 2 were found more frequently in early AD stages (sequences with the highest positive *Diff* results). Moreover, classified threads as belonging to Group 1 and Group 2 are hypothetically indicative of AD. These sequences could be used to make an EEG temporal events model of AD at early stages in order to increase the early AD diagnosis. It should be noted that the authors analyzed the temporal classification results by combinations of 4 classified threads rather than combinations of 2 or 3 because these combinations did not show clearly AD typical early sequences. It was observed that the average events propagation time in AD is 850ms, in MCI is 790ms and in Controls 650ms. There is indeed, relevant statistical significance when comparing the values distributions of average propagation time between the three groups ($p=0.0082<0.05$).

This study allowed a better understanding of EEG temporal energy dynamics between AD patients, MCI patients, and Control subjects. The results are promising because they can help to find AD characteristic events in early stages. The authors believe that the EEG may increasingly become an accurate diagnostic method to help in AD early diagnosis. Finally, The SOM demonstrated that they might be promising tools for an unsupervised detection of AD early temporal sequences.

Despite that, in future work, the authors intend to analyze the performance, accuracy, sensibility and specificity of the SOM by cataloguing the 250ms and 500ms threads for the study participants and verify the possibility that an AD event appears and does not propagate. Results should be extended to a larger population to ensure generalization. The detected increase of EEG regularity is also not specific to AD. It appears in others dementias including Parkinson's disease (Pezard, Jech, & Ruzicka, 2001; Rodrigues & Teixeira, 2010) and schizophrenia (Fell, Röschke, & Beckmann, 1995). Therefore, this kind of studies should also be followed for future research of these diseases in order to improve their diagnosis and find the differences between them.

ACKNOWLEDGMENT

The authors gratefully acknowledge the opportunity to publish this work to the editor's Book, Dr. Anastasius Moumtzoglou and to Neurological Unity of "Hospital de São João" for supplying the EEG signals used in this study.

REFERENCES

Apostol, T. M. (1988). *Calculus*. Barcelona: Reverté.

Ballard, C., Gauthier, S., Corbett, A., Brayne, C., Aarsland, D., & Jones, E. (2011). Alzheimer's disease. *Lancet*, *377*(9770), 1019–1031. doi:10.1016/S0140-6736(10)61349-9 PMID:21371747

Bird, T. (2001). Alzheimer's disease and other primary dementias. In D. Kasper, S. Hauser, D. Longo, & J. Jameson (Edits.), Harrison's Principles of Internal Medicine (pp. 2391-2399). McGraw-Hill.

Blennow, K. (2005). *Amesterdão: European College of Neuropsychopharmacology*. ECNP.

Blennow, K., Leon, M., & Zetterberg, H. (2006). Alzheimer's disease. *Lancet*, *368*(9533), 387–403. doi:10.1016/S0140-6736(06)69113-7 PMID:16876668

Blennow, K., & Zetterberg, H. (2010). Is it time for biomarker-based diagnostic criteria for prodromal Azheimer's Disease? *Alzheimer's Research & Therapy*, *2*(2), 8. doi:10.1186/alzrt31 PMID:20441609

Chen, C. H. (1988). *Signal processing handbook*. Marcel Dekker Incorporated.

Cummings, J. (2004). *La neuropsiquiatria de la enfermedad de Alzheimer y demencias relacionadas*. Altas Medical Publishing Ltd.

Fell, J., Röschke, J., & Beckmann, P. (1995). Non-linear analysis of sleep eeg data in schizophrenia: Calculation of the principal lyapunov exponent. *Journal of Psychiatric Research*, *56*(3), 257–269. doi:10.1016/0165-1781(95)02562-B

Ferri, C., Prince, M., Brayne, C., Brodaty, H., Fratiglioni, L., Ganguli, M., & Rimmer, E. et al. (2005). Global prevalence of dementia: A Delphi consensus study. *Lancet*, *366*(9503), 2112–2117. doi:10.1016/S0140-6736(05)67889-0 PMID:16360788

Gawel, M., Szmidt-Salkowska, E., & Kowalski, J. (2009). The value of quantitative EEG in differential diagnosis of Alzheimer's disease subcortical vascular dementia. *Journal of the Neurological Sciences*, *283*(1-2), 127–133. doi:10.1016/j.jns.2009.02.332 PMID:19268969

Gwyther, L. P. (2001). *Caring for People with Alzheimer's Disease: A Manual for Facility Staff*. Washington, DC: American Health Care Association.

Haykin, S. (1998). *Neural Networks*. Prentice Hall.

Haykin, S., & Veen, B. V. (2003). *Signals and Systems*. New York: John Wiley & Sons.

Jeong, J. (2004). EEG dynamics in patients with Alzheimer's disease. *Clinical Neurophysiology*, *115*(7), 1490–1505. doi:10.1016/j.clinph.2004.01.001 PMID:15203050

Jonker, C., Launer, L., Hooijer, C., & Lindeboom, J. (1996). Memory complaints and memory impairment in older individuals. *Journal of the American Geriatrics Society*, *44*(1), 44–49. doi:10.1111/j.1532-5415.1996.tb05636.x PMID:8537589

Kaiser, G. (1994). *A friendly guide to Wavelets*. Birkhäuser Verlag AG.

Kohonen, T. (2001). *Self-Organizing Maps*. New York: Springer. doi:10.1007/978-3-642-56927-2

Lahiri, D. K., Farlow, M. R., Greig, N. H., & Sambamurti, K. (2002). Current drug targets for Alzheimer's disease treatment. *Drug Development Research*, *56*(3), 267–281. doi:10.1002/ddr.10081

Machado, J. C. (2002). Doença de Alzheimer. In E. V. Freitas, L. Py, A. L. Neri, F. A. Cançado, M. L. Gorzoni, & S. M. Rocha (Eds.), Tratado de Geriatria e Gerontologia (pp. 133-147). Rio de Janeiro: Guanabara Koogan.

Mattson, M. P. (2004). Pathways Towards and Away from Alzheimer's Disease. *Nature*, *430*(7000), 631–639. doi:10.1038/nature02621 PMID:15295589

Mesulam, M. M. (2000). Aging Alzheimer Disease and Dementia. *Principies of Behavioural and Cognitive Neurology*, 439-522.

Mölsä, P. M. (1986). Survival and cause of death in Alzheimer's disease and multi-infarct dementia. *Acta Neurologica Scandinavica*, *7*, 74–103. PMID:3776457

Nestor, P., Scheltens, P., & Hodges, J. (2004). Advances in the early detection of Alzheimer's disease. *Nature Medicine*, *10*, 34–41. PMID:15298007

Pezard, L., Jech, R., & Ruzicka, E. (2001). Investigation of non-linear properties of multichannel eeg in the early stages of parkinson's disease. *Clinical Neurophysiology*, *112*(1), 38–45. doi:10.1016/S1388-2457(00)00512-5 PMID:11137659

Porth, C., & Matfin, G. (2009). *Pathophysiology: Concepts of altered health states*. Philadelphia, PA: Wolters Kluwer Health/ Lippencott Williams & Wilkins.

Rioul, O., & Vetterli, M. (1992). Wavelets and Signal Processing. *IEEE Signal Processing Magazine*, *8*(4), 14–38. doi:10.1109/79.91217

Rodrigues, P., & Teixeira, J. (2010). Classification of Electroencephalogram Signals Using Artificial Neural Networks. *3rd International Conference on Biomedical Engineering and Informatics*. doi:10.1109/BMEI.2010.5639941

Rodrigues, P., & Teixeira, J. (2011). Artificial Neural Networks in the Discrimination of Alzheimer's disease. *Communications in Computer and Information Science*, *221*, 272–281. doi:10.1007/978-3-642-24352-3_29

Rodrigues, P. M. (2011). *Diagnóstico da Doença de Alzheimer com base no Electroencefalograma*. (Master's thesis). Instituto Politécnico de Bragança, Bragança.

Rodrigues, P. M., Freitas, D. R., & Teixeira, J. P. (2013). Detection of Alzheimer's Disease Electroencephalogram Temporal Events. *International Journal of Reliable and Quality E-Healthcare*, *2*(3), 44–61. doi:10.4018/ijrqeh.2013070104

Rodrigues, P. M., & Teixeira, J. P. (2013). Alzheimer's Disease Recognition with Artificial Neural Networks. In R. Martinho, R. Rijo, M. Cruz-Cunha, & J. Varajão (Eds.), Information Systems and Technologies for Enhancing Health and Social Care (pp. 102-118). Hershey, PA: IGI Global.

Sanei, S., & Chambers, J. (2007). *EEG signal processing*. West Sussex, UK: Wiley-Interscience. doi:10.1002/9780470511923

Schiff, S. J., & Milton, J. G. (1993). Wavelet transforms for electroencephalographic spike and seizure detection.*Proceeding of the SPIE International Society for Optical Engineering*.

Shimokawa, A., Yatomi, N., Anamizu, S., Torii, S., Isono, H., Sugai, Y., & Kohno, M. (2001). Influence of deteriorating ability of emotional comprehension on interpersonal behavior in Alzheimer-type dementia. *Brain and Cognition*, *47*(3), 423–433. doi:10.1006/brcg.2001.1318 PMID:11748898

Stam, C. (2005). Nonlinear dynamical analysis of EEG and MEG: Review of an emerging field. *Clinical Neurophysiology*, *116*(10), 2266–2301. doi:10.1016/j.clinph.2005.06.011 PMID:16115797

Williams, C., Lee, S., Fisher, R., & Dickerman, L. (1999). A comparison of statistical methods for prenatal screening for Down syndrome. *Applied Stochastic Models in Business and Industry*, *15*(2), 89–101. doi:10.1002/(SICI)1526-4025(199904/06)15:2<89::AID-ASMB366>3.0.CO;2-K

KEY TERMS AND DEFINITIONS

Alzheimer's Disease: It is a neurodegenerative brain disorder. It is the most common cause of dementia among older people that causes problems with memory, thinking and behavior. There is no cure for the disease and AD has an unknown cause. Symptoms usually develop slowly and get worse over time, becoming severe enough to lead to death.

EEG Event: An Alzheimer's disease event is composed by a set of small EEG signal segments of 50ms (64 samples), characterized by a common and single dynamic energy.

EEG Early Event: An Alzheimer's disease event that it is detected in MCI patients with a high incidence.

Electroencephalogram: High resolution physiological technique that records the brain's electrical activity which originates in the neurons. It is widely used in clinical practice.

Features: Patterns that characterize a signal.

Scalp: The skin covering the top of the human head.

Shift-to-the-Left: AD EEG slowing down relatively to the control subject's EEG. It can be seen notably in Alpha band peak of Power Spectral Density.

Signal Processing: Operation or analysis of analog/digitized signals and represents time-varying or spatially varying physical quantities.

Unsupervised Classification: Type of machine learning algorithm used to draw extrapolations from datasets without labeled responses.

Chapter 8
Automatic Determination of Pauses in Speech for Classification of Stuttering Disorder

João Paulo Teixeira
Polytechnic Institute of Bragança, Portugal

Maria Goreti Fernandes
Polytechnic Institute of Bragança, Portugal

Rita Alexandra Costa
Polytechnic Institute of Bragança, Portugal

ABSTRACT

An algorithm to automatically identify segments of silence or speech is presented. The algorithm was developed to measure the silence periods in spontaneous and read speech. These silence periods are one of the parameters used to know the degree of severity of stuttered speech. For this purpose the three longer disfluent events (pauses or other disfluent events) and also the percentage of silence are useful. The algorithm is based on the evaluation of the energy and the zero crossing rate of the signal compared to the threshold values previously determined in silence. One experiment with eight subjects is described using the Stuttering Severity Instrument for Children and Adults – SSI and the percentage of silence in speech. It was concluded that the percentage of silence is good enough to separate stuttered from the normal speech but alone is not capable of measuring the degree of severity of the stuttered speech.

DOI: 10.4018/978-1-5225-1724-5.ch008

INTRODUCTION

Speech is one of the most fundamental and complex cognitive human acts. The normal speech is the final product of a complex network of linguistic, cognitive and sensorimotor processes. Its production requires the coordinated activation of distinct muscle systems and the vocal tract (Juste et al., 2012; McClean & Tasko, 2004).

Considering the analysis of the speech signal, there are three different states of the speech: silence, unvoiced speech and voiced speech. In the silence state, no speech is produced and the muscles within the vocal folds are relaxed. In the unvoiced state, the folds are closer together and tenser than in the silence state, allowing a turbulence to be generated at the folds themselves. In the voiced state, active and passive contractions of the chest and abdominal wall generate a subglottic pressure that exceeds the closure force of the adducted vocal folds. The transglottic air pressure differential produces an airflow that is modulated by the vocal folds to produce a time-varying longitudinal air pressure wave. This pressure wave is changed by the vocal tract to create the sound we hear as the normal human voice (Plant & Younger, 2000).

For a given idiom, there are a set of phonemes that characterize the language. These phonemes can be divided into vowels and consonants. The vowels group contains the oral, nasal and semi-vowels or glides. The consonants are divided in plosive, liquid, fricatives and vibrant. The plosive vowels are composed by the occlusive part (almost or completely occlusion of sound) and by the plosive part generally followed by one vowel but sometimes followed by other consonant. Anyhow, each of these consonants can be voiced or unvoiced. The voiced sounds are produced with the vibration of the vocal cord and the unvoiced sounds are produced without vibration of the vocal cords and with the glottis open. The voiced sounds generally have low frequency energy and in opposition unvoiced sounds has higher frequency energy. The frequency of vibration of the vocal cords is known as the fundamental frequency (F0), which is controlled by the states of tension and length of the vocal cords. Greater tension and length correspond to higher frequency tones, (Seeley, Stephens & Tate, 2006).

Speech disorders are human disabilities that affect millions of people worldwide and are usually treated with behavioral therapy (Barnes et al., 2016). It is estimated that 40 million Americans have a communication disorder (Ancelle, 2015). The study and evaluation of human speech disorders may lead to a wider array of treatment options and provide key insights into the genetic and neural underpinnings of human speech. Developmental stuttering is the principal disorder of fluency (Ancelle, 2015). This speech disorder is characterized by frequent occurrences of repetitions or prolongations of syllables, words, and sounds, as well as involuntary hesitations or pauses that disrupt the rhythmic flow of speech (Wieland et al., 2015). In addition to the changes in the rhythm of speech, the stuttering is commonly accompanied by body movements, such as tremors, spasms of oro-facial and laryngeal muscles, and also abnormal involuntary movements (ticks) (Mulligan et al., 2003; Riva-Posse et al., 2008; Rogić et al., 2016). Stuttering onset usually begins between the ages of two and five years, when children begin to form simple sentences (Vanhoutte et al., 2016). Recent studies have indicated that the incidence of stuttering is approximately 5%, however the majority of affected children (about 80%) recovers during the puberty (Wieland et al., 2015; Rogić et al., 2016; Ancelle, 2015). It is estimated that 1-2% of world adult population continues to suffer from severe stuttering (often called Persistent Developmental Stuttering) (Prado-Velasco & Fernández-Perunchena, 2011).

In addition to involuntary speech disruptions, stuttering can affect nearly all aspects of a person's life. Different definitions of stuttering refer to specific emotions such as fear, anxiety, embarrassment and irritation (Adriaensens, Beyers & Struyf, 2015). The importance of this subject have motivated the development of several studies. Van Lieshout, Hulstijn & Peters (2004) stated that the motor abilities (speech production system) of stutterers are limited in motion. And Peters, Hulstijn & Van Lieshout (2000) affirmed that these motor abilities could be represented in a continuous way from the normal to a deviant behavior. The cited limited motor abilities (Van Lieshout, Hulstijn & Peters 2004) means that differences between the speech of stutterers and speech from fluent persons are not permanent and happen mainly when the stutter motor system (stutterer) control is destabilized. This means that the fluent speech of persons who stutter may already have differences to the speech of fluent persons.

Another feature that can influence the stuttering level of a stutterer is the speech rate. Hirsch (2007) stated that the increase of the speech rate is a destabilizing factor of the stutter motor system. He also stated that in face of fast speech rate the stutterers do not show the 'undershoot phenomenon'. The undershoot of vowel targets in fluent persons underlies a reduction of the movement amplitude of the motor system, so as to make up for the added cost required by the accelerated speech rate.

Other authors Yaruss (1999) and Sawyer, Chon & Ambrose (2009) stated that the speech production is also perturbed by the phonological complexity. That perturbation of the motor system control was found for Spanish and English adult stutterers (Howell & Au-Yeung, 2007; Howell, Au-Yeung, Yaruss & Eldridge, 2006). A sequence of clusters at the beginning of words also increases the disfluency in adult stutterers (Howell, Au-Yeung & Sackin, 2000). Regarding these references it can also be stated that the motor behavior of stutterers may also show differences from one language to another.

Typically, the frequency of stuttering is measured by counting the number of stutters that are judged to occur in a sample and reporting this as a proportion of the total amount of speech that occurred. In other words, the percentage of syllables spoken that were stuttered (Costello & Ingham, 1984). The preferred denominator is number of syllables spoken (as opposed to words) because it more accurately depicts the amount of speech produced by controlling for variation in word length and the amount of stuttering produced by permitting counts of multiple stuttering per word. Furthermore, when data are collected in real time (i.e., concurrent with ongoing speech), the listener can more easily recognize individual syllables, the pulses of which are relatively salient, compared to words, which require more cognitive processing by the listener.

There are several counting processes of syllables and words, in order to classify the degree of stuttering. In most cases, the counting is made in real time through the listener and following a live or audio/audio-video presentation of the speech sample. This process is adequate as a sensitive indicator of stuttering frequency (Martin, Kuhl, & Haroldson, 1972; Onslow, Andrews, & Lincoln, 1994; Onslow, Costa, & Rue, 1990; Reed, & Godden, 1997; Ryan, & Ryan, 1995).

Inherent to the use of counts of stutters is the thorny issue of how stuttering is defined by the listener. Different definitions such as behavioral, perceptual, and even speaker-determined, abound in the literature (Conture, 1990; Curlee, 1981; MacDonald & Martin, 1973; Martin & Haroldson, 1981; Perkins, 1990; Wingate, 1964; Yairi, 1997; Young, 1975).

Currently, there is no research that irrefutably proves one definition more valid than the others. Therefore, it is important that researchers clearly describe the way in which stuttering was identified and recorded by listeners and include information regarding those listeners, their training, their experience, and, of course, the reliability of their counts. Readers can then judge for themselves the quality of the stuttering identification method and hence the quality of the reported findings.

In the literature, there are some specific classification instruments to evaluate the severity of stuttering speech. Riley's Stuttering Severity Instrument is one of the most common scales (Riley, 1972). Through this tool, a previous study was developed to classify the degree of severity of stuttering in a group of six subjects (Teixeira, Fernandes & Costa, 2012; Teixeira, Fernandes & Costa, 2013). The typology followed was similar to that of author Wendell Johnson (1963), since it showed episodes of stutter that fit more with the scale of measurement of the degree of severity of disfluency. These tests were implemented using spontaneous and reading speech. The behavior of the subject were observed and registered during the speech record. The evidence allowed obtaining the Frequency, which is the number of disfluent syllables divided by the total number of spoken syllables, expressed as a percentage, and the Duration, which is the average of the three longer disfluent events over both tests (spontaneous speech and reading speech). The values of these two parameters were converted to a score, using the standard scales proposed by Silva (2009). By using the Matlab® software, an algorithm was developed to automatically count the parameter for further evaluation of the degree of severity of stutter, as well as obtaining the means of the three longer disfluent events.

Finally, statements were added to the scores of the three stages of evaluation (Frequency, Duration of the three longer disfluent events and Behaviors associated with). The final value was converted into percentages for comparison with limit tabled values, allowing the classification of the degree of severity of disfluency in very low, low, moderate, severe and very severe degrees. Table 1 shows the results obtained in the above mentioned study. It should be mentioned that the 6 subjects were also used in the study of the percentage of silence. The first four subjects are known as persons with stuttering.

SCALE: STUTTERING SEVERITY INSTRUMENT FOR CHILDREN AND ADULTS

The scale "Stuttering Severity Instrument for Children and Adults" (SSI-3 and SSI-4) proposed by Riley (1972, 2009) is a common behavioral assessment tool for measuring stuttering severity among three age groups; preschool, school age and adults. This instrument provides an estimate of stuttering sever-

Table 1. Scores and degrees of severity for each of the subjects

Score									Severity Degree
#	Gender	Age	Frequency			Duration of the 3 Longer Events	Behaviors Associated	Final Score	
			Spontaneous Speech	Reading Speech	Total				
1	M	23	9	5	14	8	10	32	Serious
2	M	12	9	9	18	14	14	46	Very Serious
3	M	22	6	4	10	8	10	28	Moderate
4	F	18	5	4	9	10	6	25	Moderate
5	F	21	2	0	2	4	0	6	Not Disfluent
6	F	25	0	2	2	4	0	6	Not Disfluent

(Teixeira, Fernandes & Costa, 2012; Teixeira, Fernandes & Costa, 2013)

ity using three types of parameters: frequency (percentage of the stuttered syllables), duration (average duration of the three longest stutters) and observations of physical concomitants made at the time of the recording (i.e. distracting sounds, facial grimaces, head movements and movements of the extremities) (Todd et al., 2014). The SSI-3 has been investigated by the scientific community and classified as being a reliable scale (Ansari et al., 2010). For the application of this scale it is necessary to perform the test using spontaneous and reading speech as well as an observation and further evaluation of behaviors along the two records.

The symptoms that are considered as stutters are identical in SSI-3 and SSI-4 and are described in detail in the SSI-3 manual (Riley, 1994). All versions of the SSI scores arise from measures made on both the speech sample and observations of physical concomitants. There are standard scales that convert the percentage of stuttered syllables and duration measures into scores that are combined with raw physical concomitant scores to give the total overall SSI score (Todd et al., 2014). The scale classifies the subject in one of the five groups according to the observed behaviors (0 = none, 1 = not visible unless you're watching, 2 = barely noticeable to a casual observer, 3 = distracting, 4 = Very distracting, 5 = Severe and painful to look). The record of the two parameters over the speech will allow reaching scores of observed behaviors, using a normative scale. This score is then used to classify the degree of disfluency. Finally add up the scores of the three evaluation parameters (Frequency, Duration of the three longer diffluent events and Associated Behaviors (or Physical Concomitants)) to give a final value that is converted to a percentage, which enables, when compared to standard values, the classification of the disfluency in a severity scale in Very Low, Low, Moderate, Severe and Very Severe.

The SSI-4 includes a computer program that automates the assessment of stuttering severity (not available in SSI-3). However, according to the authors, Howell *et al.*, (2011), the program has not been assessed for reliability and validity. Also, results with the program have not been compared against the methods for obtaining stuttering severity recommended in SSI-3 (Howell *et al.*, 2011).

Some flexibility exists in the procedures that can be used to obtain speech samples. Provision is made in the SSI instrument for the assessments to be made in clinical, home, or laboratory settings.

The minimum required sample length is specified. The minimum sample length given in Riley reduced the minimum sample length from 200 to 150 syllables for SSI-4 (Todd et al., 2014).

METHODOLOGY

This section describes the methodology of the experiment to measure the stuttering severity of a group of persons in order to explore the described scale. Next section will describe the implementation of the algorithm developed to measure the duration of pauses in the speech.

Participants

This research included a total of 8 subjects of which 6 had already participated in the previous study cited in Table 1. Participants of this research were 4 male adults, 3 female adults and 1 male child who volunteered to take part in the present study. All subjects gave their informed consent prior to participation in the study. For the underaged the permission was obtained from their legal representatives. None of the study participants had presented history of head trauma, learning disabilities, dyslexia, psychiatric conditions and use of any medication. Only the child was in speech therapy. Data were acquired on eight native speakers of Portuguese Language who reported having normal hearing. Four subjects (between the ages of 11 and 23 years) reported a history of stuttering since childhood, and the other 4 subjects (between the ages of 22 and 26 years) had a normal speech production.

Speech Fluency Evaluation

The stuttering severity levels were determined from videotape recordings of spontaneous speech and reading tasks, using the Stuttering Severity Index or SSI (Riley 1972). The present analysis focuses exclusively on two tasks. The first task aimed to analyze a conversational speech (about 15 minutes of duration) between a stutterer participant and a person with normal speech, without visual contact between them. To establish communication, several similar images were given to the two participants in order to discuss the images between them (Figure 1). In the second task, the participants were invited to read a text containing 318 words and 1559 fluent syllables for analysis and comparison of the results.

Speech Signal Record

To ensure that the information obtained is reliable, it is necessary that the recording of the signal is made under adequate conditions and using the adequate equipment.

There are several processes that enable the acquisition of speech signal for later analysis. One which is commonly used is a process where the acquisition of the acoustic signal produced by the speaker is made in a soundproof room, using a unidirectional or omnidirectional microphone. This signal is amplified by a pre-amplifier with a linear frequency response and is stored on a magnetic tape with good quality, being later or immediately held for their conversion to digital signal using an anti-aliasing filter. The storage of the signal is then done in digital format, (McAulay & Quatieri, 1986; Teixeira, 2013). It

Figure 1. Example of images used to tease the spontaneous conversational speech

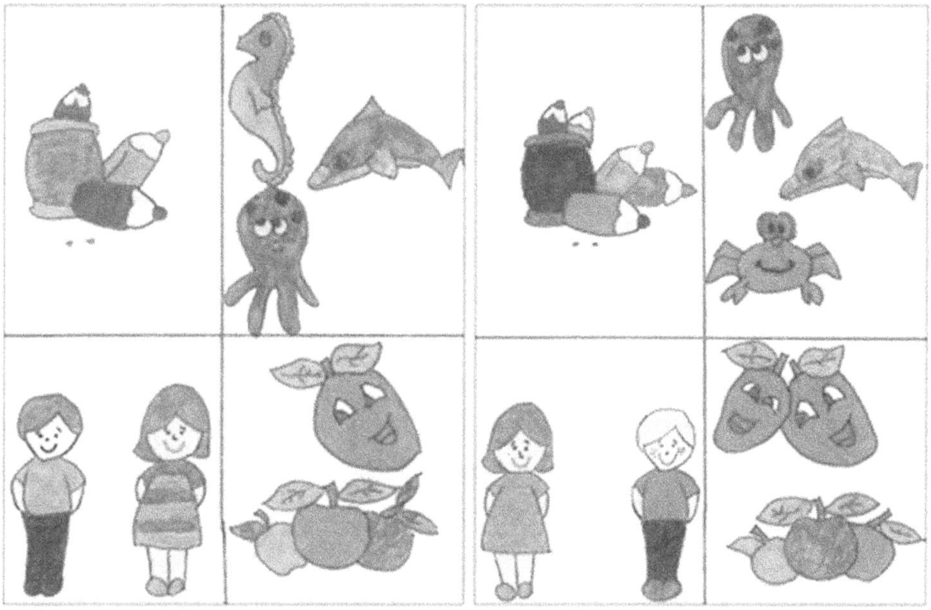

is important to use a sampling frequency high enough to guarantee a bandwidth to ensure the required quality for understanding the speech. Anyhow, once the requirements for understanding the speech do not need the higher frequencies, the sampling frequency of 11025 Hz is enough.

In the present work, the data acquisition was carried out in an appropriate and quiet room, trying to be close to a soundproof room. Participants spoke into two *Sennheiser Best e840* unidirectional microphones (frequency ranges = 40-18000 Hz) positioned directly in front of their mouths. Each trial was recorded and exported into the Praat software (Boersma & Weenink, 2009) generating .wav files. This software allowed a segmentation of the speech signal for a later use. The Record parameters were mono sound, a 16-bit resolution and a sampling frequency of 11025 Hz. Finally, MATLAB (Mathworks, Inc.) was used to develop and implement the pause measurement algorithm in each speech signal of the participants.

AUTOMATIC DETERMINATION OF PAUSES IN SPEECH

The measurement can be made using some speech signal analysis tools like Praat or SFS (Speech File System). These tools allow to represent and ear the segments of speech and label them, this allows to manually identify the silent segments in speech and measure them. Anyhow all the signals need to be manually labeled, that is a time consuming task. Alternatively an algorithm was developed in order to label and identify automatically the speech signal into silent or speech segments.

The silent segments in regular speech may occur between sentences or paragraphs, the longer segments of silence, occasionally between words, shorter segments, and also during the stop part of the stop consonants (<k>, <p>, <t>, <g>, <d> and <b>), being very short time pauses (between 40 and 70 ms in average for read speech in European Portuguese, according to Teixeira et al., 2001). Additionally, some interjections may occur during reading but mainly during spontaneous speech. Some of the interjection contains silent parts of speech. In stuttered speech several additional silent parts of speech are inserted. All these different types of silent parts of speech will be measured by the algorithm.

For the automatic determination of silence or pauses in speech some tools were used, among them the Moving Average (MA), the Moving Energy (ME) and the Zero Crossing Rate (ZCR). These tools perform processing only in the temporal domain.

The algorithm was originally developed by Teixeira (2013) for the classification of the signal in the zones of silence, voiced speech and unvoiced speech. The algorithm is based on the three mentioned tools (moving average, the moving energy and the zero crossing rate) and in one decision area. This decision is based on the result of two vectors obtained by the moving energy and zero crossing rate.

Zero Crossing Rate

Zero Crossing Rate gives the number of times the signal crosses the zero line during a defined length of signal. It can be expressed by Eq. 1 and 2.

$$ZCR(n) = \frac{1}{N+1} \sum_{m=n-N/2}^{n+N/2} \left| sign(x(m)) - sign(x(m-1)) \right| \times w_{N+1}(m) \tag{1}$$

where:

$$sign(x(m)) = \begin{cases} 1 & \text{if } x(m) \geq 0 \\ -1 & \text{if } x(m) < 0 \end{cases} \tag{2}$$

w is a window with length N+1 and x is the input signal. Different types of windows can be used. In this algorithm a rectangular window was used.

The zero crossing rate is applied to the derived signal and not directly to the original signal because the original signal often was an offset. This offset even if it is small usually leads to the noisy level of the signal above or below zero eliminating the zero crossing.

The derivative consists of a simple difference applied by the following equation:

$$d(n) = x(n) - x(n-1) \tag{3}$$

The application of the zero crossing rate to the derivative of the signal (d) consists essentially of the determination of the rate of the high and low peaks. This parameter is high inside the parts of silent speech, actually noise speech, low in voiced speech, and also high in unvoiced speech.

The advantage of using the derived signal instead of the original signal to apply the zero crossing rate is demonstrated in Figure 2. In this figure the signal corresponds to the Portuguese word "casa".

Figure 2. Application of the zero crossing rate. a) Speech signal corresponding to the Portuguese word "casa" (home); b) Zero crossing rate applied directly to the signal; c) Zero crossing rate applied to the derived signal

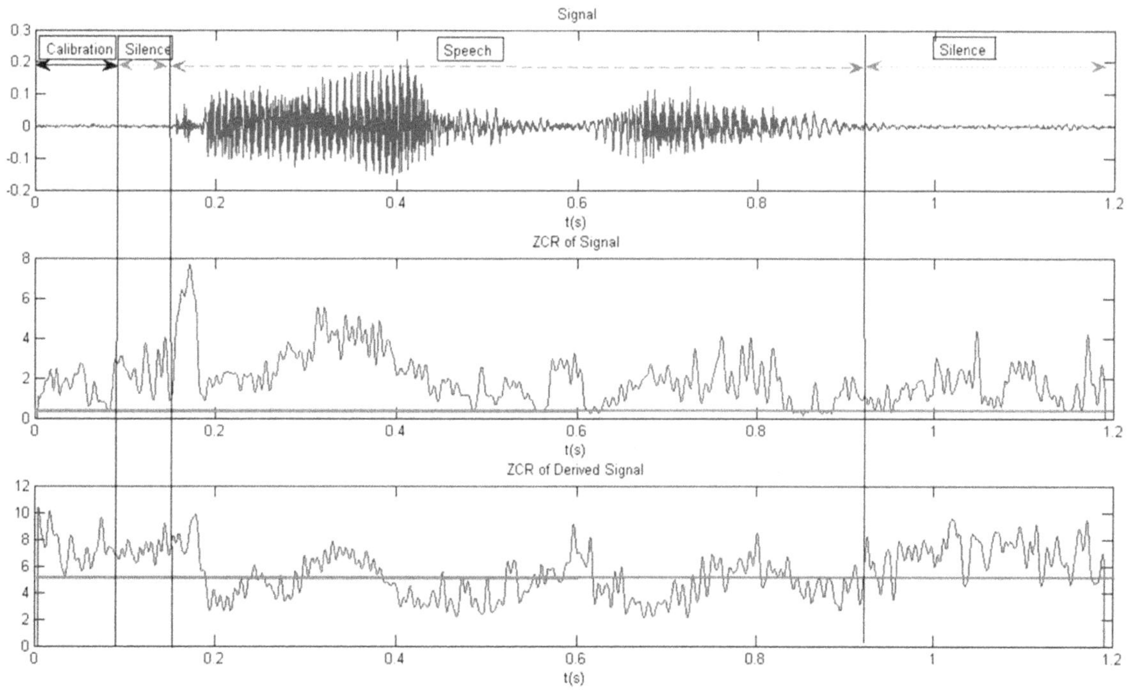

The first 150 ms correspond to a silent part of the signal, meaning high ZCR expected, then the plosive consonant <k> corresponds to unvoiced speech and therefore also high ZCR although slightly lower than in the silent part of the signal. After the consonant (about the instants of 190 ms) it follows the <a> vowel, that is a voiced sound and therefore with low ZCR. Then the next sound is the voiced fricative consonant <z>. It is expected to have low energy compared to voiced sounds, but higher energy than silence segments, and higher ZCR than in voiced segments. After the consonant comes the closed voiced vowel <a> with low ZCR and higher energy. Finally, the signal ends with a silent part corresponding to high ZCR. The upper part of Figure 2 represents the speech signal and the calibration, silence and speech segments are identified. The middle part of the figure represents the application of the ZCR to the original signal and lower part the application of the ZCR to the derived signal. The initial and final part of the signal has a very low offset, not visible in the figure, but enough to deviate the noise signal from zero line and reduce the ZCR, as it can be observed in the middle part of Fig. 2. It can be seen that the application of the zero crossing rate to the original signal do not gives high values due to this slight offset, but the application to the derived signal already detects this high values correspondent to the silent segments.

The ZCR was applied under a window of 20 samples and with a displacement of 1 sample in both cases presented in Figure 2.

Moving Average and Moving Energy

The moving average function implements Eq. 4. This function has the ability to smooth the signal. The signal is more or less smoothed according to the length of the window N+1. For this purpose the Hanning window was used for w. The indices n do not need to be of unitary space, it can be highly spaced to have higher efficiency.

$$MA(n) = \frac{1}{N+1} \sum_{m=n-N/2}^{n+N/2} x(m).w_{N+1}(m) \tag{4}$$

The moving energy function implements Eq. 5. It determines the energy of the signal and is more or less smoothed according to the length of the window N+1.

$$ME(n) = \frac{1}{N+1} \sum_{m=n-N/2}^{n+N/2} \left[x(m).w_{N+1}(m)\right]^2 \tag{5}$$

Algorithm

After reading the signal the algorithm calls the moving energy function with a window of length 20 and spaced with 10 samples allowing smoothing of the signal. This new signal, ME, will have a length 10 times lower than the original. Then, the original signal is derived to produce the d signal, and the zero crossing rate function is applied to the d signal with a window of 20 samples and a spacing of 10 (both cases correspond to a superposition of 50% of the segments). The output signal (ZCR) is smoothed out by applying the moving average function with a window length of 100 samples and unitary spacing. Also this signal will have a length ten times less than the original.

The beginning of the signal (about 100 ms) is used to calibrate the level of silence in the environment. During this period no speech should be produced and a silence is expected in order to calibrate the level of noise namely its energy and ZCR. This calibration will serve to define the threshold values for the energy and the zero crossing rate for the silence.

In Figure 3, secured silence is in the first instants of time, at least 100 ms. This beginning of the signal with silence is a noisy signal with low energy and a high zero crossing rate. This part of silent signal is used to determine the upper limit of energy (LSES) and the lower limit of zero crossing rate (LIZ) in silent part of the signal. In the second signal of Figure 3 there is a visible threshold line that relates to the maximum level of energy corresponding to the silence, called LSES (upper limit of the energy signal), and this is the maximum of the moving energy. In turn, the minimum level of zero-crossing rate after being smoothed is also established, called LIZ (Lower Limit of ZCR), which is visible by a threshold line in the third signal of Figure 3.

Continuing the follow-up of the algorithm, the variables *e* and *z* were declared for counting the number of elements below the LSES threshold and above the threshold LIZ respectively under a window of length 10. This window with 10 elements corresponds to a 100 samples of the original signal which corresponds to 9 ms long. Therefore, every 9 ms window there will be a decision about the type of signal. High values of *e* represent low-energy, high values of *z* imply high ZCR. Based on the variables *e* and *z* a decision is made to classify the original signal Silence or Speech.

Figure 3. Classification of the signal with paused read speech corresponding to "Eu moro na minha casa" (I live in my house) according to the field of decision established

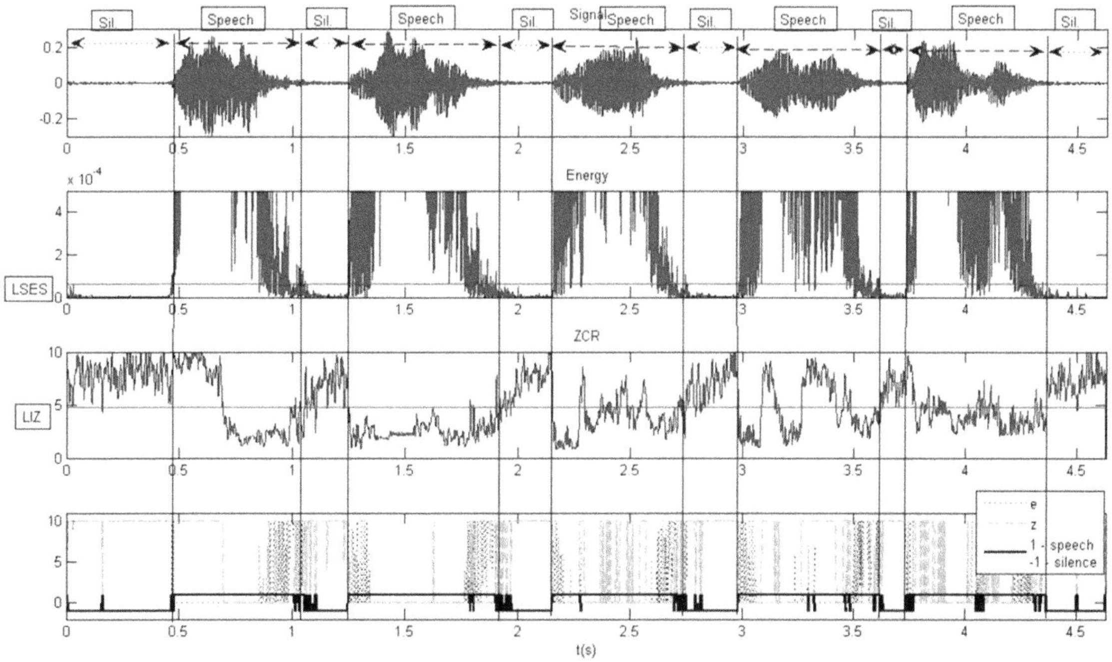

On the basis of variables e and z a "matrix of decision" was established, having the z variable in the abscissa, between 0 and 10 and the e variable in the ordinate axes, also between 0 and 10. In the matrix of decision the areas were settled for the silence and speech, as can be seen in Figure 4.

In Figure 4 the areas of classification of speech signal can be observed, where the silence corresponds to: $z \geq 8 \wedge e \geq 3$ or $z \geq 3 \wedge e \geq 8$. The first area corresponds to high ZCR and relatively low energy, the second area corresponds to relatively high ZCR and very low energy.

The second and third signals of Figure 3 present the ME (moving energy) and ZCR. The fourth signal presents the e and z and the final decision of silence/speech for each segment of 9 ms. It can be seen that the decision here correctly assumed along of the all signal in Figure 3. For this example the measured time with speech was 4.62 s, the time with silence was 1.56 s, given a percentage of silence of 33.7%, measured according to Eq. 6. It should be mentioned that this signal was read in a paused speech to show the decision between silence and speech segments and does not correspond to a stuttered speech.

Program Code

Next lines present the main algorithm to make the decision of silence or speech for each segment of the signal. Each segment has duration of 9 ms.

```
Detrend filter applied to the speech signal
Moving Energy of the signal
Determination of the threshold of energy in silent speech (LSES)
Signal is derived
```

Figure 4. "Matrix of decision" for classification of speech signals based on e and z variables

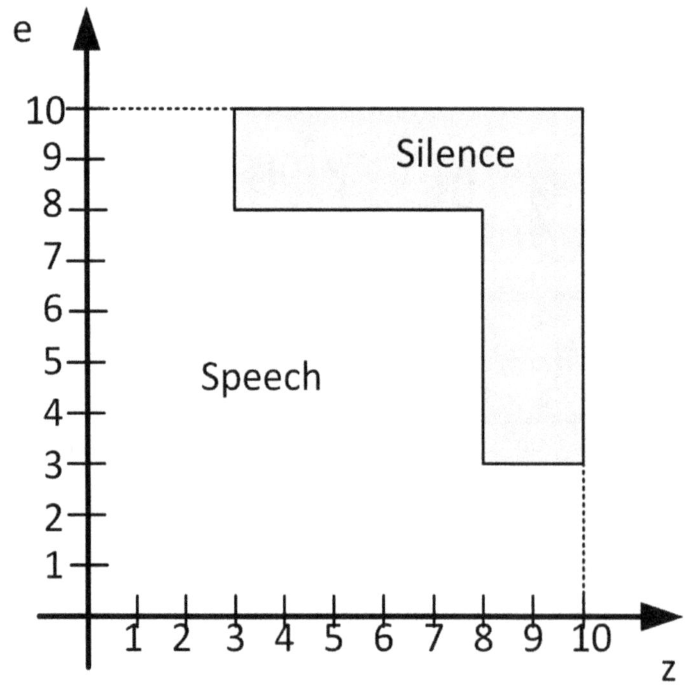

```
The zero crossing rate (ZCR) is applied to the derived signal
A moving average is applied to the ZCR
Determination of the threshold of ZCR in silent speech (LIZ)
Cycle 1, % for i=1:end - segments of 9 ms
    z=0; % number of elements above LIZ
    e=0; % number of elements below LSES
    Cycle 2 (for j=1:10)
        if ZCR(j)>LIZ,
           z=z+1;
        end
        if ME(j)<LSES,
            e=e+1;
        end
    end cycle 2
    if ((e>=8 & z>=3) or (e>=3 & z>=8)),
      decision(i)= silence
      else
      decision(i)= Speech
      end
end of cycle 1
```

ANALYSIS OF RESULTS

With the application of the algorithm to the recorded signals it was possible to make the collection of the parts of silence and parts of speech of all the segments. These results were useful to determine the percentage of silence in each of the 8 subjects. The percentage of silence was obtained based on the following equation:

$$\%\ of\ silence = \frac{Time\ of\ Silence}{Time\ of\ Speech} \times 100 \tag{6}$$

Table 2 shows the values obtained for the percentage of silence in the disfluent and control subjects. The first 6 subjects correspond to the subjects presented already in Table 1, using the same number of subject. To obtain these results, 5 tracks of the signal of each of the subjects were selected which ensured equal conditions of measurement. The segments under analysis were edited leaving an initial portion of speech signal that would guarantee at least 100 ms of silence for the determination of the LSES and LIZ, and a start and end time that corresponded to the beginning and end of the speech, respectively.

As shown in Table 2, the subjects with disfluencies present higher percentage values of silence, with an average of 26.3%. In this group the percentage of silence varies from 20.0 to 41.8%. Subject number 2, presenting 41.8% of silence is the subject among the 4 disfluent belonging to the sample under study

Table 2. Results obtained for the percentage of silence in all subjects

	Subject	% of Silence
Disfluent	1	20.0
	2	41.8
	3	23.2
	4	20.2
	Average	26.3
Control subjects	5	6.2
	6	16.2
	7	6.8
	8	14.8
	Average	11.0

that will present a disfluency more accentuated as recorded in Table 1, on the previous study (Teixeira, Fernandes & Costa, 2012; Teixeira, Fernandes & Costa, 2013). Based on results presented in Tables 1 and 2 it can be alleged that it is not a viable classification of degree of disfluency solely based on the percentages of silence. For instance, the subject 1, ranked with a degree of severity serious has the lowest percentage of silence considering the subjects 3 and 4, classified with a degree of moderate severity. This can be explained by the fact that there is a number of parameters, in addition to the silence that influence the classification of the degree of severity.

The percentage of silence in the control group (not disfluent) is minor than the ones of the disfluent subjects. For this group the percentage of silence varies from 6.2% to 16.2%, and has an average of 11.0%. All the controls have lower values than any disfluent.

One aspect that may alter results is the emotional state of the subject, because when it is under the pressure of an evaluation it may become nervous, causing a possible increase of disfluent moments throughout the speech. In addition, to being under pressure for an assessment, the fact of having to run the tests with strange people nearby can also cause changes in the occurrence of disfluent moments.

CONCLUSION

In this work an algorithm to automatically measure the silences in speech was developed. The algorithm is based on the determination of the energy and zero crossing rate for small windows of the signal. The zero crossing rate is applied to the derivate signal to recover from the eventual offset. The threshold values LSES and LIZ, the upper limit of energy and lower limit of zero crossing rate, respectively, in the silence part of speech is determined. Then the values of e and z are determined in a window with 10 samples. After that the e and z are used to decide if the segment with 10 samples, corresponding to 9 ms, is silence or speech. This algorithm was applied to determine the percentage of silence in spontaneous disfluent speech and in a normal spontaneous speech. This spontaneous speech was recorded putting two subjects discussing similar but different pictures and separately recording each subject.

The algorithm allowed the determination of the percentage of silence of each subject.

The analysis of the percentage of silence shows that this parameter clearly separates the subjects with and without disfluency. It is possible to conclude that individuals with disfluency show percentages of silence much higher compared with individuals without any kind of disturbance in speech.

Six of the eight subjects were in a previous study which was used to measure their degree of severity of the disfluency. The percentage of silence was compared to the previously determined degree of severity and it is possible to conclude that this measure alone is not able to determine the degree of severity of the disfluent speech.

REFERENCES

Adriaensens, S., Beyers, W., & Struyf, E. (2015). Impact of stuttering severity on adolescents' domain-specific and general self-esteem through cognitive and emotional mediating processes. *Journal of Communication Disorders*, *58*, 43–57. doi:10.1016/j.jcomdis.2015.10.003 PMID:26484722

Ancelle, J. A. G. (2015). Assistive Technologies at the Edge of Language and Speech Science for Children with Communication Disorders: VocalIDTM, Free SpeechTM, and SmartPalateTM. In N. R. Silton (Ed.), *Recent Advances in Assistive Technologies to Support Children with Developmental Disorders* (pp. 255–277). Hershey, PA: IGI Global. doi:10.4018/978-1-4666-8395-2.ch012

Ansari, H., Bakhtiar, M., Ghanadzade, M., Packman, A., & Seifpanahi, S. (2010). Investigation of the reliability of the SSI-3 for preschool Persian-speaking children who stutter. *Journal of Fluency Disorders*, *35*(2), 87–91. doi:10.1016/j.jfludis.2010.02.003 PMID:20609330

Barnes, T. D., Wozniak, D. F., Gutierrez, J., Han, T. U., Drayna, D., & Holy, T. E. (2016). A Mutation Associated with Stuttering Alters Mouse Pup Ultrasonic Vocalizations. *Current Biology*, *26*(8), 1009–1018. doi:10.1016/j.cub.2016.02.068 PMID:27151663

Boersma, P., & Weenink, D. (2009). *Praat Manual: doing phonetics by computer. 5.1.17.* [Computer program]. Available at: http://www.fon.hum.uva.nl/praat/download_win.html

Conture, E. (1990). *Stuttering*. Englewood Cliffs, NJ: Prentice-Hall.

Costello, J. M., & Ingham, R. J. (1984). Assessment strategies for stuttering. In R. Curlee & W. H. Perkins (Eds.), *Nature and treatment of stuttering: New directions* (pp. 303–333). San Diego, CA: College-Hill Press.

Curlee, R. F. (1981). Observer agreement on disfluency and stuttering. *Journal of Speech and Hearing Research*, *24*(4), 595–560. doi:10.1044/jshr.2404.595 PMID:7035743

Hirsch, F. (2007). *Le bégaiement Perturbation de l'organisation temporelle de la parole et conséquences spectrales*. (Ph.D dissertation). Marc Bloch Univ., Strasbourg.

Howell, P., & Au-Yeung, J. (2007). Phonetic complexity and stuttering in Spanish. *Clinical Linguistics & Phonetics*, *21*(2), 111–127. doi:10.1080/02699200600709511 PMID:17364620

Howell, P., Au-Yeung, J., & Sackin, S. (2000). Internal Structure of Content Words Leading To Lifespan Differences in Phonological Difficulty in Stuttering. *Journal of Fluency Disorders*, *25*(1), 1–20. doi:10.1016/S0094-730X(99)00025-X PMID:18259599

Howell, P., Au-Yeung, J., Yaruss, S., & Eldridge, K. (2006). Phonetic difficulty and stuttering in English. *Clinical Linguistics & Phonetics*, *20*(9), 703–716. doi:10.1080/02699200500390990 PMID:17342878

Howell, P., Soukup-Ascencao, T., Davis, S., & Rusbridge, S. (2011). Comparison of alternative methods for obtaining severity scores of the speech of people who stutter. *Clinical Linguistics & Phonetics*, *25*(5), 368–378. doi:10.3109/02699206.2010.538955 PMID:21434809

Johnson, W. (1963). *Diagnostic Methods in Speech Pathology*. New York: Herper & Row.

Juste, F. S., Rondon, S., Sassi, F. C., Ritto, A. P., Colalto, C. A., & Andrade, C. R. (2012). Acoustic analyses of diadochokinesis in fluent and stuttering children. *Clinics (Sao Paulo)*, *67*(5), 409–414. doi:10.6061/clinics/2012(05)01 PMID:22666781

MacDonald, J., & Martin, R. (1973). Stuttering and disfluency as two reliable and unambiguous response classes. *Journal of Speech and Hearing Research*, *17*(4), 691–699. doi:10.1044/jshr.1604.691 PMID:4783809

Martin, R., & Haroldson, S. (1981). Stuttering identification: Standard definition and moment of stuttering. *Journal of Speech and Hearing Research*, *24*(1), 59–63. doi:10.1044/jshr.2401.59 PMID:7253630

Martin, R. R., Kuhl, P., & Haroldson, S. K. (1972). An experimental treatment with two preschool stuttering children. *Journal of Speech and Hearing Research*, *15*(4), 743–752. doi:10.1044/jshr.1504.743 PMID:4652394

McAulay, R., & Quatieri, T. (1986). Speech Analysis/Synthesis Based on a Sinusoidal Representation. *IEEE Transactions on Acoustics Speech, and Signal Processing, 34*(4).

McClean, M. D., & Tasko, S. M. (2004). Correlation of orofacial speeds with voice acoustic measures in the fluent speech of persons who stutter. *Experimental Brain Research*, *159*(3), 310–318. doi:10.1007/s00221-004-1952-8 PMID:15248043

Mulligan, H. F., Anderson, T. J., Jones, R. D., Williams, M. J., & Donaldson, I. M. (2003). Tics and developmental stuttering. *Parkinsonism & Related Disorders*, *9*(5), 281–289. doi:10.1016/S1353-8020(03)00002-6 PMID:12781595

Onslow, M., Andrews, C., & Lincoln, M. (1994). A control/experimental trial of operant treatment for early stuttering. *Journal of Speech and Hearing Research*, *37*(6), 1244–1259. doi:10.1044/jshr.3706.1244 PMID:7877284

Onslow, M., Costa, L., & Rue, S. (1990). Direct early intervention with stuttering: Some preliminary data. *The Journal of Speech and Hearing Disorders*, *55*(3), 405–416. doi:10.1044/jshd.5503.405 PMID:2381182

Perkins, W. H. (1990). What is stuttering? *The Journal of Speech and Hearing Disorders*, *55*(3), 370–382. doi:10.1044/jshd.5503.370 PMID:2199728

Peters, H., Hulstijn, W., & Van Lieshout, P. (2000). Recent Developments in Speech Motor Research into Stuttering. *Folia Phoniatrica et Logopaedica*, *52*(1-3), 103–119. doi:10.1159/000021518 PMID:10474010

Plant, R. L., & Younger, R. M. (2000). The interrelationship of subglottic air pressure, fundamental frequency, and vocal intensity during speech. *Journal of Voice*, *14*(2), 170–177. doi:10.1016/S0892-1997(00)80024-7 PMID:10875568

Prado-Velasco, M., & Fernández-Peruchena, C. (2011). An Advanced Concept of Altered Auditory Feedback as a Prosthesis-Therapy for Stuttering Founded on a Non-Speech Etiologic Paradigm. In J. Pereira (Ed.), *Handbook of Research on Personal Autonomy Technologies and Disability Informatics* (pp. 76–118). Hershey, PA: IGI Global. doi:10.4018/978-1-60566-206-0.ch006

Reed, C., & Godden, A. (1997). An experimental treatment using verbal punishment with two preschool stutterers. *Journal of Fluency Disorders*, *2*(3), 225–233. doi:10.1016/0094-730X(77)90026-2

Riley, G. (1972). A Stuttering Severity Instrument for Children and Adults. *The Journal of Speech and Hearing Disorders*, *37*(3), 314–322. doi:10.1044/jshd.3703.314 PMID:5057250

Riva-Posse, P., Busto-Marolt, L., Schteinschnaider, A., Martinez-Echenique, L., Cammarota, A., & Merello, M. (2008). Phenomenology of abnormal movements in stuttering. *Parkinsonism & Related Disorders*, *14*(5), 415–419. doi:10.1016/j.parkreldis.2007.11.006 PMID:18316236

Rogić Vidaković, M., Jerković, A., Jurić, T., Vujović, I., Šoda, J., Erceg, N., & Dogaš, Z. et al. (2016). Neurophysiologic markers of primary motor cortex for laryngeal muscles and premotor cortex in caudal opercular part of inferior frontal gyrus investigated in motor speech disorder: A navigated transcranial magnetic stimulation (TMS) study. *Cognitive Processing*, 1–14. PMID:27130564

Ryan, B. P., & Ryan, B. V. K. (1995). Programmed stuttering treatment for children: Comparison of two establishment programs through transfer, maintenance, and follow-up. *Journal of Speech and Hearing Research*, *38*(1), 61–75. doi:10.1044/jshr.3801.61 PMID:7731220

Sawyer, J., Chon, H., & Ambrose, N. (2009). Influences of Rate, Length, and Complexity on Speech Disfluency in a Single Speech Sample in Preschool Children Who Stutter. *Journal of Fluency Disorders*, *33*(3), 220–240. doi:10.1016/j.jfludis.2008.06.003 PMID:18762063

Seeley, R., Stephens, T., & Tate, P. (2006). *Anatomy and Physiology (7th ed.)*. Mcgraw-Hill.

Silva, S. (2009). *Classificação do grau de disfluência com e sem o uso de feedback acústico modificado em adolescentes e adultos gagos portugueses*. (Unpublished undergraduate dissertation). University Fernando Pessoa, Portugal.

Teixeira, J. P. (2013). *Análise e Síntese da Fala - Modelação Paramétrica de Sinais Para Sistemas TTS*. Editorial Académica Espanhola.

Teixeira, J. P., Fernandes, M. G., & Costa, R. A. (2012). Measure and Comparison of Speech Pause Duration in Subjects with Disfluency Speech. *Procedia Technology*, *5*, 812–819. doi:10.1016/j.protcy.2012.09.090

Teixeira, J. P., Fernandes, M. G., & Costa, R. A. (2013). Pause Duration of Disfluent Speech. *International Journal of Reliable and Quality E-Healthcare*, *2*(3), 62–73. doi:10.4018/ijrqeh.2013070105

Teixeira, J. P., Freitas, D., Braga, D., Barros, M. J., & Latsch, V. (2001). *Phonetic Events from the Labeling the European Portuguese Database for Speech Synthesis, FEUP/IPB-DB*. Eurospecch.

Todd, H., Mirawwdeli, A., Costelloe, S, Cavenagh, P., Davis, S., & Howell, P. (2014). Scores on Riley's stuttering Severity Instrument Versions Three and Fur for samples os dofferent length and for different types of speech material. *Informa Healthcare, 28*(12), 912-926.

Van Lieshout, P., Hulstijn, W., & Peters, H. (2004). Searching for the weak link in the speech production chain of people who stutter: a motor skill approach. In B. Maassen, R. Kent, P. H. van Lieshout, & W. Hulstijn (Eds.), Speech motor control in normal and disordered speech. Oxford University Press.

Vanhoutte, S., Cosyns, M., van Mierlo, P., Batens, K., Corthals, P., De Letter, M., & Santens, P. et al. (2016). When will a stuttering moment occur? The determining role of speech motor preparation. *Neuropsychologia, 86*, 93–102. doi:10.1016/j.neuropsychologia.2016.04.018 PMID:27106391

Wieland, E. A., McAuley, J. D., Dilley, L. C., & Chang, S. E. (2015). Evidence for a rhythm perception deficit in children who stutter. *Brain and Language, 144*, 26–34. doi:10.1016/j.bandl.2015.03.008 PMID:25880903

Wingate, M. (1964). A standard definition of stuttering. *The Journal of Speech and Hearing Disorders, 29*(4), 484–489. doi:10.1044/jshd.2904.484 PMID:14257050

Yairi, E. (1997). Disfluency characteristics of childhood stuttering. In R. F. Curlee & G. M. Siegel (Eds.), *Nature and treatment of stuttering: New directions* (2nd ed.; pp. 49–78). Boston: Allyn & Bacon.

Yaruss, J. (1999). Utterance length, syntactic complexity, and childhood stuttering. *Journal of Speech, Language, and Hearing Research: JSLHR, 42*(2), 329–344. doi:10.1044/jslhr.4202.329 PMID:10229450

Young, M. A. (1975). Onset, prevalence, and recovery from stuttering. *The Journal of Speech and Hearing Disorders, 40*(1), 49–58. doi:10.1044/jshd.4001.49 PMID:1123928

KEY TERMS AND DEFINITIONS

Matrix of Decision: Matrix used to decide if the signal segment is silence or speech. It is based in 2 parameters related with the zero crossing rate and energy of the signal.

Moving Average: A signal with the result of the application of a moving average window along the signal. It is useful to smooth the original signal.

Moving Energy: A signal with the result of the application of a moving energy window along a signal. It gives the energy of the signal over the time.

Praat Software: Open source software to perform speech signal analysis. Useful also to phonetic studies (http://www.fon.hum.uva.nl/praat).

SSI: Stuttering Severity Instrument for Children and Adults is a common behavioral assessment tool for measuring stuttering severity.

Stuttering Disorder: Speech stuttering disorder characterized by frequent occurrences of repetitions or prolongations of syllables, words, and sounds, as well as involuntary hesitations or pauses that disrupt the rhythmic flow of speech.

Zero Crossing Rate: Gives the number of times the signal crosses the zero line during a defined period of time.

Chapter 9
Surface Segmentation:
The Case of Bronchus Anatomical Structure

S. Zimeras
University of the Aegean, Greece

ABSTRACT

Segmentation is a powerful procedure that could be used to extract relevant information of the images based on advanced techniques (like active contours, region growing, Markov random fields, and medical atlas analysis). For the procedures, the main task is the contour, or volume or surface representation of specific parts of the organs that could be used for the benefit of the patients under doctor evaluation. So, in real cases, the proposed process must be quick, accurate and easy to implement. The segmentation of the organ is another problem that must be considered. More complicated, more demanding the segmentation process. In our case (bronchus segmentation) a quick, effective and easy to implement procedure is proposed based on the combination of boundary tracking and region growing techniques.

INTRODUCTION

Image segmentation is the process of splitting a digital image into one or more regions of interest based on their organ structure (Punam, 2011). Cases where noise, unclear regions, and poor contrast make difficult the process, a human eye must be included.

Segmentation, especially in medical images, is important because based on the resulting reconstruction, the shape of the organ could be used for the measurements of the image classifications. In biomedical image segmentation, there is great interest segmenting three-dimensional anatomical structures from CT, MRI and PET data. General purpose segmentation, on the other hand, is typically a two-dimensional problem. Time complexity and storage complexity are two main problems with the implementation of the process.

From the viewpoint of the diagnosis of the chest, the bronchus is a very important organ, since a lung disease such as a tumor is often concerned with the bronchus. The bronchus has a tree structure

DOI: 10.4018/978-1-5225-1724-5.ch009

for sending air to the lungs. It starts from the trachea as the root of a tree. The trachea bifurcates the left and the right main bronchus, which enters the left and the right lung. Bronchial branches are repeatedly split toward the peripheral of the lungs and, finally, connect with alveolus, where gas exchange takes place (Netter, 1997).

Many studies on automatically extracting bronchus regions from 3D chest X-ray CT images have been reported (Mori *et al.*, 1995; Sonka *et al.*, 1996; Iseki *et al.*, 1997; Tsui and Heng, 2000; Schlathoelter *et al.*, 2002). Conventional approaches are mostly based on a region-growing method. This work is an extended work of the spinal cord segmentation analysis (Zimeras, 2012).

BACKGROUND

Based on the bronchus morphology, the segmentation procedure includes linear interpolation or B-splines between gap contour reconstructions. The common procedure is the linear interpolation where in the plane of slice i, the surface created between slice pairs 1 - i and I will usually not agree in the normal surface with the surface created between slices i and 1 + i. To avoid discontinuities in the normal surface, more than just two slices, at a given time, must be considered.

Assume that we begin with k sets of constraints, one set for each 2D data slice. Instead of considering the contours in pairs, we place the constraints for all of the k slices into 3D simultaneously. Specifically, the constraints of slices i are placed in the plane z = si, where s is the spacing between planes. Once the constraints from all slices have been placed in 3D, we invoke the implicit function interpolation once to create a single implicit function in 3D for the complete set of contours (Karangelis, 2004).

Figure 1. Implicit surface interpolation

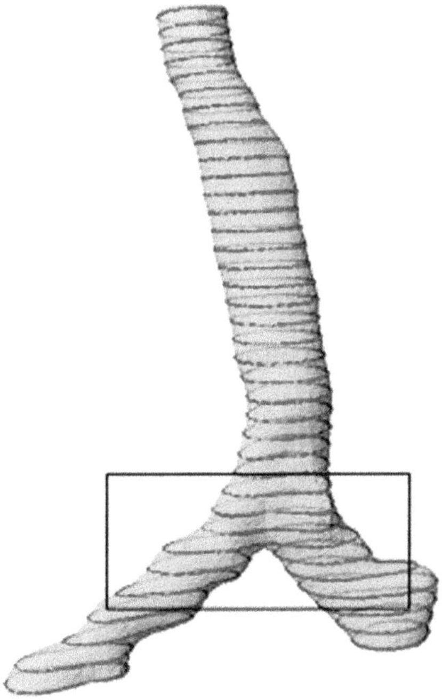

In cases where key contours between single contour shapes and split contours is usually not an option, advanced interpolation methods are required to fill the missing gaps. The main challenge for the contour interpolation of surface reconstruction algorithm is how to handle the bifurcation problem. For the implicit surfaces, the definition of bifurcation is a property that can be handled with flexibility. The degree of bifurcation is highly related to the degree of continuity of the implicit functions and the distance between the single and contour pairs.

The properties of the B-spline curves or surfaces can be extended in the image or volume reconstruction very well (Cohen et. al., 2010). The most important properties are continuity, convex hull, local control, diminishing variation and representation of multiple values. The spatial distribution result from B-spline interpolation is smooth and exhibits second order continuity C^2. One method to apply the B-spline interpolation is by estimating the control polygon of the B-spline approximation, such that the resultant case passes through the requested points. In 3D reconstruction case, the function is given by (Karangelis, 2004).:

$$S\left(z,y,x\right) = Z \cdot M \cdot \begin{bmatrix} Y_m & P'_{k-1} & X^t_m \\ Y_m & P'_k & X^t_m \\ Y_m & P'_{k+1} & X^t_m \\ Y_m & P'_{k+2} & X^t_m \end{bmatrix}$$

where: $Z=[z^3\ z^2\ z\ 1]$ an

$$P'_k = \begin{bmatrix} P_{i-1,j-1,k} & P_{i,j-1,k} & P_{i+1,j-1,k} & P_{i+2,j-1,k} \\ P_{i-1,j,k} & P_{i,j,k} & P_{i+1,j,k} & P_{i+2,j,k} \\ P_{i-1,j+1,k} & P_{i,j+1,k} & P_{i+1,j+1,k} & P_{i+2,j+1,k} \\ P_{i-1,j+2,k} & P_{i,j+2,k} & P_{i+1,j+2,k} & P_{i+2,j+2,k} \end{bmatrix}$$

with the 3D geometry of the interpolation process (Figure 2):

MAIN FOCUS OF THE CHAPTER

Segmentation (Haralick & Shapiro, 1985; Gonzales & Woods, 1992; Pal & Pal, 1993) is a powerful tool, which gives the opportunity to split the image into parts based on the importance of the regions. Especially in cases where, where parts of the medical image of the organs are involved, the importance of the final 2D or 3D reconstruction of the organs is essential for the medical diagnosis or clinical results. Organs, many times, include complicated structures which a medical expert, most of the times, can identify by manual segmentation (Karangelis and Zimeras, 2002; Zimeras, Karangelis, and Firle, 2002; Karangelis and Zimeras 2002).

In case, where reconstructed contours are parallel, and the restore of the organ is complicated (like bronchus), the segmentation procedure is difficult to achieve (Figure 3). In this case, contour shapes

Figure 2. 3D geometry of the B-slines interpolation process

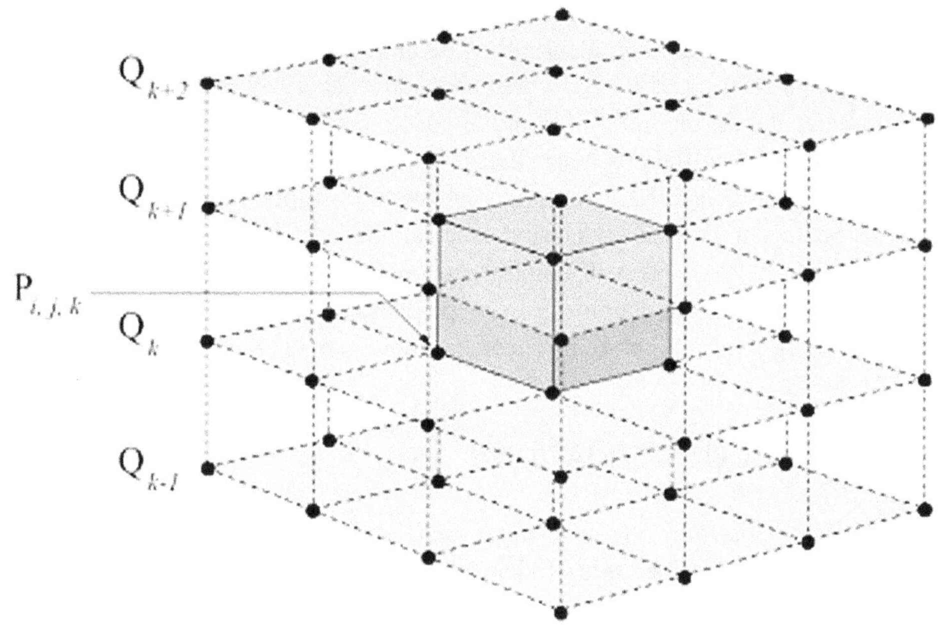

Figure 3. Contour analysis based on trachea shape

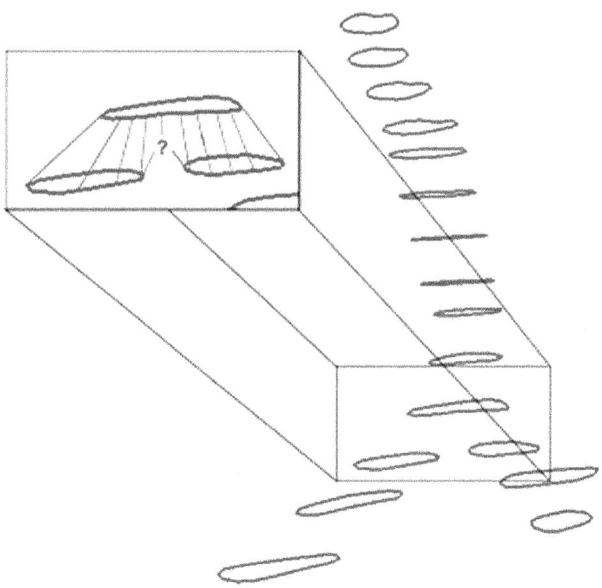

(Malik et. al., 2001) are split in different directions, and the segmentation becomes more complicated. Also, the problem with the missing gaps between contours is another problem that must be solved.

In medical images, this segmentation has traditionally been done by a human expert. Even with the aid of image processing software, manual segmentation of 3D CT images is tedious time-consuming, and thus impractical, especially in cases where a large number of objects must be specified. Many methods have been proposed to detect and segment 2D shapes, most of which is template matching (Nagel. and Rosenfield, 1972). However, their low speed has prevented the widespread use. Another technique is called snakes or active contours (Großkopf et. al., 1998; Kass et. al., 1987; Terzopoulos, 1987; Terzopoulos, and Metaxas, 1981; Blake and Isard,1998; Eviatar and Somorjai, 1996). It has been used, but the main drawbacks are associated with the initialization and poor convergence to boundary concavities which limit their utility depending on the procedure that it is used (deterministic like maximum likelihood, ICM or stochastic MCMC, simulated annealing). Substantial computational and storage requirements become especially acute when object orientation and scale have to be considered.

In this work, a quick real-time process, combining contour tracking techniques (boundary tracking) (Chalana & Kim, 1997) and threshold region growing process, is proposed. To overcome the gap problem between contours, a B-splines interpolation process is implemented (Karangelis, 2004).

SOLUTIONS AND RECOMMENDATIONS

The bronchus has a pipe structure with air inside it. Starting from the end of the trachea it extended in lungs with branching repeatedly, like a tree (Rodenwaldt, 1997; Summers, 1996; Vinnig, 1994). Because its wall is very thin, with an inner area that is filled with air, the contrast of the bronchus image is very low. If the bronchus runs across the slice, vertically its section on a slice is observed, as an approximately circular ring, but its borders are often very vague. A CT inside of bronchus presents lower contrast than that of the wall. Due to the above structure (Figure 4), segmentation, using the boundary tracking technique, is inappropriate giving unsatisfactory results.

The bronchus area is extracted as thin volumetric areas in 3D space, instead of extracting the wall of the bronchus as a curved surface (Fumikazu et. al., 1998). Tracing voxels with relatively low CT values perform for the segmentation. This process is regarded as a kind of region growing procedure. A starting point of tracking and the criterion to merge a new area to the bronchus should be selected carefully. In this work, a thresholding region growing would be performed using a constant threshold selection with levels 10 to 20 Hounsfield values. The graphical steps for the bronchus segmentation process are given in Figure 5.

Figure 4. Bronchus structure

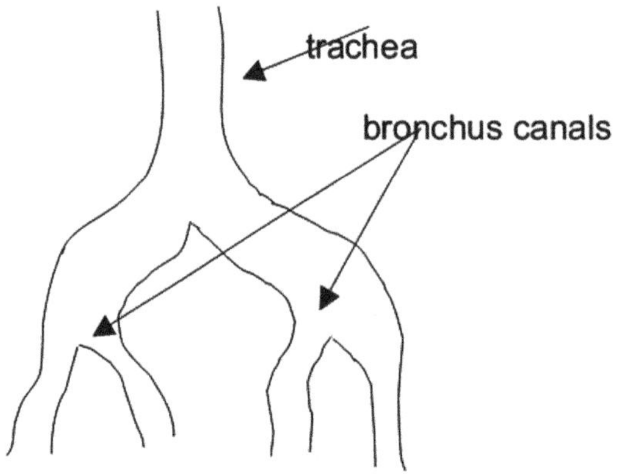

Figure 5. Whole procedure for bronchus area extraction

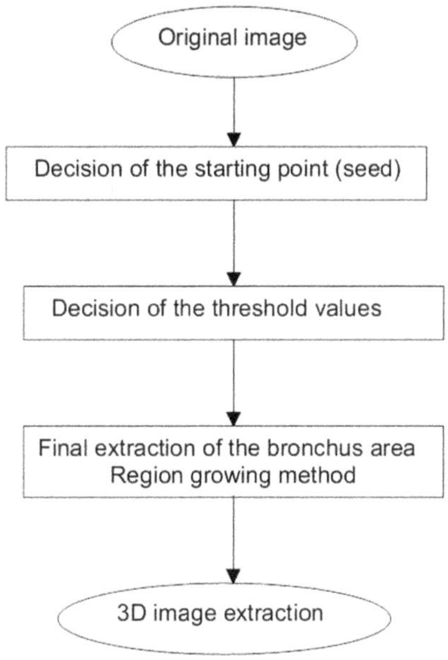

The algorithmic steps for the procedure are:

- An initial set of small areas is iteratively merged according to similarity constraints. A 4-connected model for image connectivity of most cases is considered.
- Start by choosing an arbitrary seed pixel and compare it with neighboring pixels (Figure 6).
- The region is grown from the seed pixel by adding in neighbouring pixels that are similar, increasing the size of the region (Figure 7).
- When the growth of one region stops, we simply choose another seed pixel, which does not yet belong to any region and start again.
- The whole procedure is continued until all pixels belong to some region

Figure 6. Start of growing a region

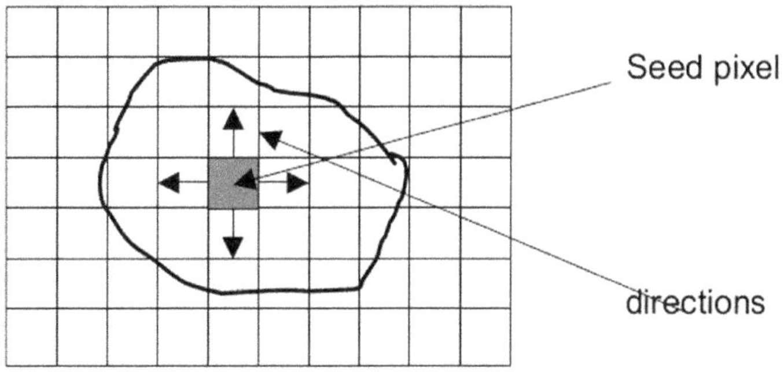

Figure 7. Growing process after a few iterations

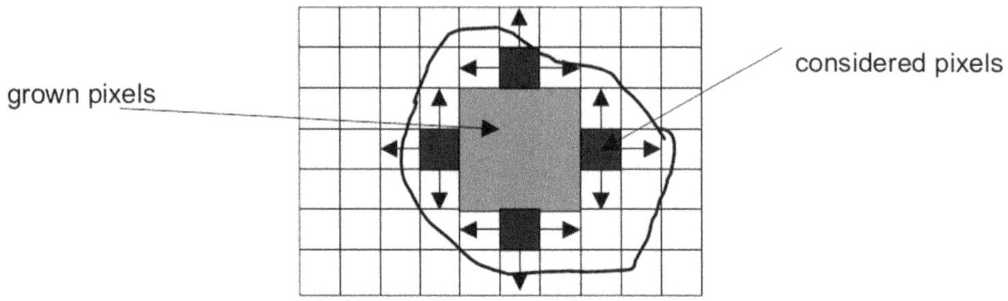

A CT tomographic sequence of 8-bit grey scale images of a size 512x512 in which we change the shape and the orientation of the objects was used. Figure 8 illustrates the 2D visual results from the segmentation method and Figure 9 the 3D visualisation of the segmentation method.

CONCLUSION

Segmentation is a powerful procedure where important information based on the shape structure of the organs could be extracted for the benefit of the patients due to the clinical diagnosis. Many times the structure of the particular organ that doctors are interested in analysing has a complicated shape that

Figure 8. Visual results for 2D bronchus segmentation at different slices: from left to right: slices 40, 45, 50, 55

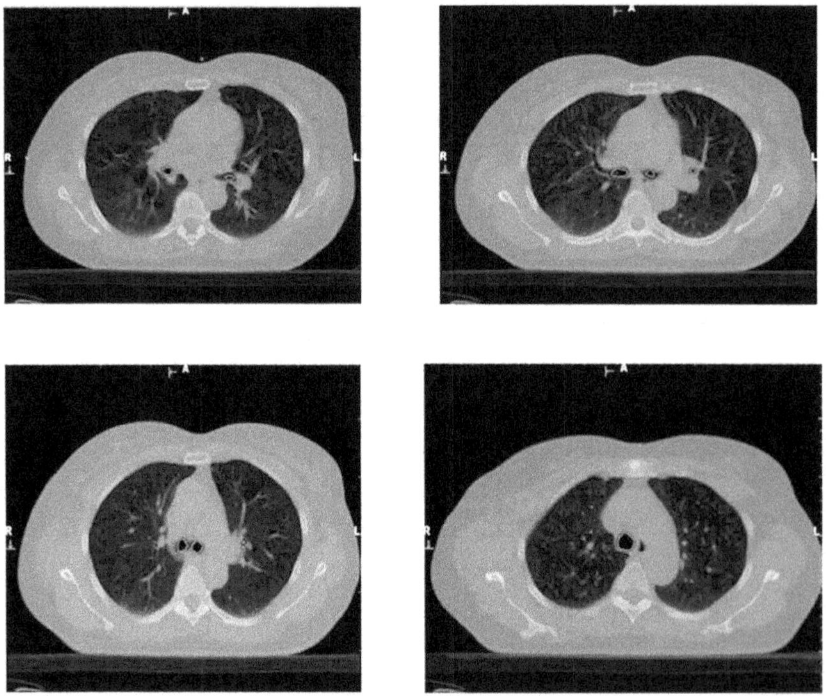

Figure 9. Visual results for 3D bronchus segmentation

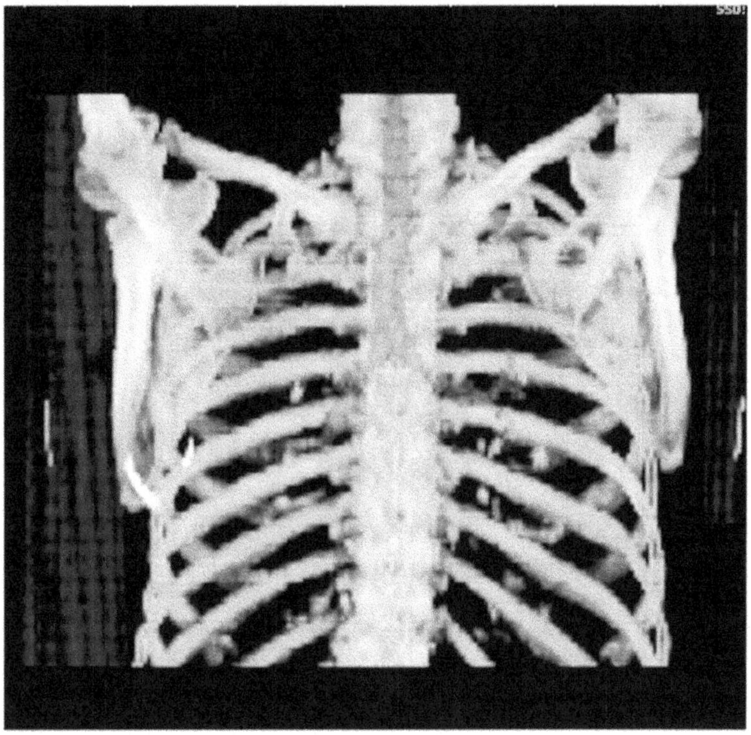

the process can be difficult. In the case of the bronchus where the organ structure is split into two parts, the proposed algorithm for the organ segmentation involves combination between tracking techniques like boundary tracking and region growing process. The algorithm is easy to implement, quick in time, especially in real- time procedures and effective for the organ reconstruction. Due to the contours gaps between different slices, two methods are proposed: the simplest linear interpolation and the B-splines interpolation.

ACKNOWLEDGMENT

The author would like to thank MedCom Company and Städtisches Klinikum Offenbach, who provided the equipment and medical data sets for the implementation of the above work. The author was supported by a Marie Curie Industry Host Fellowship Grant no: HPMI-CT-1999-00005.

REFERENCES

Adams, R., & Bischof, L. (1994). Seeded region growing. *IEEE Transaction on Pattern Analysis and Machine Learning*, *16*(6), 641–647. doi:10.1109/34.295913

Blake, A., & Isard, M. (1998). *Active contours: The application of techniques from graphics vision, control theory and statistics to visual tracking of shapes in motion*. London: Springer-Verlag. doi:10.1007/978-1-4471-1555-7

Chalana, V., & Kim, Y. (1997). A methodology for evaluation of boundary detection algorithms on medical images. *IEEE Transactions on Medical Imaging*, *16*(5), 642–652. doi:10.1109/42.640755 PMID:9368120

Cohen, E., Riesenfeld, R. F., & Elber, G. (2010). *Geometric modeling with splines: An introduction*. A.K. Peters Ltd.

Eviatar, H., & Somorjai, R. L. (1996). A fast, simple active contour algorithm for biomedical images. *Pattern Recognition Letters*, *17*(9), 969–974. doi:10.1016/0167-8655(96)00054-2

Gonzales, R. C., & Woods, R. E. (1992). *Digital Image Processing*. Addison-Wisley.

Großkopf, S., Park, S. Y., & Kim, M. H. (1998). An improved Active Contour Model for Segmentation of Medical Images. *Proc.3rd Korea-Germany Joint Conference on Advanced Medical Image Processing*.

Haralick, R. M., & Shapiro, L. G. (1985). Image segmentation techniques. *Computer Vision Graphics and Image Processing*, *29*(1), 100–132. doi:10.1016/S0734-189X(85)90153-7

Iseki, F., Kobatake, H., Omatsu, H., & Kakinuma, R. (1997). A new method to extract three dimensional tree structures of bronchus from chest CT images. *IEICE D-II*, J80-D-II, 10, 2841–2847. (in Japanese)

Iseki, F., & Baigalmaa, T. (1998). Extraction of 3D tree structure of blood vessels in lungs area from chest CT images. CARS 1998. Elsevier Science B.V.

Karangelis, G. (2004). *3D simulation of external beam radiotherapy*. (Ph.D. thesis). University of Darmstadt, Darmstadt, Germany.

Karangelis, G., & Zimeras, S. (2002). An Accurate 3D Segmentation Method of the Spinal Canal Applied on CT Images. BVM 2002, Confedrence Proceedings, Bildverarbeitung für die Medizin 2002. Springer-Verlag.

Karangelis, G., and Zimeras, S. (2002). 3D segmentation method of the spinal cord applied on CT data. *Computer Graphics Topics, 14,* 28-29.

Kass, M., Witkin, A., & Terzopoulos, D. (1987). Snakes: Active contour models. *International Journal of Computer Vision*, *1*(4), 321–331. doi:10.1007/BF00133570

Malik, J., Belongie, S., Leung, T., & Shi, J. (2001). Contour and texture analysis for image segmentation. *International Journal of Computer Vision*, *43*(1), 7–27. doi:10.1023/A:1011174803800

Mori, K., Hasegawa, J., Toriwaki, J., Anno, H., & Katada, K. (1995). Automated extraction and visualization of bronchus from 3D CT images of lung. *Proc. of 1st International Conference on Computer Vision, Virtual Reality and Robotics in Medicine (CVRMed'95)*. doi:10.1007/978-3-540-49197-2_71

Nagel, R. N., & Rosenfield, A. (1972). Ordered search techniques in template matching. *Proceedings of the IEEE*, *60*(2), 242–244. doi:10.1109/PROC.1972.8611

Netter, F. H. (1997). Atlas of human anatomy. In NOVARTIS (2nd ed.). PLATE.

Pal, N. R., & Pal, S. K. (1993). A review on image segmentation techniques. *Patt. Rec.*, *26*(9), 1277–1294. doi:10.1016/0031-3203(93)90135-J

Punam, T. (2011). A Study of Image Segmentation and Edge Detection Techniques. *International Journal on Computer Science and Engineering*, *3*(2), 899–904.

Rodenwaldt, J., Kopka, L., Roedel, R., Margas, A., & Grabbe, E. (1997). 3D Virtual Endoscopy of the Upper Airways: Optimization of the Scan Parameters in a Cadaver Phantom and Clinical Assessment. *Journal of Computer Assisted Tomography*, *21*(3), 405–411. doi:10.1097/00004728-199705000-00013 PMID:9135649

Schlathoelter, T., Lorenz, C., Carlsen, I. C., Renisch, S., & Deschamps, T. (2002) Simultaneous segmentation and tree reconstruction of the airways for virtual bronchoscopy. *Proc. of SPIE on Medical Imaging 2002*, *4684*, 103–113. doi:10.1117/12.467061

Sonka, M., Park, W., & Hoffman, E. A. (1996). Rule-based detection of intrathoracic airway trees. *IEEE Transactions on Medical Imaging*, *15*(3), 314–326. doi:10.1109/42.500140 PMID:18215912

Summers, R., Feng, D., Holland, S., Sneller, M., & Shelhamer, J. (1996). Virtual Bronchoscopy: Segmentation Method for Real-Time Display. *Radiology*, *200*(3), 857–862. doi:10.1148/radiology.200.3.8756944 PMID:8756944

Terzopoulos, D., & Metaxas, D. (1987). Dynamic 3D models with local and global deformations: Deformable superquadrics. *IEEE Trans. Pattern Anal. Mach. Int.*, *13*(7), 703–714. doi:10.1109/34.85659

Terzopoulos, D., & Metaxas, D. (1991). Dynamic 3D models with local and global deformations: Deformable superquadrics. *IEEE Transactions on Pattern Analysis and Machine Intelligence*, *13*(7), 703–714. doi:10.1109/34.85659

Tsui, Y. L., & Heng, P. A. (2000). Automated extraction of bronchus from 3D CT images of lung based on generic algorithm and 3D region growing. *Proc. of SPIE on Medical Imaging 2000*, *3979*, 906–916.

Vining, D., Shifrin, R., Haponik, E., Liu, K., & Choplin, R. (1994). Virtual Bronchoscopy (abstract). Radiology, 193, 261.

Zimeras, S. (2012). An efficient 3D segmentation method for spinal canal applied to CT volume sequence data. *International Journal of Reliable and Quality E-Healthcare*, *1*(1), 33–42.

Zimeras, S., Karangelis, G., & Firle, E. (2002). Object segmentation and shape reconstruction using computer-assisted segmentation tools. *Medical Imaging*.

KEY TERMS AND DEFINITIONS

Image Segemntation: Image segmentation is the process of splitting a digital image into one or more regions of interest based on their organ structure.

Segmentation: A powerful tool, which gives the opportunity to split the image into parts based on the importance of the regions.

Chapter 10
Migrating from ISO/IEC 9126 to SQUARE:
A Case Study on the Evaluation of Medical Speech Translation Systems

Paula Estrella
Universidad Nacional de Córdoba, Argentina

Nikos Tsourakis
University of Geneva, Switzerland

ABSTRACT

When it comes to the evaluation of natural language systems, it is well acknowledged that there is a lack of common evaluation methodologies, making the fair comparison of such systems a difficult task. Many attempts to standardize this process have used a quality model based on the ISO/IEC 9126 standards. The authors have also used these standards for the definition of a weighted quality model for the evaluation of a medical speech translator, showing the relative importance of the system's features depending on the potential user (patient or doctor, developer). More recently, ISO/IEC 9126 has been replaced by a new series of standards, the 25000 or SQuaRE series, indicating that the model should be migrated to the new series in order to maintain compliance adherence to current standards. This chapter demonstrates how to migrate from ISO/IEC 9126 to ISO 25000 by using the authors' previous work as a use case.

INTRODUCTION

Normalizing evaluations for specific contexts of use have gained increasing importance as software systems become widespread among global organizations and professionals. In particular, Natural Language Processing systems (NLP) are varied in nature and purpose, ranging from low-level applications intended to be used by developers (such as part-of-speech taggers, syntactic parsers or morphological analyzers) to complex systems targeting human end-users (such as voice-commanded booking systems (Jiao et al., 2015) or eye-commanded interfaces (Soltani et al., 2016). During the development lifecycle,

DOI: 10.4018/978-1-5225-1724-5.ch010

these systems are periodically evaluated in order to assess the level of improvement achieved, to detect, classify and recover errors or to quantify user acceptability and satisfaction. While, in the last decades numerous authors have provided evaluation results leveraging various computer and human centered metrics, it is well acknowledged that there is a lack of a methodology that would provide a fair comparison framework for different NLP systems.

Convinced that user needs and the specific context of use of NLP systems cannot be omitted in an evaluation, several initiatives emerged which decompose quality into several dimensions. The International Standards for Language Engineering (Calzolari et al., 2002) project was one of these initiatives, which aims at standardizing the evaluation of language engineering systems by relating a customized quality model based on the ISO standards 9126 (ISO/IEC, 2001) to the purpose and context of use of the system based on the ISO standard 14598 (ISO/IEC, 1999). According to these standards, software quality results in general from six categories of quality characteristics (namely functionality, reliability, usability, efficiency, maintainability and portability) that can be particularized to a given software domain and context of use; in that case such a hierarchy is called a quality model and its terminal nodes must be features of the software that can be measured using one or more metrics. Additionally, ISO proposes models to evaluate internal or external quality as well as quality in use.

These standards have been recently replaced by the new 25000 series (ISO, 2014), named SQuaRE, implying that quality models based on the 9126 standard are outdated and should be migrated to the new series. This chapter builds on previous work, where the authors applied the 9126 series to the evaluation of NLP systems in the specific area of medical speech translation systems from the perspective of doctors, patients and developers (Tsourakis & Estrella, 2013). The objective of this chapter is to propose a mapping from a previous weighted quality model to a new weighted quality model based on SQuaRE in order to reuse as much as possible from the previous evaluations, given the complex and laborious work that entails the application of international standards.

BACKGROUND

Quality Models

As quality is hard to assess and assure, several models try to address software quality issues by employing a set of quality attributes, characteristics and metrics. The Factors-Criteria-Metrics (FCM) model was one of the first proposals, extensively used in large projects in the military, space, and public domain (McCall et al., 1977). The model is described in three parts: the first part presents the quality model itself, the second part is devoted to metrics and the third part describes the evaluation process for managers. The FCM model seems more suitable to be applied at later stages of software development cycle, when at least a prototype exists. A similar model was proposed by Boehm et al. (1978), which had a four levels centered on general utility but, despite the terminology, this model is quite similar to the FCM model in structure and characteristics included. Later, the FURPS model, named after the first letters of its top-level quality characteristics, functionality, usability, reliability, performance and supportability, was developed viewing quality as the conformance of a software product to user requirements and to other requirements indirectly obtained, for example from contracts, standards, etc. (Grady, 1992). A more recent proposal took as its starting point the draft version of the ISO/IEC 9126 standard, from which a subset of top-level characteristics was retained, namely reliability, functionality, maintainability, efficiency, portability and usability (Dromey, 1995).

The proposals presented above do not represent consensus from the software engineering community: for example, each author adopts a particular terminology for the same entities or uses different definitions for the software quality. These proposals are useful to integrate quality assurance into the process of systems development but they seem difficult to compare in order to choose one quality model for the evaluation of a particular product. As stated in (ISO/IEC, 2001, p. 23), it is for this reason that the ISO/IEC began to develop the required consensus and encourage standardization world-wide.

The standard ISO/IEC 9126 defines a quality model for software products divided in two parts: the first part can be used to perform internal or external evaluation, depending on the interpretation given by the evaluator, and the second part defines a model for quality in use, necessary to determine whether the product fulfills the user's needs. The three views of quality (internal, external and in use) allow this model to be applied at different stages of the software development life cycle and they could be connected to predict quality as follows: a high level of internal quality achieved during the implementation of the software could contribute to a high level of external quality built in the final product and this, in turn, could result in acceptable quality in use levels. The quality model is shown in Figure 1.

The guidelines for the evaluation process are defined in a separate series of standards, the ISO/IEC 14598, which contains guidelines and examples to support different stakeholders during the evaluation process. When this series of standards is used in conjunction with the ISO/IEC 9126, they provide different views of the software quality depending on the role of the person designing the evaluation;

Figure 1. Quality model decomposition in ISO/IEC 9126

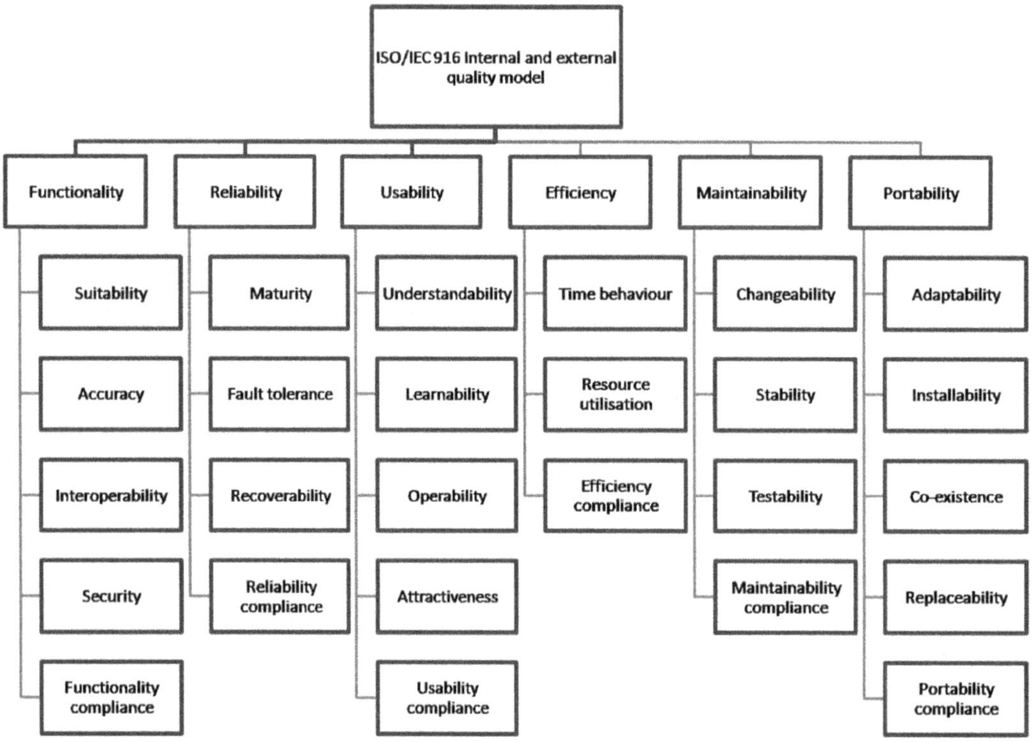

Figure 2. Organization of the SQuaRE series

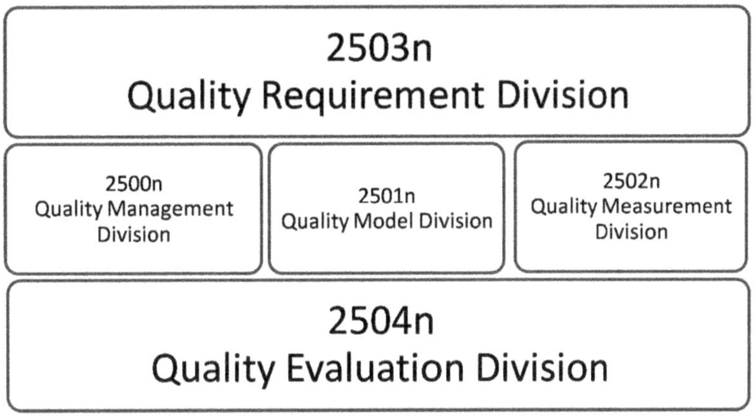

stakeholders can be users, developers, acquirers and evaluators. In 2003 a standard for internal metrics and another for external metrics were published and in 2004 a standard for quality in use metrics was published. These standards complement the ISO/IEC 9126 quality model, given that they contain examples and guidelines about applying these types of metrics. However, some inconsistencies between these series were identified during their use in practice, which motivated the creation of a unified series called Software Quality Requirements and Evaluation, SQuaRE (ISO, 2014). The main goal of SQuaRE is "to move to a logically organized, enriched and unified series covering two main processes: software quality requirement specification and software quality evaluation, supported by a software quality measurement process" (ISO, 2014, p. 5). This series is organized as shown in Figure 2 and the detailed quality model is shown in Figure 3.

As shown in Figure 3 the SQuaRE model has two more high-level characteristics than his predecessor, twelve new sub-characteristics and the rest are inherited and transformed either by renaming them to better reflect its meaning or by moving them to another level or characteristic. In particular, characteristics in group:

1. Are new, those in group
2. Have only suffered a name change and those in group
3. Have been moved to another level or branch of the hierarchy, the rest of them are inherited and remain unchanged from 9126.

Application of ISO-Based Quality Models

As the quality models defined by ISO are general, they can be applied to any software product. For example, the model in ISO/IEC 9126 (ISO/IEC, 2001) has been adapted and applied for the evaluation of systems for Business-to-Business (B2B) (Behkamal et al., 2009), platforms for blended learning (Padayachee et al., 2010; Chua and Dyson, 2004), mobile learning (Gafni, 2009), software for telecommunications (Suryn & Laverdière, 2007) and electronic commerce systems (Stefani & Xenos, 2008), among others. In the area of NLP systems, work by the ISLE group firstly produced the EAGLES 7-step recipe (EAGLES, 1999) applicable to any NLP software product, and later produced the Framework for

Figure 3. Quality model decomposition in the SQuaRE series

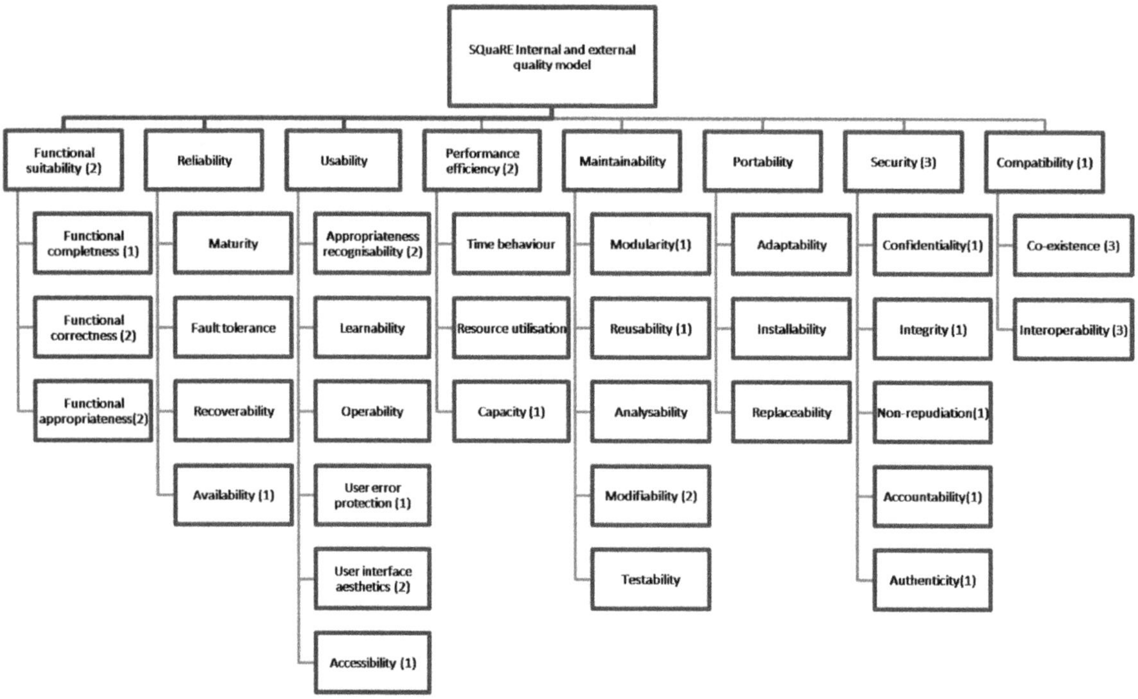

Machine Translation Evaluation in ISLE (FEMTI), which is a quality model customized for machine translation systems based on ISO/IEC 9125 with a dynamic mechanism to relate relevant quality characteristics depending on the context (Estrella et al., 2010). Other applications include customizing the 9126 model for a translation service provider, based on the premise that different types of customers have different needs (Stadler &Peter-Spörndli, 2007); applying it in the evaluation of NLP components to continuously monitor and disseminate information in almost real-time (Blench, 2008); creating an ontology to classify non-functional requirements (Rashwan et al., 2013).

While the 9126 model is the most used ISO model, the SQuaRE model has started to be adopted in a variety of situations. For example in the framework of e-government portals many quality models have been proposed but only a few are based on SQuaRE as discussed in (Fath-Allah et al., 2014); other examples are found in the process of monitoring software aging (Bombardieri et al., 2008), in the evaluation of web services quality and in Abramowicz et al. (2008), and in the evaluation of ontologies as a guide for users making informed decisions on which ontology to use under given circumstances (Duque-Ramos et al., 2011). A model applied in a closer setting to this chapter's is presented in Antonino et al. (2011), where a model is proposed for the selection of ambient assisted living platforms.

Previous work on applying ISO-based models to the evaluation of medical speech translation systems used the 9126 standard (Tsourakis & Estrella, 2013) and this chapter intends to explore how much of that laborious work can be reused and how can that previous experience be exploited to perform a new evaluation with a SQuaRE-based model. Even if special quality standards for medical devices have already been published (ISO, 2003), the authors consider this particular medical speech translator a software system instead of a medical device, therefore this work is based on the ISO/IEC series of standards. The next section details previous work, and later, a mapping from ISO/IEC 9126 to SQuaRE is proposed.

QUALITY MODEL FOR MEDICAL SPEECH TRANSLATION SYSTEMS

Medical speech-to-speech translation represents an intriguing research area as language barriers can become life-threatening when health issues come into place. For this reason professional interpreters are recruited for ensuring accurate clinical communication with foreign language-speaking patients. While interpreters are the preferred strategy they are not always available, and recent studies have shown that Google Translate (GT) is starting to be used in hospitals (Chang et al., 2014).The obvious drawback of this approach is that a system like GT can be seriously unreliable on medical language and a recent study from Patil et al. (2014) has shown that the results of GT in this domain were incorrect more than one time in three. Different researchers have also tried to create systems specialized for this area e.g. Rayner et al. (2016) and Bouillon et al. (2007).

In this respect we consider quality assurance in this domain of utmost importance and this is the reason why we decided to focus on a quality model for medical speech translation systems. Given that the target system is to be used for the communication between patients and doctors in a hospital's emergency room, the following issues were taken into account to start building the model:

1. **Quality of Translation:** The genre of the task requires safe critical high quality translation.
2. **Heterogeneous Interaction:** Users may interact with different personnel or in diverse environments.
3. **Mobility:** Interaction happens with a mobile device, which by itself involves special consideration.
4. **User Physical Constrains:** Patients' physical disabilities can pose hurdles to the efficient usage of the system.
5. **Wireless Interconnection:** The network can cause delays or even connection failures.
6. **Application Availability:** It could be preinstalled on a hospital's device or users could install it on their devices.

The entire process of evaluation design and execution consisted of three stages:

1. **Development of the Model:** Initially a tree-like hierarchy of quality characteristics was defined, either by selecting them among those proposed in ISO/IEC-9126 or by introducing new ones. In ISO terminology, the quality characteristics of a model represent the desired features of a system and are also called attributes if these are the end-nodes of the hierarchy. These characteristics were then divided into the ones that describe the external view of the software and the ones that focus on its internal aspects; each of them can be further decomposed into sub-characteristics and the end-nodes of the hierarchy must be measurable attributes of the system.
2. **Definition of the Weighting Scheme:** It is important to determine which of the quality characteristics are more important depending on the consumer of the system, therefore patients, doctors and developers were asked to assign weights of relative importance between the characteristics of the model.
3. **Weights Collection:** In the third phase different stakeholders were polled to gather the relative weights; so, for the external quality model there were two target groups of users that demonstrate different needs and goals towards the system, namely 12 doctors and 12 potential patients, and for the internal characteristics, which mainly represent a technical viewpoint, 6 developers were polled in a similar way as for the end-users.

These stages are briefly described in the following subsections, for a complete description refer to Tsourakis & Estrella (2013).

Quality Model

According to ISO/IEC 9126, when instantiating the model, both ISO characteristics and sub-characteristics can be used or a new customized hierarchy of quality attributes can be proposed, along with a mapping to the ISO hierarchy to make the resulting model ISO-compliant. To create a customized model, the attributes offered by ISO/IEC were augmented with the ones needed for the medical speech translation domain. Only the new customized definitions are summarized in Table 1, given that all the other quality characteristics were adapted from the ones proposed in ISO/IEC 9126. It is worth noting that the characteristics added are related to the particular functionalities (*Traceability, Exploitability, Controllability*) and usability issues that this kind of software product requires (*Trustability, Customizability, Privacy*).

Relative Importance of Attributes / Weight Definition

The previous section presented the quality model decomposed into quality characteristics and sub-characteristics, which were deemed pertinent for ISO-based evaluation of mobile speech translators. However, no insight was provided concerning the relative importance of each quality characteristic in the model. This relation is clearly dependent on the user and, as expected, user's perception about product quality varies across user types. For example, end-users typically value usability more than developers do. These preferences or perceptions can be incorporated in the quality model in the form of weights that will represent the relative importance of each characteristic and will allow its ranking (by importance given a specific user and context of use), helping evaluators select a subset of the most important characteristics to evaluate. In order to collect these weights a group of potential users was polled, in particular professional doctors and non-doctors (representing potential patients) were included. The analysis of their answers was based on the Analytical Hierarchy Process (AHP) (Saaty, 1994), which

Table 1. Customized quality characteristics included in the model for medical speech translation systems

Functionality
Traceability: User's activity along the pathway should be traced by the system and may be used to identify possible problems (e.g. delays), perform correct pricing of praxes, etc. *Exploitability*: Users may be forced to wait their turn for an examination or wait between examinations. This idle time can be used for familiarizing with the application, and thus fostering user's trust towards the system. *Controllability*: The system should determine the most efficient way of interaction, e.g. if the doctor gives instructions he should also be control of the dialog flow but during diagnosis the weight of control should be equilibrated between the two parties. This also conforms to current clinical theory of patient-centered medicine (Stewart et al., 2003).
Usability
Trustability: The system should offer results that are predictable and do not engender any surprise to end-users, so that patients establish trustful relations towards the system that works as a mediator for human-to-human interaction. *Customizability*: As users may vary in a range of literate to complete illiterate, the system should take this into account as well as other special needs (weak sight, hearing problems, etc.). It can therefore present the output in different ways, for example with images or voice instead of text. *Privacy*: The system should contemplate issues of privacy, e.g. patients can be reluctant to talk in front of other, even in front of relatives, be embarrassed when using the system unsuccessfully, etc.

models a problem in a hierarchical structure, where each level represents the relationship between the overall goal (level 1), criteria (level 2), sub-criteria and alternatives (level 3). Accordingly, we shape the ISO model in three levels, where the goal (first level) is to evaluate a mobile speech translator; the top-level quality characteristics of the ISO model constitute the second level (e.g. functionality) and the sub-characteristics the third one (e.g. suitability). The result of applying the AHP methodology to the questionnaires gathered is a weighted quality model, i.e. an ISO-compliant model augmented with preference judgments.

Methodology Used to Poll Subjects

As briefly described before, each participant was asked to fill in a questionnaire consisting of pair-wise comparisons of the characteristics in the model. By the juxtaposition of statements for each sub-characteristic they were asked to express their opinion by choosing a number in a scale of 1-9 favoring the feature they liked most. For each pair in the questionnaire, they had to answer to which statement they agreed the most and how strongly. An example is shown in Figure 4 where the left statement corresponds to *Learnability* and the right one to *Attractiveness*. Note that the focus of the statement was underlined in each case and the comparisons were limited to attributes under the same quality characteristic.

For completeness, developers were asked to quantify the relative importance of some internal characteristics using a survey similar to that sent to end-users; they were asked to evaluate *Maintainability* that was not included in the previous analysis, and also *Efficiency* and *Portability*.

Results for Internal and External Characteristics

In order to collect the weights as explained in the previous section, a number of subjects were asked to fill in a questionnaire consisting of pair-wise comparisons of the characteristics in the model. For the external quality model, it was sent to different doctors and potential patients from which 16 and 20 completed surveys were returned, respectively; for the internal quality model, 9 developers were polled. The resulting weighted models for external and internal quality are depicted in Tables 2 and 3, respectively.

As in every human assessment, coherence and consistency are important to support the reliability of the results; in APH this is calculated with the Consistency Ratio (CR). For the external evaluation participants with the highest CR (outliers) were eliminated, so the overall CR dropped to an acceptable 10% (approximately). Hence, the weights presented in Table 2 were obtained from the answers of the 12 most consistent physicians and of the 12 most consistent patients. Similarly, for the internal evaluation the 6 most consistent developers according to their CR were retained. However, in the internal

Figure 4. Example of pair-wise comparison of attributes: Learnability vs. attractiveness

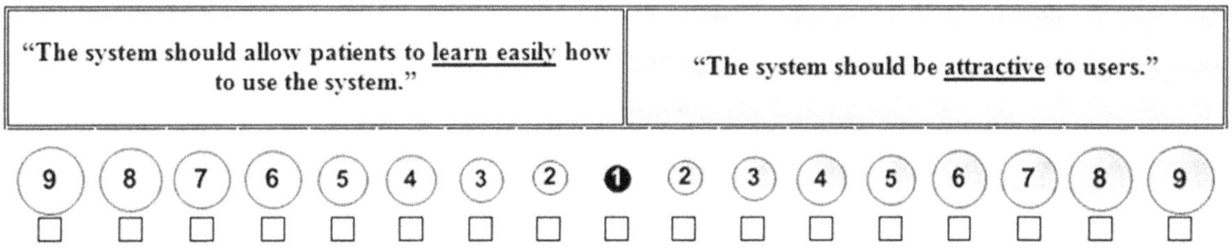

Table 2. Weighted quality model for external characteristics

Quality Factor	Weight % Doctors	Weight % Patients	Quality Sub-Factor	Weight % Doctors	Weight % Patients
Functionality	38.53	10.88	Suitability Accuracy Interoperability Security Traceability Exploitability Controllability	18.18 26.29 10.38 22.27 9.26 5.40 8.22	12.28 39.17 13.37 17.01 8.61 4.26 5.30
Reliability	18.04	13.47	Maturity Fault tolerance Recoverability	55.80 38.50 5.70	48.70 6.20 45.10
Usability	17.47	9.53	Understandability Learnability Operability Attractiveness Uniformability Trustability Customizability Privacy	4.31 10.24 15.83 2.37 9.43 11.87 23.32 22.63	7.63 9.61 17.42 3.30 3.97 19.91 23.26 14.90
Efficiency	5.64	30.32	Time behavior Resource utilization	78.38 21.62	69.70 30.30
Portability	6.40	15.74	Adaptability Installability Co-existence Replaceability	22.14 14.31 40.08 23.47	18.95 15.54 26.65 38.86
Compliance	13.92	20.06			

Table 3. Weighted quality model for internal characteristics

Quality Factor	Quality Sub-Factor	Weight %
Efficiency	Time behavior Resource utilization	82.35 17.65
Maintainability	Analyzability Changeability Stability Testability	20.30 10.03 58.95 10.72
Portability	Adaptability Installability Co-existence Replaceability	28.11 11.27 50.40 10.22

evaluation more inconsistencies among subjects were found and the authors speculate that it might stem from the use of scale with many points (as shown in Figure 4 it had 9 points), so one future venue for the present work is to re-run the internal evaluation both to apply the new SQuaRE-based model and to obtain more reliable results.

The following sections address the issues of adapting this 9126 weighted model for external quality and of generating the weights for the SQuaRE-based model.

SOLUTIONS AND RECOMMENDATIONS: MIGRATING FROM 9126 TO SQUARE

In order to upgrade the quality model to the new series the authors proceeded in two steps: by firstly mapping characteristics form the old to the new model and, secondly, by defining a set of rules to re-use and distribute the weights. These steps are described in the following subsections.

Mapping the Characteristics to SQuaRE

For the first step, the authors identified the quality characteristics in the new model that correspond to each characteristic in our 9126-based model; this step was supported by the ISO standards, given that SQuaRE devotes a section to explain the changes from one model to the new one, and therefore, it was only needed to map the customized characteristics (those not part of the ISO standard). As described in the previous section the added characteristics pertain to *Functionality* (*Traceability*, *Exploitability, Controllability)* and to *Usability* (*Trustability*, *Customizability, Privacy)*. From these characteristics, only three of them could be mapped to SQuaRE as their definition was very close; the mapping was made in the following way: *Functionality → Traceability* was mapped to *Security → Accountability; Usability → Trustability* was mapped to *Usability → User error protection*; *Usability → Customizability* was mapped to *Usability → Accessibility*. The remaining characteristics were placed under *Functional suitability* and *Usability*, as these are the equivalent characteristics under which they were in ISO/IEC 9126. The mapped characteristics along with the ISO and customized definitions are summarized in Table 4 while the complete list of characteristics with their definitions is provided in the appendix.

Reusing the Weights

As shown in Figure 3, the quality characteristics in SQuaRE have suffered a number of changes and consequently, the weights they previously had will also need alterations that reflect their new relative weight more accurately. Intuitively, the idea is to "move the characteristics around" as stated by SQuaRE and let them "carry their weight" to their new position. In order to implement this intuition, four types of transformations were identified (Categories 1 to 4) and each one of the characteristics was grouped

Table 4. Customized quality characteristics mapped to SQuaRE

Customized Definition	SQuaRE Definition
Functionality – Traceability: User's activity along the pathway should be traced by the system and may be used to identify possible problems (e.g. delays), perform correct pricing of praxes, etc.	*Security – Accountability*: Degree to which the actions of an entity can be traced uniquely to the entity.
Usability – Trustability: The system should offer results that are predictable and do not engender any surprise to end-users, so that patients establish trustful relations towards the system that works as a mediator for human-to-human interaction.	*Usability – User error protection:* Degree to which a system protects users against making errors.
Usability – Customizability: As users may vary in a range of literate to complete illiterate, the system should take this into account as well as other special needs (weak sight, hearing problems, etc.). It can therefore present the output in different ways, for example with images or voice instead of text.	*Usability – Accessibility*: Degree to which a product or system can be used by people with the widest range of characteristics and capabilities to achieve a specified goal in a specified context of use.

under one of these categories depending on the transformation it went through form 9126 to SQuaRE. Examples of characteristics in each category are presented in Table 5. Additionally, these transformations are treated separately if the characteristic is a top-level one or a sub-characteristic. The weights in each category are adapted as follows:

Category A: The same characteristic is present in both models in the same position of the hierarchy. In this case there are no changes on the weight. For example, *Functionality* suffers a name change becoming *Functional suitability* but remains a top-level characteristic, so its weight is the same:

$$Weight_{Functional\ suitability} = Weight_{Functionality} = 38.53\%,$$

which corresponds to the weight presented in Table 2.

Category B: A sub-characteristic in the old model becomes a characteristic in the new one, that is, it moved up in the ISO hierarchy. In this case its weight should be proportional to the one it had in the old model; in other words its contribution to the higher-level characteristic will be calculated and that mass will be deducted from that characteristic. For example *Functionality→Security* becomes a top-level characteristic and therefore using the weights presented in Table 2, we can calculate its new weight as follows: $Weight_{Functionality} * Weight_{Security} = 38.53*22.27 = 8.5\%$; then this amount is subtracted from the weight of *Functional suitability:*

$$Weight_{Functional\ suitability} = Weight_{Functionality} - Weight_{Functionality} * Weight_{Security} = 29.95\%$$

Category C: A characteristic is discarded, so it is not present in the new model. In this case its weight is distributed proportionally among the other characteristics. *Compliance* is an example of this category, which had a weight of *13.92%* according to Table 2. This is equally distributed among the top-level characteristics of the SQuaRE model, for example *Functional suitability* was modified before to deduct the weight of *Security* and now its weight should be augmented with the proportion of *Compliance* in this manner:

Table 5. Categorization of all top-level characteristics

ISO 9526	SQuaRE	Category
Functionality	Functional suitability	A
Efficiency	Performance efficiency	A
Usability	Usability	A
Reliability	Reliability	A
Portability	Portability	A
Compliance		C
	Compatibility	D
	Security	B

$$Weight_{Functional\ suitability} = Weight_{Functionality} - Weight_{Functionality} * Weight_{Security} + 1/7*Weight_{Compliance} = 31.94\%$$

Category D: a new characteristic is introduced with sub-characteristics obtained from the old one. In this case its weight is determined by the proportional weights of these sub-characteristics. For example, *Compatibility* contains *Portability→Co-existence* and *Functionality→Interoperability* and its weight is:

$$Weight_{Compatibility} = Weight_{Portability} * Weight_{Co\text{-}existence} + Weight_{Functionality} * Weight_{Interoperability} + 1/7*Weight_{Compliance} = 8.55\%.$$

Following the specific methodology, the final calculation for the weight of *Functional suitability* becomes*:*

$$Weight_{Functional\ suitability} = Weight_{Functionality} - Weight_{Functionality} * Weight_{Security} - Weight_{Functionality} * Weight_{Interoperability} - Weight_{Functionality} * Weight_{Traceability} + 1/7*Weight_{Compliance} = 24.37\%.$$

New Weights for the Sub-Characteristics

This section shows how the reassignment of weights took place for the sub-characteristics. To redistribute the weights among sub-characteristics, a set of rules were defined in order to obtain the final new weight for each characteristic in the new model. The following rules were applied sequentially in descending priority order:

Rule 1: If a sub-characteristic remained in its initial position, keep its weight. Example: *Functionality→Accuracy* renamed to *Functional suitability→Functional correctness.*

Rule 2: If a new sub-characteristic was introduced, assign an initial weight equal to zero. Example: *Performance efficiency→Capacity.*

Rule 3: If a characteristic contains previously compared sub-characteristics, assign them weights according to their previous proportional weights. Example: *Compatibilty→Co-existance, Interoperability.*

Rule 4: If a characteristic does not contain previously compared sub-characteristics, assign them equal weights. Example: *Security→Confidentiality, Integrity, Non-repudiation, Accountability, Authenticity.*

Rule 5: If a sub-characteristic was removed from its initial position, redistribute its weight to the remaining ones. Example: *Functionality→Interoperability* redistributed to *Functional suitability→ Functional completeness, Functional correctness, Functional appropriateness, Exploitability, Controllability.*

Rule 6: If a characteristic was removed from the new model, redistribute its weight to each one of the sub-characteristic. Example: 1/7 of *Compliance* was added to all sub-characteristics.

After applying the two-step methodology described in this section, which proposes the mapping of quality characteristics form ISO/IEC 9126 to SQuaRE and the recalculation of weights guided by the above-mentioned rules, the result is a migrated (upgraded) weighted quality model. For the particular use case of the medical speech translation system, the resulting weighted model is presented in Table 6.

FUTURE RESEARCH DIRECTIONS

It has already been suggested that one natural continuation of this work, is to apply the new model to an internal evaluation, given that the results obtained in the past have evidenced a number of issues regarding the consistency of the evaluators. Other venues for future research include the application of specific user-centric metrics for each quality characteristic in the model and the definition of an aggregation criterion to obtain global scores of a system's quality. A particularly interesting topic would be to integrate additional sources of data that could provide more insights into the evaluators' perception of a system's quality; for example, one could think of integrating wearable devices in usability evaluations, such as sensors or eye-tracking devices combined with key-logging.

Table 6. Upgraded weighted quality model for medical speech translation systems

Quality Factor	Weight % Doctors	Weight % Patients	Quality Sub-Factor	Weight % Doctors	Weight % Patients
Functional suitability	24.37	9.5	Functional completeness	9.43	9.33
			Functional correctness	33.35	43.59
			Functional appropriateness	25.97	20.07
			Exploitability	14.34	13.05
			Controllability	16.91	13.96
Performance efficiency	7.63	33.19	Time behavior	75.84	66.82
			Resource utilization	22.28	30.54
			Capacity	1.88	2.64
Compatibility	8.55	8.52	Co-existence	39.49	72.94
			Interoperability	60.51	27.06
Usability	19.46	12.4	Appropriat. recognizability	5.43	8.54
			Learnability	10.55	10.15
			Operability	15.37	16.5
			User error protection	11.96	18.53
			User interface aesthetics	3.76	5.02
			Accessibility	21.83	21.25
			Uniformability	9.85	5.56
			Privacy	21.25	14.45
Reliability	20.03	16.33	Maturity	53.53	46.26
			Availability	1.84	2.57
			Fault tolerance	37.51	8.14
			Recoverability	7.12	43.03
Security	14.14	5.65	Confidentiality	20	20
			Integrity	20	20
			Non-repudiation	20	20
			Accountability	20	20
			Authenticity	20	20
Portability	5.82	14.41	Adaptability	35.38	28.27
			Installability	27.99	25.13
			Replaceability	36.63	46.6

CONCLUSION

This chapter focuses on the evaluation of complex systems that are to be used in critical situations, such as in the communication of patients and doctors. The main problem that developers face when evaluating such systems is that there is a lack of standardized methodology that would provide a fair comparison framework for different systems. A first approach to overcome this problem was the use of international standards developed by ISO, namely ISO/IEC 9126 and ISO/IEC 14598, which when used together provide a view of quality from a particular stakeholder perspective, that is, how an evaluator, a developer or an end-user would perceive the quality of the software product being evaluated. While this was a breakthrough in the quest for a fair evaluation methodology, these standards have been replaced by a new series (ISO 25000 or SQuaRE) rendering obsolete the quality models and evaluations designed if they are based on ISO/IEC 9126. Performing ISO-compliant evaluations benefits from being a standardized methodology but it has the drawback of being a time-consuming and laborious task. Therefore, this chapter proposes a methodology for the migration or upgrade of quality models to the new SQuaRE series. This methodology is presented through the use case: converting a 9126-compliant weighted quality model for medical speech translation systems into a SQuaRE-compliant weighted quality model. Previous work by the authors defined an ISO-compliant quality model for mobile medical speech translation systems by taking as a starting point the quality characteristics defined in the ISO/IEC 9126 standard; the top-level nodes of the hierarchy that defines the model are ISO characteristics while some of the sub-characteristics and attributes are new ones introduced for the specific application domain (called customized quality characteristics). That model was upgraded in this chapter, proceeding in two stages: first, a mapping of quality characteristics has to be done to find out if those custom characteristics can be replaced by ISO characteristics, and second, the weights assigned to each characteristic shall be recomputed to be consistent with the resulting model. The outcome of this process is a weighted quality model compliant with the new ISO standards that preserves most of the work done by the evaluators, saving much time and effort that would have been necessary if building the model from nothing. Finally, this chapter provides a set of general rules that can be followed to repeat the process for any other case, serving as guidelines for other evaluators interested in recycling previous evaluation efforts.

REFERENCES

Abramowicz, W., Hofman, R., Suryn, W., & Zyskowski, D. (2008). SQuaRE based web services quality model. *Proceedings of the International MultiConference of Engineers and Computer Scientists, 2008*, 827–835.

Antonino, P. O., Schneider, D., Hofmann, C., & Nakagawa, E. Y. (2011). Evaluation of AAL platforms according to architecture-based quality attributes. In *Ambient Intelligence* (pp. 264–274). Springer Berlin Heidelberg. doi:10.1007/978-3-642-25167-2_36

Behkamal, B., Kahani, M., & Akbari, M. K. (2009). Customizing ISO 9126 quality model for evaluation of B2B applications. *Journal of Information and Software Technology*, *51*(3), 599–609. doi:10.1016/j.infsof.2008.08.001

Blench, M. (2008). Global public health intelligence network (GPHIN). In *Proceedings of the conference of the American machine translation association (AMTA)*. Waikiki, HI: AMTA.

Boehm, B. W., Brown, J. R., & Kaspar, H. (1978). *Characteristics of software quality*. North Holland.

Bombardieri, M., & Fontana, F. A. (2008, September). A specialisation of the SQuaRE quality model for the evaluation of the software evolution and maintenance activity. In *Automated Software Engineering-Workshops, 2008. ASE Workshops 2008. 23rd IEEE/ACM International Conference on* (pp. 110-113). IEEE. doi:10.1109/ASEW.2008.4686328

Bouillon, P., Flores, G., Starlander, M., Chatzichrisafis, N., Santaholma, M., Tsourakis, N., & Hockey, B. A. et al. (2007). A Bidirectional Grammar-Based Medical Speech Translator.*Workshop on Grammar-Based Approaches to Spoken Language Processing* (pp. 41–48). doi:10.3115/1626333.1626341

Calzolari, N., McNaught, J., Palmer, M., & Zampolli, A. (2002). International Standards for Language Engineering. Final Report.

Chang, D., Thyer, I., Hayne, D., & Katz, D. (2014). Using mobile technology to overcome language barriers in medicine. *Annals of the Royal College of Surgeons of England*, *96*(6), e23–e15. doi:10.1308/003588414X13946184903685 PMID:25198966

Cote, M. A., Syryn, W., Martin, A. R., & Laport, Y. C. (2004). Evolving a Corporate Software Quality Assessment Exercise: A Migration Path to ISO/IEC-9126. *Software Quality Professional*, *6*(3), 1–17.

Dromey, G. R. (1995). A model for software product quality. *Software Engineering. IEEE Transactions on*, *21*(2), 146–162.

Duque-Ramos, A., Fernández-Breis, J. T., Stevens, R., & Aussenac-Gilles, N. (2011). OQuaRE: A SQuaRE-based approach for evaluating the quality of ontologies. *Journal of Research and Practice in Information Technology*, *43*(2), 159.

EAGLES. (1999). *The EAGLES 7-step recipe EAGLES Evaluation Working*. ISSCO, UNIGE. Retrieved May 2016 from http://www.issco.unige.ch/en/research/projects/eagles/ewg99/7steps.html

Estrella, P., Popescu-Belis, A., & King, M. (2010). The FEMTI guidelines for contextual MT evaluation: Principles and resources. *Evaluation of Translation Technology*, *8*, 43.

Fath-Allah, A., Cheikhi, L., Al-Qutaish, R. E., & Idri, A. (2014). A Comparative Analysis of E-Government Quality Models. *International Journal of Social, Behavioral, Educational, Economic Business and Industrial Engineering*, *8*(11), 3526–3530.

Gafni, R. (2009). Quality Metrics for PDA-based M-Learning Information Systems. *Interdisciplinary Journal of E-Learning and Learning Objects*, *5*, 359–287.

Grady, R. B. (1992). *Practical software metrics for project management and process improvement*. Prentice-Hall, Inc.

ISO. (2003). *ISO 13485: Medical devices - Quality management systems - Requirements for regulatory purposes*. Geneva: International Organization for Standardization.

ISO. (2011). *ISO 25000: Systems and software engineering– Systems and software Quality Requirements and Evaluation (SQuaRE)–System and software quality models*. Geneva: International Organization for Standardization.

ISO. (2014). *ISO 25000: Systems and software engineering– Systems and software Quality Requirements and Evaluation (SQuaRE)–Guide to SQuaRE*. Geneva: International Organization for Standardization.

ISO/IEC. (1999). *ISO/IEC 14598-1: Information Technology, Software Product Evaluation*. Geneva: International Organization for Standardization.

ISO/IEC. (2001). *ISO/IEC, 9126: Software engineering–Product quality–Part 1: Quality model*. Geneva: International Organization for Standardization.

Jiao, Z., Wang, Z., Wang, G., Tian, H., Wu, H., & Wang, H. (2015). On the Granularity of Dialog Strategies: Insights from Large-scale Analyses of Two Commercial Travel Information Spoken Dialog Systems. In *AAAI 2015 Spring Symposium*.

McCall, J. A., Richards, P. K., & Walters, G. F. (1977). *Factors in software quality. Concept and definitions of software quality: final technical report*. Springfield: National Technical Information Service (NTIS), Report nr. RADC-TR-77-369 (I, II and III).

Padayachee, I., Kotze, P., & van der Merwe, A. (2010). ISO 9126 external systems quality characteristics, sub-characteristics and domain specific criteria for evaluating e-Learning systems. In *SACLA 2010 Conference*.

Patil, S., & Davies, P. (2014). Use of Google Translate in medical communication: evaluation of accuracy. British Medical Journal,349.

Rashwan, A., Ormandjieva, O., & Witte, R. (2013). Ontology-based classification of non-functional requirements in software specifications: A new corpus and SVM-based classifier. In *Computer Software and Applications Conference (COMPSAC), 2013 IEEE 37th Annual* (pp. 381-386). IEEE. doi:10.1109/COMPSAC.2013.64

Rayner, M., Armando, A., Bouillon, P., Ebling, S., Gerlach, J., Halimi, S., & Tsourakis, N. et al. (2016). Helping domain experts build phrasal speech translation systems. *Lecture Notes in Computer Science*, *9577*, 41–52. doi:10.1007/978-3-319-33500-1_4

Saaty, T. L. (1994). How to make a decision: The Analytic Hierarchy Process. *Interfaces*, *24*(6), 19–43. doi:10.1287/inte.24.6.19

Soltani, S., & Mahnam, A. (2016). A practical efficient human computer interface based on saccadic eye movements for people with disabilities. *Computers in Biology and Medicine*, *70*, 163–173. doi:10.1016/j.compbiomed.2016.01.012 PMID:26848728

Stadler, H. U., & Peter-Spörndli, U. (2007). The quest for machine translation quality at CLS Communication. *MT Summit XI*, 435-442.

Stefani, A., & Xenos, M. (2008). E-commerce system quality assessment using a model based on ISO 9126 and Belief Networks. *Software Quality Journal*, *16*(1), 107–129. doi:10.1007/s11219-007-9032-5

Stewart, M., Brown, J. B., Weston, W. W., McWhinney, I. R., McWilliam, C. L., & Freeman, T. R. (2003). *Patient-centered Medicine: Transforming the Clinical Method.* Radcliffe Medical Press.

Suryn, W., & Laverdière, F. (2007). The Applicability Analysis of ISO/IEC 9126 Series of Standards in Telecom Sector: The Example of Softswitch Category of Software. *Software Quality Journal, 15*(4), 417–448. doi:10.1007/s11219-007-9024-5

Tsourakis, N., & Estrella, P. (2013). Evaluating the quality of mobile medical speech translators based on ISO/IEC 9126 series: Definition, weighted quality model and metrics. *International Journal of Reliable and Quality E-Healthcare, 2*(2), 1–20. doi:10.4018/ijrqeh.2013040101

KEY TERMS AND DEFINITIONS

External Evaluation: Systematic assessment of a set of quality characteristics considered relevant from the point of view of an end-user.

Internal Evaluation: Systematic assessment of a set of quality characteristics considered relevant from the point of view of a developer.

ISO-Based Evaluation: Systematic assessment of a set of quality characteristics adapted from an ISO standard, including external and internal evaluations. Execution of an evaluation based on a quality model defined by an ISO standard.

Quality Characteristic: Attribute of a software product or system that can be further decomposed into sub-characteristics and that contributes to the overall quality of the system. Top-level node in a hierarchical quality model.

Quality Model: Hierarchical decomposition of the quality attributes of a system; this hierarchy is composed of quality characteristics and sub-characteristics and the end-nodes of the hierarchy are measurable attributes.

Quality Sub-Characteristic: Attribute of a software product or system that contributes to the definition of a top-level attribute. Internal node or end-node in a hierarchical quality model.

Weight: Value from a scale assigned to quality (sub-)characteristics to make them comparable with each other in order to state their relative importance in a quality model.

Weighted Quality Model: Quality model augmented with a weight for each of its (sub-)characteristics.

APPENDIX: DEFINITIONS OF THE SQUARE-BASED QUALITY MODEL

Table 7. Quality characteristics for medical speech translation systems

Functionality
Functional completeness. The tasks and objectives that the system needs to cover should be defined from the beginning. There is a clear distinction between a system aiming for a full medical diagnosis and a tool for determining the priority of patients based on the severity of their condition in the emergency department (triage).
Functional correctness. In this specific application domain the translation between languages needs to be produced in the most reliable and robust way, achieving high quality. Also, the Text-to-Speech (TTS) should replicate human voice as natural and clear as possible.
Functional appropriateness. The system can be seen either as a replacement when no interpreters are available or as a palliative before resorting to an interpreter. It should therefore support as many languages, diagnosis domains and diverse usage environments as possible.
Exploitability (added attribute). Users may be forced to wait their turn for an examination or wait between examinations. This idle time can be used for familiarizing with the application, and thus fostering user's trust towards the system.
Controllability (added attribute). The system should determine the most efficient way of interaction, e.g. if the doctor gives instructions he should also be control of the dialog flow but during diagnosis the weight of control should be equilibrated between the two parties. This also conforms to current clinical theory of patient-centered medicine (Stewart et al., 2003).
Performance Efficiency
Time behavior. Time management is very important as the diagnosis should be made as quickly as possible. It should also be dependent on the usage scenario, e.g. it may be more urgent to complete a task at the welcome reception than at the laboratory.
Resource utilization. The system should target efficient utilization of resources (e.g. battery life, wireless connectivity, position tracking, storage and access of user data, etc.) to allow unhindered usage and also fair sharing among users.
Capacity. In the case when the system exceeds its capacity limits in terms of bandwidth, storage, etc. the users should be informed for possible alternative actions (e.g. wait for a certain time interval, address to the personnel, etc.).
Compatibility
Co-existence. The system should successfully co-exist with other independent systems working in a common environment and sharing common resources. Issues of conflicts may include the bandwidth usage, interference problems, other wearable medical devices, etc.
Interoperability. The system should facilitate interoperability of the different nodes in the pathway seamlessly, e.g. information about prescribed medication or special treatment must be available to the corresponding personnel or system.
Usability
Appropriateness recognizability. One important aspect is to make users understand what the system is supposed to do. Short introductions should be provided along with context dependent prompts. Cultural limitation or physical disabilities should also be addressed. In this way users can form a concrete theory of the machine's mind (ToM), and update it as they interact.
Learnability. As in any spoken dialogue application, it should give users immediate feedback on the system's intended coverage, particularly when recognition fails. This can be achieved through an intelligent help module, which tries to identify user's requests and propose possible alternatives.
Operability. As end-users may use a system like this only once in their life the interaction should be based on simplicity. A basic interaction pattern should be adopted, based on modality synergies.
User error protection. The system should offer results that are predictable and do not engender any surprise to end-users, so that patients establish trustful relations towards the system that works as a mediator for human-to-human interaction.
User interface aesthetics. Due to the limited lifecycle of the application (used only in a hospital environment), the issue of attractiveness becomes of lesser importance. However, when subjective judgments are involved, the success of the system may depend on relevant factors.
Accessibility. As users may vary in a range of literate to complete illiterate, the system should take this into account as well as other special needs (weak sight, hearing problems, etc.). It can therefore present the output in different ways, for example with images or voice instead of text.

continued on following page

Table 7. Continued

Uniformability (added attribute). Following the path of healthcare each user should experience a uniform interaction. This will minimize the effort of learning how the system works in different situations and will cause less confusion.
Privacy (added attribute). The system should contemplate issues of privacy, e.g. patients can be reluctant to talk in front of other, even in front of relatives, be embarrassed when using the system unsuccessfully, etc.
Reliability
Maturity. The special nature of the application demands zero faults therefore the system should aim to minimize the frequency of failures.
Availability. The system should be able to handle operational and accessibility issues by offering to users alternative ways to access it, e.g. the system can be preinstalled on a number of hospital's devices.
Fault tolerance. In case of any faults the system should resort to a backup plan, e.g. trained personnel could take over control and interact with the patient.
Recoverability. The software should be able to recover after a failure either by incorporating a logging mechanism or by storing user's data in a database locally or remotely.
Security
Confidentiality. The system should guarantee that the information gathered during the interaction is stored and accessed in a restricted manner.
Integrity. The treatment of sensitive medical data should be carefully considered and any attempt to access or modify it, even by authorized personnel, should be registered.
Non-repudiation. As the system can be used by more than one peers, administrative personnel, physicians and patients, it should be made clear which actions and events took place and by whom.
Accountability. User's activity along the pathway should be traced by the system and may be used to identify possible problems (e.g. delays), perform correct pricing of praxes, etc.
Authenticity. Each involved party (administrative personnel, physicians and patients) should be assigned the proper credentials that uniquely and authentically identify them.
Maintainability
Modularity. "Degree to which a system or computer program is composed of discrete components such that a change to one component has minimal impact on other components" (ISO, 2011).
Reusability. "Degree to which an asset can be used in more than one system, or in building other assets" (ISO, 2011).
Analyzability. "Degree of effectiveness and efficiency with which it is possible to assess the impact on a product or system of an intended change to one or more of its parts, or to diagnose a product for deficiencies or causes of failures, or to identify parts to be modified"(ISO, 2011).
Modifiability. "Degree to which a product or system can be effectively and efficiently modified without introducing defects or degrading existing product quality" (ISO, 2011).
Testability. "Degree of effectiveness and efficiency with which test criteria can be established for a system, product or component and tests can be performed to determine whether those criteria have been met" (ISO, 2011).
Portability
Adaptability. The system should be adaptable to a number of platforms. Proprietary solutions may narrow the possible options, so the design should take into account forthcoming technologies and open source alternatives.
Installability. If end-users decide to install the system on their own device this should be as transparent as possible considering that the application's life time could be limited to just the time the patient stays in the hospital.
Replaceability. As most of the times upgrading the existing software should not be performed by end-users, issues of replaceability are not a subject of their concern. Technical personnel should be responsible for the specific task on the offered devices.

Chapter 11
Digital Medicine:
The Quality Standpoint

Anastasius Moumtzoglou
Hellenic Society for Quality and Safety in Healthcare, Greece

ABSTRACT

Individualizing care must take into account the diversity of patient values and perspectives while attending to the specific needs of people must take into account the multifaceted nature of culture. Digital medicine enables digital proximity and self-care, challenges the traditional paternal model of medicine, reshapes the nature and expectations of health care delivery, emphasizes the active involvement of patients and has an enormous potential to empower patients. Moreover, the concepts of bio-objects, cultural competence, and patient-centered care could be apparently thought on a continuum with one pole representing the bio-objects and the other representing one of the health care quality dimensions, patient-centered care. All-embracing, digital medicine affects the core values of cultural competence, which are shared by patient-centered care, one of the health care quality dimensions.

INTRODUCTION

Ubiquitous computing is a concept coined by Mark Weiser in 1988, who largely defined ubiquitous computing and sketched out its prime concerns. He also stressed that the increase of processing power would necessitate understandings of social, cultural and psychological phenomena. Overall, there is not a single definition for ubiquitous computing but a taxonomy of its features. However, it is described as pervasive computing, ambient intelligence, ambient media, and everyware. It also touches on a broad spectrum of research topics, including:

- Mobile computing.
- Mobile networking.
- Context-aware computing.
- Sensor networks.
- Human-computer interaction.

DOI: 10.4018/978-1-5225-1724-5.ch011

- Artificial intelligence.
- Distributed computing.
- Location computing.

With progress in technology and data communications, ubiquitous healthcare systems such as mobile health applications are becoming the quickest solution to the overwhelming problem of the healthcare system issues. In addition to easier management, ubiquitous technology has the potential to motivate users to take an active role and manage their conditions. Likewise, wearable health monitoring systems integrated into a ubiquitous mobile health system (mHealth), emerged as a technology of choice for ambulatory monitoring. They facilitate continuous monitoring, optimal maintenance of a chronic condition or computer assisted rehabilitation.

The first generation of ubiquitous systems used wearable computers that were integrated into clothes or worn on the body. However, the need for ubiquitous connectivity and unification of multiple devices on a single platform created the need for smartphones. Furthermore, health and medical apps are one of the newest developments in the digitizing of health and medical information. The evolution and mass access to the Internet led to a proliferation of health and medical websites and online discussion groups. The first websites were mostly static, infrequently updating their information offering little opportunity for sharing of information by patients or contribution of experience details.

Technological advances in low-power integrated circuits have also facilitated the design of Body Area Networks which integrate, lightweight, low-cost intelligent sensors and networking platforms. They connect nodes attached to the body surface, implanted into the body, or dispersed in clothing. From this angle, context-awareness, in Body Area Networks, describes the system capability to understand the user's state and change its behavior. Current technology provides context awareness, such as light, noise level, position, proximity, activity, social interaction, connectivity, and GPS location.

On the whole, the health and medical apps currently span an ample range of content sophistication. Many provide information on a specific medical condition or treatments while others involve highly detailed anatomical visualizations or assist in diagnosing, identifying risks, self-tracking fitness, and self-care. An assortment of apps that are currently on the market includes versions of medical training and education. They accommodate:

- Detailed anatomical and visual information.
- Digital versions of medical dictionaries and textbooks.
- Drug prescribing information.
- Training videos.

As a result, the digital technologies that emerged in the past decade have augmented the access opportunities and the sharing of health and medical information. Moreover, they offer patients the opportunity to be responsible for their health and engage in self-monitoring and self-care practices (Lupton, 2013; Sosnowy, 2014; Greenhalgh, 2012). Patients can describe their experiences, rate healthcare providers and medical treatments using social media platforms, and create and upload images or videos. Moreover, these apps have proliferated in recent years as part of a constellation of current digital health technologies which generate knowledge about healthcare, health behaviors and disease patterns (Lupton, 2014). However, social analysts have yet to commit energy and thoughts to the role played and the contribution of health and medical apps to the digitized landscape taking into account the issue of medical information validity and quality of apps. In this context, the chapter substantiates that the concepts of bio-objects, cultural competence, and patient-centered care could be apparently thought on a continuum with one pole representing the bio-objects and the other representing one of the health care quality dimensions, patient-centered care. All-embracing, it concludes that digital medicine affects the core values of cultural competence, which are shared by patient-centered care, one of the health care quality dimensions.

BACKGROUND

Digital health is a term that encompasses a variety of products, including consumer-focused mobile apps with no clinical validation or approved by FDA. It also consists of potentially disruptive technologies whose full impact has yet to be realized. In the past five years, a multitude of wearable sensor technologies has emerged placing the fast moving, user-centric, focused tech sector on a fascinating collision course with the much-slower-moving, and highly regulated world of medicine. Digital health can be envisaged as the convergence of the digital and genomic revolutions with health, healthcare, living, and society. It is empowering people to track, improve, and manage their health while also helping to cut down inefficiency in healthcare delivery, increase access, and quality and contribute to more personalized and precise medicine.

Eric Topol first recited the principal components of digital health in his book "The Creative Destruction of Medicine: How the Digital Revolution Will Create Better Health Care" (Topol, 2012). According to Topol, converging elements are comprising digital health which include:

- Health information technology.
- The Internet.
- Wireless devices.
- Microprocessors and integrated circuits.
- Hardware sensors, and software sensing technologies.
- Mobile and body area networks.
- Genomics.

Furthermore, the underlying lexicon of Digital Health is extensive and includes:

- mHealth.
- Wireless Health.
- Health 2.0.
- eHealth.
- e-Patient(s).
- Healthcare IT / Health IT (information technology).
- Big Data.
- Health Data.
- Cloud Computing.
- Quantified Self.
- Wearable Computing.
- Gamification.

- Telehealth / Telemedicine.
- Precision Medicine and Personalized Medicine.
- Connected Health.

In the quest to individualized medicine, it is essential to know the biology of a person via genomics, proteomics, metabolomics, epigenomics, and biomarkers. The other critical step is the understanding of an individual's physiology which has only become possible through the growth of wearable wireless sensor technology. Physiology metrics can now be measured at home during everyday activities with an intensive care unit level of accuracy and continuity, as mobile technologies allow for greater convenience and also increase the ability to understand the daily variability. This capability allows for the largest refinement of existing phenotypes allowing for higher individualization in the management of acute and chronic conditions.

The subset of products with potential in disease management that could have a significant impact on the healthcare ecosystem is differentiated under the umbrella term digital medicine (Elenko, Underwood & Zohar, 2015). In the coming digital medicine era, for some conditions, there is the potential to deviate toward earlier interventions using both continuous temporal monitoring and prevention tools. Moreover, in the future, the line between diagnosing and monitoring could blur, as constant patient monitoring allows diagnosis on an on-going basis. Such an approach could detect outbreaks and acute disease before the onset of analytical symptoms that require hospitalization. As frequent monitoring becomes more of reality, it will be substantial to balance the positives of early intervention against the downside of false-positive signals.

Additionally, with multiple passive monitoring tools and sensors capturing an unprecedented amount of data about patients and treatments, digital medicine is also changing the way we think about clinical studies. Digital medicine platforms empower patients in several ways. They allow communities of engaged patients monitor their signs of illness and submit data on experiences associated with conditions and various treatments. They also enable information sharing and connection with other individuals who may be suffering similar symptoms. Finally, likewise to information collected by sensors, communities of engaged patients are proactively submitting data on their experiences with conditions and various treatments.

However, patient-reported data lack objective validation and include biases arising from variable data sampling schedules. Furthermore, the meta-analysis of the literature raises the issue of medical information validity and quality of apps, as a literature major concern. The viewpoint is that any developer can release a health or medical app, which conforms to the guidelines required by the publishing app store. In this context, several studies identifying significant problems with the medical accuracy of apps' content have been published (Mosemghvdlishvili & Jansz, 2012; Buijink, Visser, Marshall, 2013; Bender et al., 2013). They argue that many developers do not nominate specific medical experts in contributing to the content. They also suggest that developers are vague in their attribution of authorship (Wolf et al., 2013; Hamilton & Brady, 2012; Rosser & Eccleston, 2011, Stevens et al., 2014; O'Neill, S.; Brady, 2012) while there are conflicts of interest and legal and regulation difficulties (Ozdalga E, Ozdalga A, Ahuja, 2012; Wallace & Dhingra, 2014; Visvanathan, Hamilton & Brady, 2012; Yetisen et al., 2014; McCartney, 2013). Finally, health and medical apps deviate in the accuracy of their content and the credibility of information resources while some app developers appear to draw on little or no direct medical expertise.

Given this background, quality control data of medical applications for 4G mobile phones is not available, although some of the applications have received FDA 510(k) clearance. The FDA 510(k) process or premarket notification is similar to the 'generic' drug concept, and it is used to allow marketing authorization for a device, which is similar to effectiveness and safety to another promoted device. The 510(k) clearance means that the new device must demonstrate almost the same safety and effectiveness characteristics as the device to which the new one is being compared. The essential qualities of this comparison depend on the degree of risk associated with its use, including physical or performance characteristics measured by standardized methods. In some instances, a premarket notification submission for a new device is based on evidence that the device, under existing conditions, has the same effectiveness and safety characteristics as the predicate. A successful 510(k) submission means, as a result, the FDA clearance to promote the new device, which does not translate into an approval process by legal sense. The premarket approval process is based on inherent evidence of effectiveness and safety, which results in approval of the new device. It is the FDA's review, which evaluates the safety and effectiveness of Class III medical devices, conforming to scientific principles. To gain approval, the manufacturer must submit adequate scientific evidence to prove that the device is effective and safe in its use.

QUALITY CONTROL OF MEDICAL APPLICATIONS

Quality control is a process, which includes the necessary actions to verify the characteristics of a product or service in order to ensure its quality (Ishikawa, 1976). In simple terms, quality control is the process of ensuring conformance of all products and services to a set standard of quality. It involves several steps in the process, encompassing a system of technical activities to evaluate quality that ensure data integrity, correctness, and completeness. The objective of quality control is to ensure that products and services comply with specific requirements. Essentially, quality control involves the testing of a product, service, or procedure for conformance with minimum levels of quality. A quality control team stops production temporarily if it identifies products that do not comply with the specified standards of quality. Quality control activities cover standard methods such as precision checks on data collection and standardized procedures for measurements.

An effective quality control program begins with setting the standards of quality, which will serve, as the guideline, to determine whether the products pass the quality control. After setting detailed standards, quality control turns to the sample of tested products and the extent of inspections. At this stage, the manufacturer has to determine the exact percentage of products, thought as the representative sample. At this point, the quality control must be able to gather relevant information from existing production processes. The data should reflect what percentage of products fails to meet the specified standards and help learn ways of avoiding errors that lead to costly repairs.

Quality control is closely related to the Six Sigma initiative, a business strategy developed by Motorola (Tennant, 2001) with Bill Smith formulating the particulars of the methodology. The term originated from terminology associated with statistical modeling of manufacturing processes and relates to a process that produces 3.4 defective parts per million opportunities. As a result, it refers to an exceptionally high percentage of production within specification and seeks to improve the quality of a process output. It uses quality and statistical methods to create a distinctive infrastructure of people within the organization.

Six Sigma projects followed DMAIC and DMADV methodologies, composed of five phases each, and were inspired by Deming's Plan-Do-Check-Act cycle (Tennant, 2001). DMAIC aims at improving an existing business process, while DMADV at creating new product or process designs. DMAIC project methodology incorporates the following phases:

- *D*efine the problem.
- *M*easure key aspects.
- *A*nalyze the data.
- *I*mprove the current process.
- *C*ontrol the future state process.

The DMADV project methodology, also known as DFSS (Design for Six Sigma) features the following phases:

- *D*efine design goals.
- *M*easure and identify critical characteristics to quality.
- *A*nalyze to develop and design alternatives.
- *D*esign details.
- *V*erify the design.

A distinction has to be made between quality control, which refers to the product, and quality assurance, which is process oriented. The main concern of quality control is the quality evaluation of the product or service, while quality assurance is focused on ensuring the processes conform to the manufacturer's specifications. As a result, quality assurance focuses on production processes, while quality control on the end product. Quality assurance activities include a planned system of review procedures, preferably by independent third parties, which are performed after the implementation of the quality control procedures. Finally, it is worthwhile mentioning that information technology has made it possible to use automated quality control tools to great effect. Tools of this type are constantly gathering and arranging data in formats that quality control and assurance personnel can evaluate.

TOTAL QUALITY CONTROL AND TOTAL QUALITY MANAGEMENT (TQM)

Total quality control, often referred as total quality, originated from Armand V Feigenbaum (1961), who defined it as 'an effective system for integrating the quality development, quality maintenance, and quality improvement efforts of the various groups in an organization so as to enable production and service at the most economical levels'. Feigenbaum conceptualized it as a business strategy and proposed quality leadership, modern quality technology, and organizational commitment, as the three steps to quality. Total quality control provides a total approach to quality control, emphasizes the importance of management, includes socio-technical thinking and promotes participation by all staff. On the other hand, it does not differentiate between different kinds of quality context, and does not bring together the different management theories into one coherent whole.

Total quality control was discussed during the 70's, as a companywide quality control that involves all employees. However, the next decade was marked by the new wave of quality control, known as Total Quality Management (TQM). TQM, a logical extension of quality control, is a philosophy, which considers the whole organization as a unit of quality. Quality was initially achieved by inspection with quality control creating the systematic approach to detecting and treating the quality problems. Quality assurance broadened the authority to highlight processes, and TQM incorporated both but also developed its own distinctive features. TQM emphasizes meeting of customers' needs and expectations, development of systems and procedures that promote quality improvement.

As a result, we can no longer conceptualize quality as only relating to quality control, as there are several approaches to improving the quality of care. These approaches include evidence-based practice (EBP) and evidence-based clinical practice guidelines, professional education and development, assessment and accountability, patient-centered care, and total quality management (Grol, 2001). The underlying principle for all of these approaches is that if we want to improve the quality of care, healthcare professionals must be able to evaluate their performance. Nevertheless, healthcare providers have limited ability to obtain feedback regarding performance in their daily work, due in part to a lack of information systems and to a lack of consistency on how to measure qua1ity of care (McGlynn & Ashe, 1998).

The premise of EBP and evidence-based clinical practice guidelines is that we can improve clinical decision making and patient care by incorporating the best available evidence with provider preferences and patient values (Sackett et al., 1996). Professional education and development strategies address the complexity of clinical practice and propose improvement based on professional self-regulation and ownership by clinicians (Grol, 2001). Interactive forms of education and small group learning have been successful for changing clinical behavior (Davis et al., 1999). The third approach to improving the quality of care emphasizes regular assessments of clinical performance and public accountability. The assumption is that healthcare professionals will change practice when their performance is compared to their peers or presented for others to see. Moreover, patient-centered care emphasizes the need to empower patients participate in medical decision making. The essential elements of patient-centered care include human interactions and relationship-centered caring, access to information, healing partnerships, nutrition, spiritual and cultural diversity, complementary and alternative practices into conventional care, effects of viewing art on health outcomes, healing environments, and healthy communities (Frampton & Charmel, 2009). Methods employed include patient satisfaction surveys, needs assessments, decision aids, and risk tables for shared decision making (Grol, 2001). Total quality management (TQM) and continuous quality improvement (CQI) offer an integrated approach to improving patient care. They emphasize that the greatest opportunity for improvement is found by focusing on the health system's organizational characteristics rather than on individuals. The quality improvement model developed by Nolan is the most widely accepted conceptual framework. It includes a reflective component and a dynamic component (Berwick, 1998), with the reflective component seeking to identify aims and measures, and refine strategies by asking: What is our goal? How will we know when we reach our goal? What changes will we make to achieve our goal? The dynamic component uses learning cycles to develop and evaluate changes in systems and processes that we usually refer to as Plan-Do-Study-Act (PDSA) cycles. This quality improvement model attempts to analyze and improve processes, initially testing the change on a small scale prior to wide dissemination.

Finally, we have to refer to patient safety because efforts to improve patient safety have become a global priority. Despite focused efforts, we have to acknowledge that the boundaries between the broader concept of quality and patient safety remain poorly defined, and patient safety is an evolving science. So far, we interpret patient safety not as a characteristic of individuals, but a system property. As a result, in order to minimize risk and ensure safety, clinicians must focus on designing systems that help prevent errors or that mitigate harm from errors that cannot be entirely prevented.

DIGITAL MEDICINE AND PERSONALIZED MEDICINE

The quest to provide personalized medicine involves awareness of the individual's biology and understanding of the intricacies of its physiology. Both have become possible through the development of wearables and mobile health (mHealth) technologies which are defined as medical and public health practice supported by mobile devices, such as mobile phones, patient monitoring devices, personal digital assistants (PDAs), and other wireless devices. It involves the use and capitalization on a mobile phone's core utility of voice and short messaging service as well as more complex functionalities and applications including general packet radio service (GPRS), third and fourth generation mobile telecommunications (3G and 4G systems), global positioning system (GPS), and Bluetooth technology. By definition (Istepanian et al., 2006), mHealth can better reach areas, people, and healthcare professionals with limited exposure to certain aspects of healthcare. As a result, it enables personalized care, which relates to the integrated practice of medicine and patient care based upon one's unique life characteristics, behavior, and surroundings. Internet-based applications allow individuals to shape the application based on their individual needs (Nijland et al., 2009), while autonomous and adaptive Web applications encourage individual 'participation' in the medical decision-making and self-management (American College of Physicians, 2008). However, although we might easily endorse the concept of personalization, its effective implementation in the health care setting can be difficult. Standardization rather than personalization has been the norm for decades. Therefore, even if there are no written policies, many traditional perceptions form the dominant organizational culture at many institutions (Frampton & Charmel, 2009). An important aspect of personalized care is the burgeoning field of patient advocacy, which acts as a support structure and relationship between the patient and health care provider. The patient advocate may be an individual or a nonprofit organization focusing on a health care aspect or disease.

Personalized care relates to personalized medicine, which emphasizes customization of healthcare. However, personalized medicine is a conceptual paradigm, with only a few clinical practices. Nevertheless, personalized treatment is anticipated because of the increased consciousness of the shortcomings in the delivery of drugs, molecular understanding, and an increased demand for integrating genetic information into the drug development process (Lesko, 2007). The core issue of personalized medicine is tailoring individualized therapies by using an individual's specific biological characteristics. Consumer personalized medicine is the additional level of collecting, synthesizing, and using personal data to proactively manage your health. In this framework, we might consider four areas of consumer personalized medicine (Swan, 2009):

- Direct-to-consumer personalized genomics services.
- Blood and other biomarker testing.
- Environmental testing.
- Predictive biosimulation.

Personalized genomics is the key input to consumer personalized medicine. Genomic testing has been available for some time, but was ordered by the physician as an only once test for a specific condition. The qualitative change is in the formation of companies focusing on direct-to-consumer genetic testing. The second area to consider is blood and other biomarker data since there is a growing consumer demand for more granular information than the yearly check of a few regularly used biomarkers. An increasing number of individuals would like to pursue a wider range of personalized indicators on a regular ongoing basis. The benefits to direct access blood testing for the ongoing self-quantifier include precision, low cost, and consolidated network statistics of the current and recent results. At some time it might be possible for individuals to upload data to their data storage facilities at health social networks and health portals. Environmental data, screening for body burden and the cumulative effect of exposure to toxic substances in the environment are the third area to consider in consumer personalized medicine. Personalized chemical testing services focus on pollutants while environmental screening may also be conducted by hair analysis tests, which perform nutritional analysis and assess exposure to toxic substances. The fourth area, which is crucial to consumer personalized medicine, is predictive biosimulation, which translates into using biological data as well as mathematical modeling to create an electronic interpretation of an individual. The virtual patient may be used to evaluate simulated treatments, but predictive biosimulation is not targeted at consumers yet.

DIGITAL MEDICINE AND HEALTH CARE QUALITY

The medical applications provide various types of capabilities and responsibilities which significantly affect medical authority, the doctor-patient relationship, the practice of medicine, the delivery of healthcare, public health work, and the doctor-patient relationship. They also have the potential to reshape the ways in which we visualize, understand and treat the human body as they are, not only, traditional forms of human body representation but also new ways of the digitised embodiment, which are generated using self-monitoring. They also create a cybernetic relationship between the bio-object and the user (Lupton, 2012; Haggerty, K. & Ericson, 2000) which is based on liveliness, vitality, and the social life of the data they provide (Latour, 2005; Ruckenstein, 2014; Beer, 2013). In addition, they represent the changes of the human embodiment as amenable to vigilance and self-responsibility. When behaviours and body functions are digitised as quantifiable data, indicators and concepts of health and fitness become compressed representations represented by certain numbers that are collected by a self-tracking device (Lash, 2007). In this sense, they comprise new forms of patienthood and embodiment which make visible the body dimensions that were previously hidden. Most importantly, they are cultural artefacts, described as 'bio-objects' or 'data doubles' (Johnson, 2014), which provide information about the types of illnesses and health conditions at a particular moment. As a result, they affect cultural competence which is defined as a set of attitudes, congruent behaviors, and policies that come together in the healthcare system.

However, many aspects of the cultural competence formulation are also central aspects of patient-centeredness, as at the core of patient centeredness lies the ability of the healthcare provider to:

- See the patient as a unique person.
- Maintain unconditional positive regard.
- Build effective rapport.

- Use the biopsychosocial model.
- Explore patient beliefs, and values.
- Find consensus regarding treatment plans.

As a result, it has been argued that the essence of cultural competence is a 'patient-centered approach'.

However, patient-centered care is one of the six dimensions of health care quality. It focuses on patients' preferences, experienced needs, and values, in decisions about care and treatment. It has a broadened perspective of illness, in which patients' experiences and control are prominent. It also focuses on interactions, striving for an alliance between patients and professionals working together and having common grounds and goals (Epstein et al., 2005; Glasgow et al., 2008; Mead et al., 2000; Michie et al., 2003; Stewart et al., 2000; Swedish Agency for Health and Care Services Analysis, 2012). Howie et al. (2004) reported that patient-centeredness is based on the patients' concerns, putting emphasis on giving the patients time to express these concerns.

Patient-centeredness also pertains to patient empowerment which is grounded in equality and respect. As a result, It features self-determining agents with some control over their health and health care and conceptualizes personal monitoring and self-efficacy. For patient empowerment, it is important that patients have knowledge and skills to define and achieve their goals (Funnell et al., 2003; Nyatanga et al., 2002). It is furthermore important that care be planned and performed from this perspective (Ekman et al. 2011; Funnell & Anderson, 2003).

Overall, patient-centeredness involves patients in decision making as well as in their health and health care. Involving patients in decisions relates to the concept of shared decision making while involving patients in their health and health care implies the concepts of self-management support, and support planning (Ahmad, Ellis, Krelle, & Lawrie, 2014).

Conclusively, the concepts of bio-objects, cultural competence, and patient-centered care could be apparently thought on a continuum with one pole representing the bio-objects and the other representing one of the health care quality dimensions, patient-centered care. Acknowledging the overlapping of the ideas of digital medicine and bio-objects, digital medicine affects health care quality.

CONCLUSION

Taking account all its main features, digital medicine not only facilitates care but also interacts with other technologies and shapes the ways in which patients are treated. It emphasizes the active involvement of patients (Chetney, 2003; Montfort & Helm, 2006) and can be thought as an active transformer of health care (Berg & Mol, 1998; Webster, 2002). Its principal characteristic is that health care can be provided at a distance, thus replacing face-to-face contacts by technology-mediated interactions. Consequently, it affects the key dimensions of traditional health care delivery, physical proximity and narrative proximity (Malone, 2003). Physical proximity refers to the vicinity within which health professionals physically touch and care for patients while narrative proximity is used to refer to practices in which health professionals appear to 'know the patient' by hearing and trying to understand the patient story.

On the other hand, it challenges the traditional paternal model of medicine by facilitating digital proximity that provides patients with practical tools for self-care (Oudshoorn, 2009). As a result, it promotes a co-diagnosis, co-care, collaborative model of health care delivery (Charles et al., 1999). The physician is a partner and advisor while the patient is an informed participant, an active responsibility-taker, the owner, director and coordinator of his health data (Charles et al., 1999). In this context, the provider-patient encounter involves knowledgeable patients, performing self-testing and self-tracking activities and doctors approaching the doctor-patient relationship from a neuroscientist perspective (Benedetti, 2011) and co-interpreting the results.

However, individualizing care must take into account the diversity of patient values and perspectives while attending to the specific needs of people must take into account the multifaceted nature of culture. Digital medicine enables digital proximity and self-care, challenges the traditional paternal model of medicine, reshapes the nature and expectations of health care delivery, emphasizes the active involvement of patients and has an enormous potential to empower patients.

All-embracing, it affects the core values of cultural competence, which are shared by patient-centered care, one of the health care quality dimensions.

REFERENCES

Akhtar, S. (2008). 2G-5G Networks: Evolution of Technologies, Standards, and Deployment. In Encyclopedia of Multimedia Technology and Networking (2nd ed.). Idea Group Publisher.

American College of Physicians. (2008). *E-health and its impact on Medical Practice. Position paper.* Author.

Anderson, P., & Blackwood, A. (2004). *Mobile and PDA technologies and their future use in education. JISC TechWatch*. Bristol: JISC.

Anya, O., Tawfik, H., Nagar, A., & Amin, S. (2009). E-workbench: A Case for Collaborative Decision Support in E-health. Paper presented at the 11th International Conference on Computer Modelling and Simulation.

Apple Inc. (2011). *iPhone Facetime*. Retrieved from http://www.apple.com/iphone/features/facetime.html

Beer, D. (2013). *Popular Culture and New Media: The Politics of Circulation*. Houndmills, UK: Palgrave Macmillan. doi:10.1057/9781137270061

Bender, L. J., Yue, K. R. Y., To, J. M., Deacken, L., & Jadad, R. A. (2013). A lot of action, but not in the right direction: Systematic review and content analysis of smartphone applications for the prevention, detection, and management of cancer. *Journal of Medical Internet Research*, *15*(12), e287. doi:10.2196/jmir.2661 PMID:24366061

Benedetti, F. (2011). *The Patient's Brain: The neuroscience behind the doctor-patient relationship*. Oxford, UK: Oxford University Press.

Berg, M., & Mol, A. (Eds.). (1998). *Difference in Medicine; Unravelling Practices, Techniques, and Bodies*. Durham, NC: Duke University Press.

Berwick, D. M. (1998). *Examining Errors in Health Care: Developing a Prevention, Education, and Research Agenda*. Paper presented at the American Hospital Association and Centennial Regional Leadership Forum, Cleveland, OH.

Buijink, A. W. G., Visser, B. J., & Marshall, L. (2013). Medical apps for smartphones: Lack of evidence undermines quality and safety. *Evidence-Based Medicine*, *18*(3), 90–92. doi:10.1136/eb-2012-100885 PMID:22923708

Charles, C., Whelan, T., & Gafni, A. (1999). What do we mean by partnership in making decisions about treatment? *British Medical Journal*, *319*(7212), 780–782. doi:10.1136/bmj.319.7212.780 PMID:10488014

Chetney, R. (2003). The Cardiac Connection Program. *Home Healthcare Nurse*, *21*(10), 680–686. doi:10.1097/00004045-200310000-00007 PMID:14557707

Chlamtac, I., Conti, M., & Liu, J. J.-N. (2003). Mobile ad hoc networking: Imperatives and challenges. *Ad Hoc Networks*, *1*(1), 13–64. doi:10.1016/S1570-8705(03)00013-1

Davis, D., O'Brien, M. A., Freemantle, N., Wolf, F. M., Mazmanian, P., & Taylor-Vaisey, A. (1999). Impact of formal continuing medical education: Do conferences, workshops, rounds, and other traditional continuing education activities change physician behavior or health care outcomes? *Journal of the American Medical Association*, *282*(9), 867–874. doi:10.1001/jama.282.9.867 PMID:10478694

Elenko, E., Underwood, L., & Zohar, D. (2015). Defining digital medicine. *Nature Biotechnology*, *33*(5), 456–461. doi:10.1038/nbt.3222 PMID:25965750

eMobility. (2007). In D. Bourse & R. Tafazolli (Eds.), *Beyond 3G / 4G Radio Access Technologies (RATs) and Standards Roadmaps* (eMobility Technology Platform Whitepaper). Retrieved from http://www.ist-emobility.org/

Feigenbaum, A. (1961). *Total Quality Control*. New York: McGraw-Hill.

Frampton, S., & Charmel, P. (2009). *Putting Patients First: Best Practices in Patient-Centered Care*. San Francisco: Jossey-Bass.

Frattasi, S., Fitzek, F., & Prasad, R. (2005). Cooperative Services for 4G. In *Proceedings of the 14th IST Mobile & Wireless Communications Summit*. European Association for Signal Processing (EURASIP).

Fu, X., Hogrefe, D., Narayanan, S., & Soltwisch, R. (2004). QoS and Security in 4G Networks. In *Proceedings of the 1st CIC/IEEE Global Mobile Congress (GMC 2004)* (pp. 117-122).

Gani, A., Li, X., Yang, L., & Zakaria, O. (2008). Radio Frequency Combination for TCP/IP Suite Protocol Improvement in 4G Mobile Internet Networks. *International Journal of Communication*, *2*(1), 27–36.

Grami, A., & Schell, B. H. (2004). Future Trends in Mobile Commerce: Service Offerings, Technological Advances and Security Challenges. In *Proceedings of the Second Annual Conference on Privacy, Security and Trust*.

Greenhalgh, T., Procter, R., Wherton, J., Sugarhood, P., & Shaw, S. (2012). The organising vision for telehealth and telecare: Discourse analysis. *BMJ Open*, *2*(4), e001574. doi:10.1136/bmjopen-2012-001574 PMID:22815469

Grol, R. (2001). Improving the quality of medical care: Building bridges among professional pride, payor profit, and patient satisfaction. *Journal of the American Medical Association*, *286*(20), 2578–2585. doi:10.1001/jama.286.20.2578 PMID:11722272

Haggerty, K., & Ericson, R. (2000). The surveillant assemblage. *The British Journal of Sociology*, *51*, 605–622. doi:10.1080/00071310020015280 PMID:11140886

Hamilton, A., & Brady, R. (2012). Medical professional involvement in smartphone 'apps' in dermatology. *The British Journal of Dermatology*, *167*(1), 220–221. doi:10.1111/j.1365-2133.2012.10844.x PMID:22283748

He, L., & Zhao, C. (2008). 4G Technology Promote Mobile Learning for New Development. In *Proceedings of the 2008 International Symposium on Knowledge Acquisition and Modeling* (pp. 486-490). IEEE Computer Society. doi:10.1109/KAM.2008.151

Higashino, T., Yamaguchi, H., Yasumoto, K., & Shimada, K. (2005). Toward Future Innovation of Mobile Communication Systems - Current Requirements for Research -. In *Proceedings of the 2nd International Conference on Mobile Computing and Ubiquitous Networking (ICMU 2005).*

Hong, J. W., & Leon-Garcia, A. (2005). Requirements for the Operations and Management of 4G Networks. In *Proceedings of the 19th International Telegraffic Congress* (pp. 981-990).

Huang, C.-Y., Yang, Y.-L., Tzeng, G.-H., Cheng, S.-T., & Lee, H.-Y. (2010). 4G Mobile phone consumer preference predictions by using the Rough Set Theory and flow graphs. In Proceedings of Technology Management for Global Economic Growth (PICMET'10) (pp. 1 - 10).

Hwang, J.-S., Consulta, R. R., & Yoon, H.-Y. (2007). 4G Mobile Networks–Technology Beyond 2.5G and 3G. In *Proceedings PTC'07.*

Ishikawa, K. (1976). *Guide to Quality Control*. Tokyo: Asian Productivity Organization.

Istepanian, R., Laxminarayan, S., & Pattichis, C. (Eds.). (2006). *M-Health: Emerging Mobile Health Systems*. New York: Springer. doi:10.1007/b137697

Janevski, T. (2009). 5G Mobile Phone Concept. In *Proceedings of the 6th IEEE Consumer Communications and Networking Conference, 2009* (CCNC 2009). IEEE.

Johnson, S. (2014). "Maternal devices", social media and the self-management of pregnancy, mothering and child health. *Societies*, *4*(2), 330–350. doi:10.3390/soc4020330

Lash, S. (2007). Power after hegemony: Cultural studies in mutation? *Theory, Culture & Society*, *24*(3), 55–78. doi:10.1177/0263276407075956

Latour, B. (2005). *Reassembling the Social: An Introduction to Actor-Network-Theory*. Oxford, UK: Clarendon.

Lesko, L. J. (2007). Personalized Medicine: Elusive Dream or Imminent Reality? *Clinical Pharmacology and Therapeutics*, *81*(6), 807–816. doi:10.1038/sj.clpt.6100204 PMID:17505496

Lupton, D. (2012). M-health and health promotion: The digital cyborg and surveillance society. *Social Theory & Health*, *10*(3), 229–244. doi:10.1057/sth.2012.6

Lupton, D. (2013). The digitally engaged patient: Self-monitoring and self-care in the digital health era. *Social Theory & Health*, *11*(3), 256–270. doi:10.1057/sth.2013.10

Lupton, D. (2014). Health promotion in the digital era: A critical commentary. *Health Promotion International*. doi:10.1093/heapro/dau091

Malone, R. E. (2003). Distal nursing. *Social Science & Medicine*, *56*, 2317–2326.

McCartney, M. (2013). How do we know whether medical apps work? *BMJ (Clinical Research Ed.)*. doi:10.1136/bmj.f1811 PMID:23516158

McGlynn, E. A., & Asche, S. M. (1998). Developing a clinical performance measure. *American Journal of Preventive Medicine*, *14*(3), 14–21. doi:10.1016/S0749-3797(97)00032-9 PMID:9566932

MIM Software Inc. (2011). Retrieved from www.mimsoftware.com

MobiSante. (2011). Retrieved from http://mobisante.com/

Montfort, A.P.W.P. & Helm, M.H.J. (2006). Telemonitoring of Patients with Chronic Heart Failure. *Disease Management & Health Outcomes*, *14*(1), 33–35.

Mosemghvdlishvili, L., & Jansz, J. (2012). Negotiability of technology and its limitations. *Information Communication and Society*, *16*(10), 1596–1618. doi:10.1080/1369118X.2012.735252

Nijland, N., Seydel, E. R., van Gemert-Pijnen, J. E. W. C., Brandenburg, B., Kelders, S. M., & Will, M. (2009). *Evaluation of an Internet-Based Application for Supporting Self-Care of Patients with Diabetes Mellitus Type 2*. Paper presented at the International Conference on eHealth, Telemedicine, and Social Medicine. doi:10.1109/eTELEMED.2009.33

O'Neill, S., & Brady, R. R. W. (2012). Colorectal smartphone apps: Opportunities and risks. *Colorectal Disease*, *14*(9), e530–e534. doi:10.1111/j.1463-1318.2012.03088.x PMID:22646729

Oudshoorn, N. (2009). Physical and digital proximity: Emerging ways of health care in face-to-face and telemonitoring of heart-failure patients. *Sociology of Health & Illness*, *31*(3), 390–405. doi:10.1111/j.1467-9566.2008.01141.x PMID:19144084

Ozdalga, E., Ozdalga, A., & Ahuja, N. (2012). The smartphone in medicine: A review of current and potential use among physicians and students. *Journal of Medical Internet Research*, *14*(5), e128. doi:10.2196/jmir.1994 PMID:23017375

Perrucci, G. P., Fitzek, F. H. P., Zhang, Q., & Katz, M. D. (2009). Cooperative Mobile Web Browsing. *EURASIP Journal on Wireless Communications and Networking*, *2009*, 1–9. doi:10.1155/2009/543054

Rosser, B., & Eccleston, C. (2011). Smartphone applications for pain management. *Journal of Telemedicine and Telecare*, *17*(6), 308–312. doi:10.1258/jtt.2011.101102 PMID:21844177

Roussos, G., Marsh, A., & Maglavera, S. (2005). Enabling pervasive computing with smart phones. *IEEE Pervasive Computing / IEEE Computer Society [and] IEEE Communications Society*, *4*(2), 20–27. doi:10.1109/MPRV.2005.30

Ruckenstein, M. (2014). Visualized and interacted life: Personal analytics and engagements with data doubles. *Societies*, *4*(1), 68–84. doi:10.3390/soc4010068

Sackett, D. L., Rosenberg, W. M., Gray, J. A., Haynes, R. B., & Richardson, W. S. (1996). Evidence based medicine: What it is and what it isn't. *British Medical Journal*, *312*(7023), 71–72.

Santhi, K. R., & Kumaran, G. S. (2006). Migration to 4 G: Mobile IP based Solutions. In *Proceedings of the Advanced International Conference on Telecommunications and International Conference on Internet and Web Applications and Services* (AICT/ICIW 2006). IEEE Computer Society.

Shim, J. P., & Shim, J. M. (2003). M-commerce Around the World: Mobile Services and Applications in Japan, Korea, Hong Kong, Finland, and the United States. *Decision Line*, *34*(5), 9–13.

Sosnowy, C. (2014). Practicing patienthood online: Social media, chronic illness, and lay expertise. *Societies*, *4*(2), 316–329. doi:10.3390/soc4020316

Srirama, S. (2006). Publishing and Discovery of Mobile Web Services in Peer to Peer Networks. In *Proceedings of First International Workshop on Mobile Services and Personalized Environments (MSPE'06)*.

Srirama, S., Jarke, M., & Prinz, W. (2007). Mobile Web Service Discovery in Peer to Peer Networks. In *Proceedings of the 5th International Workshop on Ubiquitous Mobile Information and Collaboration Systems*.

Srirama, S. N., Jarke, M., Zhu, H., & Prinz, W. (2008). Scalable Mobile Web Service Discovery in Peer to Peer Networks. In *Proceedings of the 2008 Third International Conference on Internet and Web Applications and Services*, 2008 (pp. 668-674). IEEE Computer Society.

Stevens, D. J., Jackson, J. A., Howes, N., & Morgan, J. (2014). Obesity surgery smartphone apps: A review.[PubMed]. *Obesity Surgery*, *24*(1), 32–36. doi:10.1007/s11695-013-1010-3

Subversus Interactive. (2011). Retrieved from http://subvers.us/

Swan, M. (2009). Emerging Patient-Driven Health Care Models: An Examination of Health Social Networks, Consumer Personalized Medicine and Quantified Self-Tracking. *International Journal of Environmental Research and Public Health*, *6*, 492–525.

Tachikawa, K. (2003). A perspective on the evolution of mobile communications. *Communications Magazine, IEEE*, *41*(10), 66–73.

Tennant, G. (2001). *Six Sigma, SPC and TQM in Manufacturing and Services*. Hampshire, UK: Gower Publishing, Ltd.

Topol, E. (2012). *The Creative Destruction of Medicine*. New York, NY: Basic Books.

Toye, E., Sharp, R., Madhavapeddy, A., Scott, D., Upton, E., & Blackwell, A. (2007). Interacting with mobile services: An evaluation of camera-phones and visual tags. *Personal and Ubiquitous Computing*, *11*(2).

Valtonen, E., Addams-Moring, R., Virtanen, T., Järvinen, A., & Moring, M. (2004). Emergency announcements to mobile user devices in geographically defined areas. In *Proceedings of the first International Workshop on Information Systems for Crisis Response and Management*.

Visvanathan, A., Hamilton, A., & Brady, R. (2012). Smartphone apps in microbiology—Is better regulation required? *Clinical Microbiology and Infection, 18*(7), E218–E220. doi:10.1111/j.1469-0691.2012.03892.x PMID:22563840

Wallace, L. S., & Dhingra, L. K. (2014). A systematic review of smartphone applications for chronic pain available for download in the united states. *Journal of Opioid Management, 10*, 63–68. doi:10.5055/jom.2014.0193 PMID:24604571

Webster, A. J. (2002). Innovative health technologies and the social: Redefining health, medicine and the body. *Current Sociology, 50*, 443–457.

Wilson, J. (2006). 3G to Web 2.0? Can Mobile Telephony Become an Architecture of Participation? *The International Journal of Research into New Media Technologies, 12*(2), 229–242.

Wolf, J., Moreau, J., Akilov, O., Patton, T., English, J., Ho, J., & Ferris, L. (2013). Diagnostic inaccuracy of smartphone applications for melanoma detection. *JAMA Dermatology, 149*, 422–426.

Yetisen, A. K., Martinez-Hurtado, J., da Cruz Vasconcellos, F., Simsekler, M. C. E., Akram, M. S., & Lowe, C. (2014). The regulation of mobile medical applications. *Lab on a Chip, 14*(5), 833–840. doi:10.1039/c3lc51235e PMID:24425070

KEY TERMS AND DEFINITIONS

Bio-Objects: Contested socio-technical objects which depend on the existence and manipulation of living entities that have some coherent biological form and agency.

Cultural Competence: Refers to the ability of healthcare systems to demonstrate cultural competence toward patients. It includes the consideration of the individual social, cultural, and linguistic needs of patients.

Digital Medicine: The subset of products with potential in disease management that could have a significant impact on the healthcare ecosystem.

Mobile Health: It describes the use of a broad range of telecommunication and multimedia technologies within wireless care delivery design and can be broadly defined as the delivery of healthcare services via mobile communication devices.

Patient-Centered Care: It is more than a method of communication which focuses on patients' preferences, experienced needs and values in decisions about care and treatment.

Quality: There are many definitions of healthcare quality. However, the definition of the Institute of Medicine (IOM) which captures the features of many other definitions has received wide acceptance. According to the Institute of Medicine (IOM), quality is the "degree to which health services for individuals and populations increase the likelihood of desired health outcomes and are consistent with current professional knowledge." A following IOM report specified several aims of a high-quality medical care system: 1) Safe: Avoiding injuries to patients, 2) Effective: Providing services based on scientific knowledge, 3) Patient-centered: Providing respectful care which is responsive to individual patient preferences, 4) Timely: Reducing waits and sometimes harmful delays, 5) Efficient: Avoiding waste, 6) Equitable: Providing care that does not vary according to personal characteristics.

Ubiquitous Computing: Ubiquitous computing is a concept coined by Mark Weiser in 1988, who largely defined ubiquitous computing and sketched out its prime concerns. He also stressed that the increase of processing power would necessitate understandings of social, cultural and psychological phenomena. Overall, there is not a single definition for ubiquitous computing but a taxonomy of its features. However, it is described as pervasive computing, ambient intelligence, ambient media, and everyware.

Chapter 12
ICT for Enabling the Quality Evaluation of Health Care Services:
A Case Study in a General Hospital

Alexandra Pomares-Quimbaya
Pontificia Universidad Javeriana, Colombia

Rafael A. González
Pontificia Universidad Javeriana, Colombia

Alejandro Sierra
Pontificia Universidad Javeriana, Colombia & Hospital Universitario San Ignacio, Colombia

Alvaro Bustamante
Pontificia Universidad Javeriana, Colombia & Hospital Universitario San Ignacio, Colombia

Julián Camilo Daza
Pontificia Universidad Javeriana, Colombia & Hospital Universitario San Ignacio, Colombia

Olga Milena García
Pontificia Universidad Javeriana, Colombia & Hospital Universitario San Ignacio, Colombia

Oscar Muñoz
Pontificia Universidad Javeriana, Colombia & Hospital Universitario San Ignacio, Colombia

Wilson Ricardo Bohórquez
Pontificia Universidad Javeriana, Colombia & Hospital Universitario San Ignacio, Colombia

Angel García
Pontificia Universidad Javeriana, Colombia & Hospital Universitario San Ignacio, Colombia

ABSTRACT

Medical practice, monitoring and control guidelines enable standardization, assessment and quality improvement in healthcare. This often implies collecting and analyzing electronic medical records (EMRs) in order to calculate compliance metrics and support evidence-based decision-making. However, for these benefits to materialize a set of challenges must be overcome, including the complexity required to represent guidelines in such a way that compliance can be automatically determined with the aid of software; the combination of both structured and unstructured (narrative text) data; and cultural or political barriers. In this chapter, we present a strategy to overcome these challenges using three case studies in chronic disease for a developing country. As such, this work contributes an approach to enable the use of ICT-supported medical guideline evaluation, in order to contribute to a more reliable and context-dependent way of improving healthcare in developing countries in particular.

DOI: 10.4018/978-1-5225-1724-5.ch012

INTRODUCTION

Medical guidelines have been widely used by governments and institutions to assess and improve the quality of healthcare services. They are typically developed through an evidence-based decision-making process and address elements for effective delivery of healthcare services considering a variety of settings, contexts and populations. For an institution, compliance with government regulation and internal standards of quality is the main priority, followed by an analysis for quality improvement as well as an input for detecting opportunities to generate new services. Once indicators have been aggregated over a set of institutions, region or countrywide analysis is possible conducing to recommendations in terms of public health policy.

The method used for evaluating compliance with a medical guideline depends on the institution, but is usually highly dependent on manual processes that involve selecting and checking a sample of medical records for where the guideline is applicable. Even though automatic evaluation of facts contained in Electronic Medical Record (EMR) systems should be a more effective strategy for evaluating whether an institution is following a guideline, the real complexity behind this strategy limits the possibilities. Such complexity results in the following set of challenges:

1. The first difficulty is structuring the guideline itself. Most guidelines are defined for human medical experts, so in order for them to be used as standards for automatically calculating an institution's compliance, they need to be structured for computer readability as well. Part of the issue is how to support the mechanical step-by-step procedure for structuring the guideline, but also checking that the guideline is complete, accurate, and easy to register and edit.
2. The second challenge stems from the fact that once a guideline is defined for direct, computer-supported analysis it will then have to be applied over a set of existing EMRs. However, often each EMR is a mix of structured and unstructured data. This means that there will be an initial problem in identifying the set of EMRs over which to calculate compliance. Furthermore, once the set of EMRs has been properly identified, calculating compliance will need to include structured data as well as narrative text contained in each record to verify compliance with the guideline.
3. Last but not least, there remains a non-technical hurdle. Cultural or political barriers may be at least as critical. On the preparation stage, there may be resistance or insufficient capability for the information to be properly recorded in the EMR system; there may be insufficient incentives; there may be lack of awareness or fear; and there may be disagreement or inconsistency with respect to the accuracy, depth or method that each institution is using and a consequent concern that aggregate indicators may be incomplete, incoherent, misused or strategically manipulated by others.

This chapter focuses on the first challenge and in doing so provides an initial strategy for dealing with the other two, especially in developing countries where unstructured data and immature EMR systems are more widespread. As such, it proposes a data structure for enabling the quality evaluation of health care services. This data structure allows the definition of an assessment tool for any medical guideline that can be applied semi-automatically to a set of EMR contained in an existing EMR system. The completeness of the proposed data structure was validated using it to describe a sample of medical guidelines recommendations related to prevalent diseases in a general hospital of a developing country.

The chapter is structured as follows: Section 2 reviews how the evaluation process is currently done and which projects have been proposed already to structure the guidelines, then Section 3 describes our approach using a data structure for describing clinical practice guidelines. In Section 4 we present a set of guidelines used to validate the proposed structure and we describe why we choose them, and finally we move on to Section 5 where we present our conclusions and propose future work.

MEDICAL GUIDELINE EVALUATION

Current Status, Approaches, and Challenges

Medical guidelines are syntheses of the best available evidence that support decision making by clinicians, managers, and policy makers. Numerous population-based studies demonstrate low compliance with guidelines produced by prominent government and professional agencies for chronic and acute conditions (Gagliardi, Brouwers, Palda, Lemieux-Charles, & Grimshaw, 2011). Several studies have evaluated different guideline dissemination and implementation strategies targeting medically qualified health care professionals that reported objective measures of provider behaviour and/or patient outcome. It is now clear that passive dissemination of educational materials is largely ineffective, whereas, audit and feedback, reminders and educational outreach and multifaceted interventions are more effective (Grimshaw et al., 2006).

Audit and feedback is widely used as a strategy to improve professional practice, either on its own or as a key component of multifaceted quality improvement interventions. Audit and feedback generally leads to moderate, but potentially important improvements in professional practice (N. Ivers et al., 2012; N. M. Ivers et al., 2014). The effectiveness of audit and feedback seems to depend on baseline performance and feedback provided more than once, and delivered in both verbal and written formats, including both explicit targets and an action plan (N. Ivers et al., 2012). In order to support feedback it is important to develop tools able to reduce the burden associated with the audit information recollection process. This section presents first the current audit process of medical guidelines compliance in healthcare providers in a developing country, then it explores the current works to structure medical guidelines, and finally, exposes the main challenges related to the assessment of medical guidelines.

Medical Guideline Evaluation Process

As part of the continuous quality improvement processes and the procedures required by the region healthcare secretaries and the Colombian Ministry of Health and Social Protection, it is mandatory for Health Care Providers (called IPS in Colombia) the development, presentation and update of institutional clinical practice guidelines and its compliance evaluation. Such guidelines must be developed for the treatment of the main diseases associated to the specific institution, and the compliance evaluation must be done for their own guidelines and for the nationwide guidelines and indicators designed for the country's most frequent pathologies (gpc.minsalud.gov.co). This complex process requires the continuous development and evaluation of adherence indicators for such guidelines; these indicators are designed by each IPS according to its own institutional goals and to comply with different healthcare standards proposed inside the national healthcare policies.

The process of compliance evaluation involves first the analysis and extraction of information from the medical records to obtain the data that is going to be used for the indicators evaluation. This process assumes that the healthcare providers involved in writing those records, perform such task in a proper manner and using the right fields. In Colombia the evaluation is done by manually inspecting the medical records in the cases where they are in paper (physical version). When the records are stored in an EMR system they can be evaluated by checking manually such electronic records (electronic version). These processes frequently consume a lot of time, economic and human resources in order to completely accomplish the aforementioned tasks. Additionally, it requires a variety of skills for the people involved in the analysis and evaluation (Johansen, Pedersen, & Ellingsen, 2015).

Although recently EMRs have been used for the evaluation of indicators and the conformity of healthcare goals (Downing et al., 2007; Garzon et al., 2012; Gonzalez et al., 2012; Van der Ent, 2008), in some cases this information is obtained late, delaying the implementation of improvements and adjustments to the processes necessary to accomplish optimal healthcare results.

Related Works on the Evaluation of Guidelines

Defining a structured language, which supports the definition of clinical practice guidelines, is a partially studied topic in which different approaches have been proposed. Those approaches partially cover the definition of machine-readable guidelines, but they have different purposes or are restricted to specific diseases.

PROforma (Fox, Patkar, & Thomson, 2006) is a process-modelling language in which the guidelines can be defined when they are related to well-defined processes. To model the processes PROforma makes use of four different types of task: Decisions, Actions, Enquiries and Plans. Decisions represent choices performed during the process, Actions are meant to be used for the different procedures performed during the process, Enquiries are used for representing the task of asking for information to an external entity and finally, Plans permit the representation of complex tasks composed of other tasks.

Arden (Samwald, Fehre, de Bruin, & Adlassnig, 2012), part of the HL7 standards, provides a language to structure MLMs (Medical Logic Module). Each MLM represents a clinical rule specified with great detail. In the context of using the guideline representation to be evaluated against an EMR, Arden lacks a clear connection to the EMR making the adherence test more complicated. This is due to the goal of Arden, which is to share knowledge among clinicians.

GEM (Shiffman et al., 2000), proposes an XML based schema definition intended to describe recommendations to be translated from a free-text representation to a structured representation. GEM represents in great detail the recommendations including their evidence and their strength.

Table 1, taken from our previous work (Pomares-Quimbaya, et al., 2015), renders for each approach the compliance of representing the necessary aspects related to a medical guideline recommendation. Although Arden represents the most complete language, it fails in our context of evaluating the adherence of EMRs.

Challenges of Medical Guideline Evaluation

Medical guidelines contribute to standardization of healthcare practices, response to recurring health issues (e.g. infection), fostering patient safety or improving quality of care (Pearson, 2001). However, in order for these benefits to materialize, a few hurdles need to be addressed.

The first difficulty is structuring the medical guideline itself. Most guidelines are defined for human medical experts, so in order for them to be used as standards for automatically calculating an institution's compliance, they need to be structured for computer readability as well (Hewelt & Kunde, 2014;

Table 1. Indicators used by PROforma, Arden and GEM

	PROforma	ARDEN
Phase		x
Diagnosis	x	x
Time	x	x
Risk Factor	x	x
Antecedents	x	x
Severity Level		

(Pomares-Quimbaya et al., 2015)

Serban, ten Teije, van Harmelen, Marcos, & Polo-Conde, 2007; Simalatsar, You, Gotta, Widmer, & De Micheli, 2014). Part of the issue is how to support the mechanical step-by-step procedure for structuring the guideline, but also checking that the guideline is complete, accurate, and easy to register and edit.

The second challenge stems from the fact that once a guideline is defined for direct computer-supported analysis, it will then have to be applied over a set of existing EMRs. However, often each EMR is a mix of structured and unstructured data (Macedo & Isaías, 2011). This means that there will be an initial problem in identifying the set of EMRs over which to calculate compliance. Furthermore, once the set of EMRs has been properly identified, calculating compliance will need to include structured data as well as narrative text contained in each record to verify compliance with the guideline. This comparison between a well-structured guideline and a record which combines structured and unstructured attributes is problematic, with potential incompleteness, ambiguity or incoherence to be found.

Last but not least, there remains a non-technical hurdle. Cultural or political barriers may be at least as critical and in some cases major barriers for more effective calculation of medical guideline compliance (Gajanayake, Sahama, & Iannella, 2014; Heath & Appan, 2014). On the preparation stage, there may be resistance or insufficient capability for the information to be properly recorded in the EMR system. On top of the aforementioned presence of unstructured data, usually narrative (e.g. progress notes, nursing notes), there may be insufficient incentives for filling in accurate and complete data, or in doing so when and where it is supposed to be recorded. In addition, there may be lack of awareness or fear that the analysis will be used for individual monitoring of health professionals. Also, there may be disagreement or inconsistency with respect to the accuracy, depth or method that each institution is using and, as a consequence, indicators may be incomplete, incoherent, misused or strategically manipulated by others.

MEDICAL GUIDELINE DEFINITION

Considering that one important challenge related to the implementation of a medical guideline is the compliance evaluation in the healthcare institution, this chapter proposes an innovative data structure to formally define the medical guideline indicators that should be assessed. The structure of this definition is intended to be machine-readable in order to allow the semi-automatic compliance evaluation using as input the facts contained in an EMR system. This section presents first an overview of the data structure, emphasizing on the decisions made in order to describe a medical guideline, and then each subsection describes the specific parts of the assessment tool.

Overview

The main purpose of the proposed data structure is to enable the quality department of a healthcare institution to define the indicators related to a medical guideline, and then support the automatic evaluation of them using as input the facts consigned in the EMR system. Figure 1 illustrates the medical guideline decomposed in a set of conditions. Each one of them describes one recommendation, using a consequent, and the characteristics of the patients to whom the recommendation applies, using a precedent. For instance, a precedent can be: patient with chronic renal failure who is hospitalized, and the consequent can be: estimation of GFR (Glomerular filtration rate).

The recommendation, described in the consequent, may involve a temporal restriction. This kind of restriction represents the periodicity or duration of the recommendation. For instance, the consequent must occur every 6 hours. Similarly, in order to evaluate the recommendation compliance the consequent has a relationship with an evaluation context that describes when a condition can be evaluated as positive. For the example, the evaluation context defines that the consequent must be true during all the hospitalizations of the patient in order to set as true the compliance.

Formally, the definition 1 represents the medical guideline. The following sections will describe in detail the conditionals and its components: the precedent and the consequent.

Definition 1. Medical Guideline Evaluation Instrument

A medical guideline evaluation instrument M is composed by a set of conditionals $M = \{C_1, C_2, \ldots, C_n\}$ *where* $C_i = \{ExpP, ExpC\}$, *ExpP represents the precedent and ExpC the consequent.*

Figure 1. Medical guideline overview

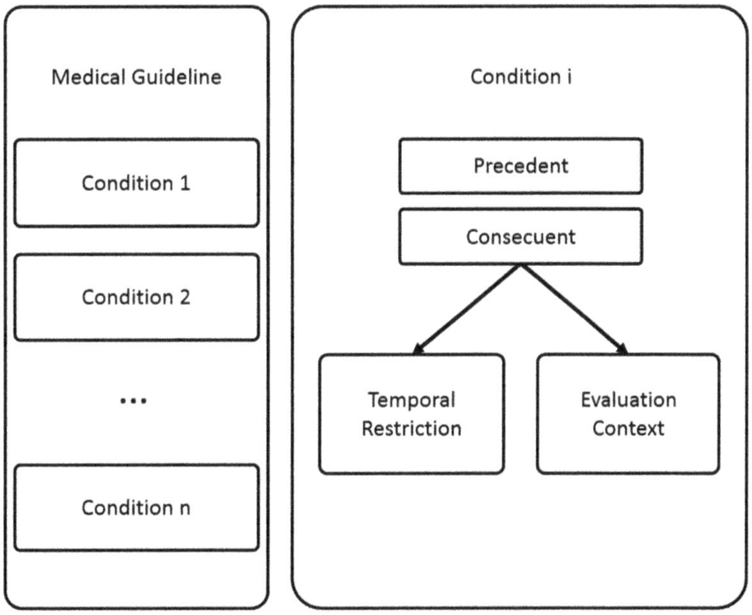

Conditional

The objective of the conditional is to represent the recommendations of a medical guideline using expressions connected by logical operators OP = (∧, ∨). The first part of the conditional called Precedent allows the definition of the characteristics of the patients to whom the recommendation applies. The second part, called Consequent describes the recommendations itself. The conditional is formally described in definition 2.

Definition 2. Conditional

A conditional C represents logically the recommendations described in a medical guideline and the context of evaluation where it must be evaluated. A conditional is composed by a precedent expression ExpP = {ExpPOPExpP|ExpP} where ExpP = {(ConceptI =Value)} and a consequent expression ExpC = {(ExpCOP ExpC)|ExpC}where ExpC={(ConceptII=Value), (tempRest), EvalContext}

The conditional uses a set of ConceptI and ConceptII to describe the characteristics of the patient and the recommendations, respectively. These concepts were identified through the analysis of global, national and institutional medical guidelines. They are described in detail in our previous work (Pomares-Quimbaya, et al. 2015.) and are summarized in the following list:

1. Conduct or Medical Intervention is the act, fact or method of interfering with the outcome or course of a medical condition. This concept is specialized in Laboratory Test, Medical Education, Medicine Supply, Procedure, Formulated Exams, and Formulated Medicine.
2. Location is the place where a medical act, fact or method occurs.
3. Risk Factor represents all the elements that can increase the likelihood of developing a disease.
4. Severity Level describes the categories that measure the relative impact of a disease on a patient.
5. Adverse Event is an injury related to medical management.
6. Diagnosis is the identification of the possible patient disease or disorder.
7. Moment during the attention of the patient. For example admission, hospitalization, hospital discharge, etc.
8. Antecedent is a relevant patient fact that occurs before and may be linked to subsequent events.
   ConceptI may have expressions using: {ConductoOrMedicalIntervention|Location|RiskFactor|SeverityLevelL|Adverse Event|Diagnosis|Moment|Antecedent}.
   ConceptII may have expressions using: {ConductoOrMedicalIntervention|Location|SeverityLevelL}.

The optional element of a consequent expression called tempRest represents the temporal restrictions defined in some medical recommendations. This temporal restriction describes the duration or the periodicity of the recommendation. For instance, a patient may have medicine supply each 8 hours. Definition 3 describes it.

Definition 3. Temporal Restriction

A temporal restriction describes the temporal boundaries of a medical recommendation within the medical history of a patient. This restriction can be expressed as follows:

tempRest = {Duration,Periodicity}
Duration = {value, UnitofMeasure}
Periodicity = {value, UnitofMeasure}
UnitofMeasure = {minute,hour,day,month,year,life}

The last part of the consequent expression ExpC is the evaluation context EvalContext. Due to its importance this element is going to be described in the following section.

Evaluation Context Definition

Based on the large number of attentions that can be gathered by the analysis of the conditional definition using ExpP, we have to create a mechanism able to select the best candidates for executing the evaluation based on the conditional definition. We defined an Evaluation Context as some additional criteria. This context allows the system to select the patients who qualify for the evaluation (e.g. only patients who were in the emergency room). Additionally, this context includes an accomplishment level that defines the times that a recommendation must be true in a medical record for considering it correct. An evaluation context is expressed as:

EvalContext = {EvalType, When}
EvalType = {Chronic|Acute}
When = {TempRelation,Situation,AccomplishmentLevel}
TempRelation = {During,before,after,start,end,M}
$Situation = \{ExpS,(keyword_1,...,keyword_n)\}$
$ExpS = \{(Concept_L = Value)\}$
$AccomplishmentLevel = \{All|AtLeast1|AtLeast_n\}$

The EvalType describes the granularity to which the evaluation is going to be made. In the Chronic case the granularity is the whole medical record. In the acute case the granularity level is the medical attention.

The TempRelation expresses the temporal relationship of a medical event and the recommendation. Sometimes a recommendation must be accomplished during the execution of a medical event, no matter when, other times it must be accomplished at the beginning, others at the end, or a time after the end. The possible relationships are illustrated in Figure 2 and are based on the definition of temporal events presented in (Pomares-Quimbaya, et al. 2015).

The Situation allows the definition of the specific characteristics that must have the medical events where the recommendation is going to be evaluated. The situation may have the same ConceptI, presented previously, plus some keywords that will be searched on the narrative texts of the medical records.

Finally, the AccomplishmentLevel defines how many times the recommendation must be true or in what kind of situations. It is important to notice that the AccomplishmentLevel is associated to the Situation. In some guidelines there is no need to use the Situation field, in those cases the default value associated to the Situation field it is the precedent expression ExpP itself.

Figure 2. Temporal relationship

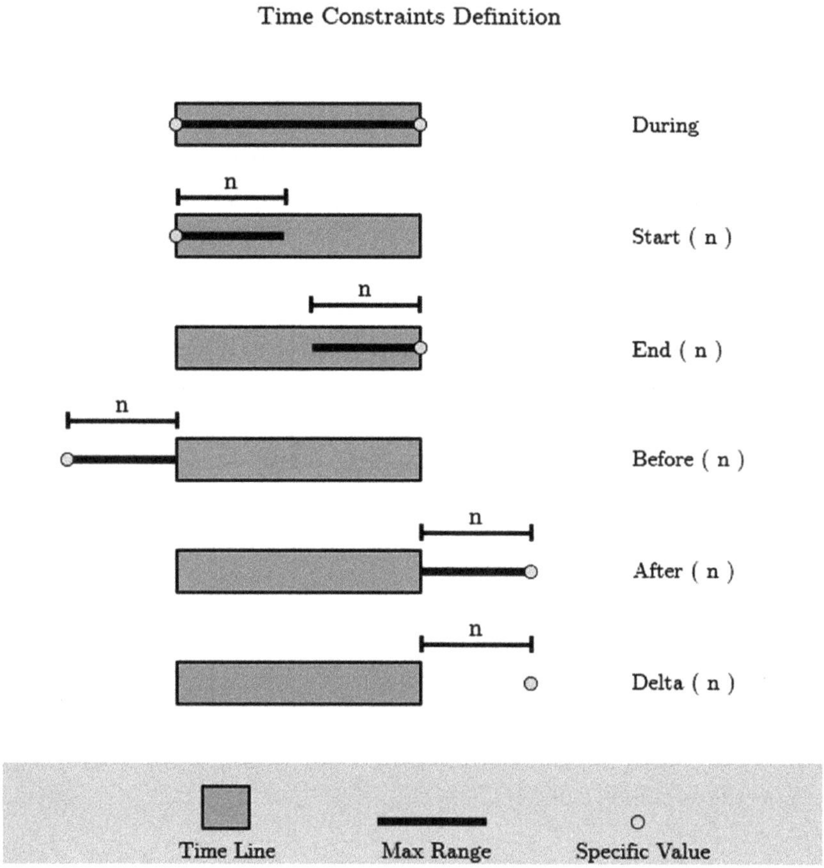

VALIDATION

Selection of Medical Guidelines

In order to select the clinical practice guidelines for validation, we take into account the prevalence of the disease, the costs generated to the healthcare system and the application in local, national and international levels. Subsequently we evaluated the process and outcome indicators on these guidelines.

In a local context, we consider evaluating the guideline for community-acquired pneumonia, given the acute nature of the disease and the incidence rates ranging from 1.0 per 1,000 to 11 per 1,000 inhabitants.

Nationally, we adopt the guideline developed by the Colombian Ministry of Health and Social Protection for chronic obstructive pulmonary disease (COPD), given the chronic nature of the disease and its prevalence of 8.9% in the Colombian population.

From an international point of view, we select the guidelines for the acute coronary syndrome developed by the international organization American Heart Association (AHA), given the high diffusion of these guidelines and the fact that the acute coronary syndrome is the most prevalent cause of death worldwide.

Assessment Tools Related to Chronique Conditions

In this section we proceed to model the selected Clinical Practice Guidelines using the proposed medical guideline definition notation. These guidelines defined by medical doctors after a training process on the notation.

Coronary Syndrome

The international guideline for acute coronary syndrome states that all patients with diagnostic impression of acute myocardial infarction, an ECG should be performed 12 lead as soon as possible, with a limit of time between first medical contact with a target delay equal or minor to 10 min.

Based in the narrative guideline we define the following precedent expression:

MedGuideline = {ExpP, ExpC,}
ExpP = {ExpP1, ExpP2, ExpP3,ExpP4,ExpP5,ExpP6,ExpP7,ExpP8}
ExpP1 = {(DIAGNOSTIC = (Acute myocardial infarction, unspecified I219))}
ExpP2 = {(DIAGNOSTIC = (Acute transmural myocardial infarction of anterior wall I210))}
ExpP3 = {(DIAGNOSTIC = (Acute transmural myocardial infarction of inferior wall I211))}
ExpP4 = {(DIAGNOSTIC = (Acute transmural myocardial infarction of unspecified site I213))}
ExpP5 = {(DIAGNOSTIC = (Subsequent myocardial infarction of anterior wall I220))}
ExpP6 = {(DIAGNOSTIC = (Subsequent myocardial infarction of inferior wall I221))}
ExpP7 = {(DIAGNOSTIC = (Subsequent myocardial infarction of other sites I228))}
ExpP8 = {(DIAGNOSTIC = (Subsequent myocardial infarction of unspecified site I229))}

The consequent expression is defined by:

$ExpC = \{ExpC_1\}$
$ExpC_1$ *= {(FORMULED EXAMS = Normal conventional electrocardiogram),*
(tempRest),EvalContext} tempRest = {Duration}
Duration = {10,minute}

For this case the Evalcontext is used to specify a situation where medical act, fact or method occurs.

EvalContext = {EvalType,When}
EvalType = {Acute}
When = {TempRelation,Situation,AccomplishmentLevel}
TempRelation = {During}
Situation = {ExpS}
ExpS = {(LOCATION = 1 Floor - Urgencies)} AccomplishmentLevel = {All}

Community-Acquired Pneumonia

In the guideline of the Community-acquired pneumonia, the Hospital states that patients with this suspected diagnosis in the emergency department, based on clinical findings, should have an x-ray method diagnostic. The precedent expression is defined as:

MedGuideline = {ExpP,ExpC,}
ExpP = {ExpP1,ExpP2,ExpP3}
ExpP1 = {(DIAGNOSTIC = (Bacterial pneumonia, unspecified J159))}
ExpP2 = {(DIAGNOSTIC = (Other bacterial pneumonia J158))}
ExpP3 = {(DIAGNOSTIC = (Other pneumonia, organism unspecified J188))}

Now we define the consequent, for this case a keyword field is used for CURB-65 and CRB-65 as the assessment of severity of and the required formulated exam.

ExpC = {ExpC1, ExpC2}
ExpC1 = {(SEVERITYLEVEL = RISKFACTOR),(KEYWORDS =(CURB-65,CRB-65),
ExpC2 = {(FORMULED EXAMS = X-RAY), EvalContext

In this case the EvalContext doesn't have a specific Situation, as a consequence the default Situation is used and it is the same ExpP.

EvalContext = {EvalType,When}
EvalType = {Acute,Situation,AccomplishmentLevel}
When = {TempRelation}
TempRelation = {During}
Situation = {ExpP}
AccomplishmentLevel = {AtLeastn = 1}

Chronic Obstructive Pulmonary Disease

The national guideline for Chronic Obstructive Pulmonary Disease states that all patients diagnosed with COPD should have pre- and post-bronchodilator spirometry confirmation as confirmatory diagnostic method.

The precedent expression is defined as:

MedGuideline = {ExpP,ExpC,}
ExpP = {ExpP1}
ExpP1 = {(DIAGNOSTIC = (Chronic obstructive pulmonary disease, unspecified J449))}

The consequent expression is defined as:

ExpC = {ExpC1, ExpC2}
ExpC1 = {(FORMULED EXAMS = (Pre and Post spirometry)),EvalContext}

ExpC2 = {(FORMULED EXAMS = (Pre and Post bronchodilator spirometry)),EvalContext}

In this case the Evalcontext is used to specify another situation where medical act, fact or method occurs.

EvalContext = {EvalType,When}
EvalType = {Chronic}
When = {TempRelation,Situation,AccomplishmentLevel}
TempRelation = {after}
Situation = {ExpS}
ExpS = {(LOCATION = External consulting)}
AccomplishmentLevel = {AtLeastn = 1}

The definition of these conditionals extracted from accepted medical guidelines, as well as others not included in this chapter, allowed us to validate the ability of our proposal to represent diverse medical guidelines related to different diseases and varied evaluation contexts.

CONCLUSION

In this chapter we have shown some of the most pressing challenges related to evaluating compliance against standard medical guidelines. These include: a difficulty in expressing the guideline in a computer-readable format; the combination of structured and unstructured data from EMRs, in order to evaluate compliance; and cultural or political difficulties related to ICT-supported guideline evaluation.

With respect to the first challenge, namely representing guidelines in computer-readable format, we have started from a description of how this is being done, paying special attention to the process carried out in a developing country university hospital. Through a collaborative effort between medical and informatics researchers, the chapter has proposed a strategy and a notation that can accomplish a computer-readable definition. The guiding principles have been to use expressions that are machine-readable, while being expressed in a notation that can also be understood by trained users without adding unnecessary complexity, as well as reducing the risk of ambiguity in the resulting expressions. We also describe the way in which further guidelines can be elaborated and validated against the original guideline.

Once the guideline has been properly expressed, the chapter presents the validation in three cases where the presence of structured data as well as unstructured narrative text is present in order to move to the second stage: calculating compliance at an institutional level.

The third challenge, which is often hardest, is not technological, but related to cultural or political barriers. The first premise is that instead of neglecting or attempting to reduce the amount of unstructured data, the strategy opts for exploiting the information already contained in EMRs, regardless of whether it is structured or not. This reduces the difficulty of forcing or assuring an already structured set of EMRs, which may not be an option. In addition, we present the way in which guidelines can be selected for automation, in order to create the necessary conditions for social acceptance of the results. Moreover, this selection helps in focusing the efforts where they can have a higher impact in terms of local conditions and needs. As a result, the intention is to be able to increase the potential that ICT-. support can have in improving healthcare in developing countries.

As future work, the calculation and validation of compliance are in the pipeline for the very near future. Later, aggregate results from various institutions can be articulated in order to provide policy recommendations for healthcare in developing countries. Finally, issues related to performance, privacy and distributed data can also provide interesting research paths.

ACKNOWLEDGMENT

This work is part of the project entitled "Sistema de análisis de indicadores de adherencia a las guías de práctica clínica" funded by Pontificia Universidad Javeriana and Hospital Universitario San Ignacio

REFERENCES

Downing, A., Rudge, G., Cheng, Y., Tu, Y.-K., Keen, J., & Gilthorpe, M. S. (2007). Do the uk government's new quality and outcomes framework (qof) scores adequately measure primary care performance? a cross-sectional survey of routine healthcare data. *BMC Health Services Research*, *7*(1), 166. doi:10.1186/1472-6963-7-166 PMID:17941984

Fox, J., Patkar, V., & Thomson, R. (2006). Decision support for health care: The proforma evidence base. *Informatics in Primary Care*, *14*(1), 49–54. PMID:16848966

Gagliardi, A. R., Brouwers, M. C., Palda, V. A., Lemieux-Charles, L., & Grimshaw, J. M. (2011). How can we improve guideline use? a conceptual framework of implementability. *Implementation Science; IS*, *6*(1), 26. doi:10.1186/1748-5908-6-26 PMID:21426574

Gajanayake, R., Sahama, T., & Iannella, R. (2014). The role of perceived usefulness and attitude on electronic health record acceptance. *International Journal of E-Health and Medical Communications*, *5*(4), 108–119. doi:10.4018/ijehmc.2014100107

Garzon, G., Gil, A., Alvaro, A., Rodrigo, R., Cerezo, M., & Dominguez, C. (2012). Relationship between process indicators measured using electronic records and intermediate health outcomes in patients with diabetes. *Revista de calidad asistencial: organo de la Sociedad Espanola de Calidad Asistencial, 28* (4), 207–216.

González, G. G., Morales, D. R., Palomino, M. Á. R., Gómez, D. T., Barrera, V. H., & De Miguel, Á. G. (2012). Evaluación sobre historia clínica electrónica. asociación entre indicadores de proceso medidos sobre historia electrónica y resultados intermedios en salud, en pacientes con hipertensión. *Atencion Primaria*, *44*(12), 709–719. doi:10.1016/j.aprim.2012.06.004 PMID:22980946

Grimshaw, J., Eccles, M., Thomas, R., MacLennan, G., Ramsay, C., Fraser, C., & Vale, L. (2006). Toward evidence-based quality improvement. *Journal of General Internal Medicine*, *21*(S2), S14–S20. PMID:16637955

Heath, M., & Appan, R. (2014). *Impact of information technology culture conflict on meaningful use of electronic health records system: A conceptual framework*. Academic Press.

Hewelt, M., & Kunde, A. (2014). *Integration of documentation task into medical treatment processes in the hospital*. Academic Press.

Ivers, N., Jamtvedt, G., Flottorp, S., Young, J. M., Odgaard-Jensen, J., French, S. D., & Oxman, A. D. et al. (2012). Audit and feedback: Effects on professional practice and healthcare outcomes. *The Cochrane Library*. PMID:22696318

Ivers, N. M., Grimshaw, J. M., Jamtvedt, G., Flottorp, S., O'Brien, M. A., French, S. D., & Odgaard-Jensen, J. et al. (2014). Growing literature, stagnant science? systematic review, meta-regression and cumulative analysis of audit and feedback interventions in health care. *Journal of General Internal Medicine*, *29*(11), 1534–1541. doi:10.1007/s11606-014-2913-y PMID:24965281

Johansen, M., Pedersen, Å., & Ellingsen, G. (2015). The role of medical transcriptionists in producing high-quality documentation. *Studies in Health Technology and Informatics*, *218*, 114. PMID:26262537

Macedo, M., & Isaías, P. (2011). A methodology to develop a clinical ontology for healthcare business. *Human Interface and the Management of Information. Interacting with Information*, 285–291.

Pearson, M. (2001). The role of national guidelines in the prevention of healthcare-associated infections. *Japanese Pharmacology and Therapeutics, 29*(10), 667-679.

Pomares-Quimbaya, A., Amórtegui, M. P., González, R. A., Muñoz, O., Bohórquez, W. R., García, O. M., & Ascanio, M. M. (2015). A system for the semi-automatic evaluation of clinical practice guideline indicators. *International Journal of Reliable and Quality E-Healthcare*, *4*(1), 1–10.

Roncancio, C. (1997). Toward duration-based, constrained and dynamic event types. In *Active, real-time, and temporal database systems, second international workshop, proceedings* (pp. 176–193). doi:10.1007/3-540-49151-1_10

Samwald, M., Fehre, K., de Bruin, J., & Adlassnig, K.-P. (2012). The arden syntax standard for clinical decision support: Experiences and directions. *Journal of Biomedical Informatics, 45*(4), 711 - 718. Retrieved from http://www.sciencedirect.com/science/article/pii/S1532046412000226

Serban, R., ten Teije, A., van Harmelen, F., Marcos, M., & Polo-Conde, C. (2007). Extraction and use of linguistic patterns for modelling medical guidelines. *Artificial Intelligence in Medicine*, *39*(2), 137–149. doi:10.1016/j.artmed.2006.07.012 PMID:16963241

Shiffman, R. N., Karras, B. T., Agrawal, A., Chen, R., Marenco, L., & Nath, S. (2000). Gem: A proposal for a more comprehensive guideline document model using xml. *Journal of the American Medical Informatics Association*, *7*(5), 488–498. doi:10.1136/jamia.2000.0070488 PMID:10984468

Simalatsar, A., You, W., Gotta, V., Widmer, N., & De Micheli, G. (2014). Representation of medical guidelines with a computer interpretable model. *International Journal of Artificial Intelligence Tools*, *23*(03), 1460003. doi:10.1142/S0218213014600033

Suarez-Coloma, J., Verdier, C., & Roncancio, C. (2014). Quality indices in medical alert systems. In *ICEIS 2014 - Proceedings of the 16th international conference on enterprise information systems,* (pp. 81–89). Retrieved from doi:10.5220/0004893900810089

Van der Ent, C. (2008). Quality assessment: Is the truth in the outcome? *The European Respiratory Journal*, *31*(1), 6–7. doi:10.1183/09031936.00141507 PMID:18166589

KEY TERMS AND DEFINITIONS

Electronic Medical Record: It is a record in a digital format that contains the health-related information of an individual. Typically, one health care institution manages the set of electronic medical records of the patients that have had a medical interaction with their medical staff.

Electronic Medical Record System: It is a system in charge of managing electronic medical records.

Medical Guideline: It is a document that contains the set of guidelines and recommendations around the diagnosis, management and treatment of a specific healthcare service. Medical guidelines have been widely used by governments and institutions to assess and improve the quality of healthcare services. They are typically developed through an evidence-based decision-making process and address elements for effective delivery of healthcare services considering a variety of settings, contexts and populations.

Medical Guideline Evaluation Instrument Conditional: Represents logically the recommendations described in a medical guideline and the context of evaluation where it must be evaluated. A conditional is composed by a precedent expression and a consequent expression.

Medical Guideline Evaluation Instrument: It is the set of recommendations defined in a medical guideline expressed using a structured language that can be processed by a machine.

Structured Attribute: In the context of electronic medical records, a structured attribute is an attribute that has a predefined set of values; for instance, the diagnosis coded using the ICD10 codes.

Unstructured Attribute: In the context of electronic medical records, an unstructured attribute is an attribute that does not have a predefined set of values. Examples of unstructured attributes are those that contain narrative texts or images.

Chapter 13
Informed Consent in Healthcare:
A Study Case of Genetic Services

Bo Yu
George Mason University, USA

Duminda Wijesekera
George Mason University, USA

Paulo Costa
George Mason University, USA

ABSTRACT

Informed consents, either for treatment or sensitive information use/disclosure, that protect the privacy of patient/participant information subject to law that in certain circumstances may override patient wishes, are mandatory practice in healthcare. Similarly, for protecting and respecting research participants, informed consents are also prerequisite for human subjects research. Although the healthcare industry has widely adopted Electronic Medical Record (EMR) systems, consents are still obtained and stored primarily on paper or scanned electronic documents. Integrating a consent management system for different purposes into an EMR system involves various implementation challenges. A case study, informed consent for genetic services, is used to show how genetic informed consents placed new challenges on the traditional ethical standards of informed consent, and how appropriate consents can be electronically obtained and automatically enforced using a system that combines medical workflows and hierarchically, ontologically motivated rule enforcement. Finally, this chapter describes an implementation that uses the open-source software-based addition of these components to an open-source EMR system, so that existing systems do not need to be scrapped or otherwise rendered obsolete.

DOI: 10.4018/978-1-5225-1724-5.ch013

INTRODUCTION

The healthcare industry seeks quality improvement strategies to provide standardized, safer and more efficient patient services as well as medical research, focusing on patient safety, quality of care, risk management, data security and privacy preservation. The term "informed consent", first used by a California appeals court in 1957 (Cal. App. Ct. 1957), has become a vital ethical doctrine in medical practice. The American Medical Association states that "obtaining informed consent is an ethical obligation of the practice of medicine and a legal requirement per statute and case law in all 50 States" (O'Leary, 2010). In healthcare domain, informed consent has been considered one of the effective strategies to achieve the above goals. Herein the authors focus on three different categories: consent for medical treatment; consent for sensitive medical information use and disclosure; and consent for human subjects research.

In the last several decades, evolving computer-based Information Technology (IT) in healthcare has changed how computing systems support healthcare service delivery, with examples including Electronic Medical Record (EMR) systems and Personal Health Record (PHR) systems. The U.S government plays a major role in promoting healthcare IT, including EMR systems. The healthcare industry has adopted EMR systems widely. Nonetheless, nearly all EMR systems do not have an integrated electronic informed consent management system to support obtaining and automatically enforcing, patients' or participants' informed consents during treatment or medical research. In current practice, nearly all medical or research facilities use paper-based informed consent forms. The common approach used for managing informed consent forms in EMR systems is to scan paper consent forms and store them in electronic media, thereby restricting it to basic record keeping. Scanned consents are difficult to use by electronic information systems during medical processes, which makes caregivers responsible for enforcing the consents the same way it was done before introducing the EMR systems. Advanced automated features such as consistent enforcement of informed consent pursuant to statutes, regulations and guidelines are missing. In addition, hospitals spend on average $80,000 per year (Anonymous, 2007) scanning consent forms to perpetuate an inefficient, less than perfect consent system that results in subpar enforcement in the form of wrong or inapplicable consents. Failure to obtain informed consent is a top-ten reason for generating medical malpractice claims; "a properly completed consent form would have prevented 45% of errors on surgery wrong sites" (Compbell, 2004). Furthermore, studies concerning enforcement of medical informed consent in existing EMR systems reveal that no EMR systems support dynamically obtaining, and automatically enforcing, patients' informed consents when implementing medical processes. Consequently, a mechanism to implement and enforce e-consent is needed.

Informed consents in healthcare are governed by statutes and regulations that change over time. For example, a medical lawsuit that establishes precedent may trigger a new or amended statute or regulation or alter how a law is interpreted. Nevertheless, studies on consent laws are scarce, perhaps because ever changing laws would cause such studies to have a short shelf life. Issuing proper medical consent demands to evaluate all consent rules and to determine the type of consent to be obtained from the appropriate consent provider. Yet, no implementation method or modeling changes to consent laws are available that govern specific institutional practices (Beauchamp, & Childress, 1989). Consent is rendered unreliable without adhering to corresponding changes in laws. Moreover, consent statutes and regulations are complex. At times, ambiguous and complex laws (e.g., precedent changing interpretations of the law that, due to ambiguity, is subject to multiple interpretations) result in having gaps between user's understanding and the mechanized enforcements. Thus, a methodology for acquiring proper consent based on evolving law must be able to accommodate the dynamism inherent in changing regulations.

Authors' approach incorporates a medical consent management component into an existing EMR system to obtain and automatically enforce dynamically e-consent by using workflow technologies. More specifically, the authors use ontology-based knowledge representation and reasoning mechanisms to obtain required informed consents based on requester role, request purposes, each unique patient situation to ensure compliance with consent laws pertaining to the applicable sub-discipline. This technique also enforces protection of patient privacy in EMR systems. A case study, informed consent for genetic services, is used to show authors' work.

Following this Introduction, Section 2 describes informed consent in healthcare domain; Section 3 provides a case study, to show detailed models of authors' approach; Section 4 displays an implementation and, finally, Section 5, entitled "Conclusion," summarizes the proposed EMR system and briefly identifies future improvements.

MEDICAL INFORMED CONSENT

Categories of Consent

As mentioned above, medical informed consent has become the bedrock of medical practice. It majorly falls into three categories:

Treatment Consent

Patient safety, quality of care is the first major concern in practice medicine. Currently, every provider must obtain consent from a patient or guardian before commencing treatment, terminating treatment and choosing among alternative treatments. Nonetheless, the forms of treatment consent are various. In some cases, the patient or legal guardian must consent and/or sign a document memorializing that consent has been given. And yet, in most care providing entities, the patient showing up or requesting diagnosis or treatment constitutes default consent.

Informed treatment consent– either expressed or derived– is an important aspect of proper medical treatment, including but not limited to undertaking alternative treatments or terminating treatment. That process includes providing an unbiased risk/benefit analysis; explaining alternative treatments in a way that the patient understands, accurately communicating the care provider's understanding of the appropriateness of the treatment; advantages and disadvantages of obtaining the treatment or not obtaining it; and available alternatives (Appelbaum, & Thomas, 1995). The informed aspect of consent requires care receiver's awareness of he/she is willing to consent without undue influence by caregivers, insurers, or other involved actors.

Another requirement is caregiver acknowledgment that the patient and/or guardian have the mental capacity to consent. This makes psychiatric consents and consent given under anesthesia particularly difficult. Many federal, state and local governments have developed laws and regulations, and healthcare organizations have developed guidelines, for obtaining and memorializing informed treatment consent. Traditionally, the care seeker or his/her legal consent holder sign consent forms.

Much literature shows that researchers focus their research on different informed treatment consent requirements. For the standards of disclosing treatment benefits, risks, and alternatives, Studdert, D. M., et al. (2007) analyzed geographic variation in informed consent law. Authors in (Boonstra, & Nash,

2000; Bourgeois et al., 2008; Buchanan, 2004; Grisso, & Appelbaum, 1998; Holder, 1987) assessed patients' decisional capability to assent to treatment. In (Fisher, 2002), authors described four psycho-legal standards, communicating a choice, factual understanding, appreciation of the situation, and rational manipulation of information, all used to evaluate a patient's competence in giving consent. However, to date, this aspect of consent lacks a widely accepted standard.

Advances in medicine and technologies bring new challenges to treatment consent. For example, advantages in genetics being adopted as medically acceptable indicators to provide preventive and pre-emptive treatment for hereditary diseases. Gene therapy inserts genetic material into patients' targeted cells to treat disease. Up to date, gene therapy has been used to treat cardiovascular disease and cancer. Thomas Wirth (Wirth, Parker, & Ylä-Herttuala, 2013) made projections that "Gene therapy… will sooner or later be part of the standard care for a variety of different diseases". Unlike common treatment, informed consent delivers explicit risks/benefits of treatment to help patients in making a decision; it has been very difficult to determine precisely immediate benefits from gene therapy. Without full awareness patients' interests and choice may become compromised. Therefore, the contents of automatically generated consent forms should be dynamic, clear and explicit to the individuals.

Although less research has been devoted to managing treatment consent in EMR systems compared to protecting identifiable patient information, many researchers continue to improve consent treatment management. See for example, papers "Informed consent for clinical treatment" (Hall, Prochazka, & Fink, 2012) and "Informed Consent for Medical Treatment and Research: A Review" (Del Carmen, & Joffe, 2005) that introduced the basic concepts of informed treatment consent and made several practical suggestions for processing treatment consents effectively. However, none of those suggestions or analysis provides approaches to obtain dynamically or enforce automatically informed treatment consent in EMR systems. Even though, many healthcare organizations have attempted to include electronic consent management in their EMR systems. Veterans Administration Medical Centers use iMedConsent™ (VHA HANDBOOK 1004.05, 2005) that supports electronic access, completion, signing and storage of informed consent forms and advanced directives. iMedConsent has two parts: Software application and clinical content library. iMedConsent generates consents on each procedure without workflows, so the system is limited; it neither dynamically gains informed consents at the point of providing treatments nor enforces consents on medical procedures.

Some medical treatments are procedure-oriented, established by specialty boards as practice standards consisting of activities that caregivers must complete. Required informed treatment consents are embedded in some of those activities, which is an important factor that can change the medical treatment workflow. Standardized treatment procedures, documented in guidelines, usually require multiple checks. However, current EMR systems do not truly support and enforce pre-defined treatment workflow in run-time. To surmount this challenge, the authors proposed using workflow technologies to develop a Workflow-based EMR system in authors' previous work "Building Dialysis Workflows into EMRs" (Yu, & Wijesekera, 2013).

Authors' Workflow-based EMR system provides procedural choreography for treatment regimens using a Workflow Management System (WfMS). Authors' Workflow-based EMR system directly controls the progression of predefined and prebuilt care procedures that comply with local and national standards and policies; and also by providing flexibility that caregivers may need to continue treatment when, in their judgment, superior care compels moving to the next or alternate methods. Inability to obtain consent in emergencies is an example of an exception to a predefined workflow. Authors' system is also well suited to study healthcare delivery safety and quality care issues: Workflow logs perform an ongoing audit trail to satisfy accountability requirements and can also be used to improve the workflow. Furthermore, to enforce consent requirements, EMR systems must conditionally grant permissions upon prior receipt of valid, appropriate consent. Therefore, a Consent Management System (CMS) should be introduced in existing EMR systems. By leveraging the fact that medical consents accompany medical procedures, the best way to implement a CMS is by incorporating a medical consent management component into a Workflow-based EMR system. Without changing the Workflow-based EMR system architecture, the authors treat a CMS as an additional component of WfMS. Informed consents obtained by authors' CMS are stored in the EMR as part of patient medical records. The authors also designed additional user interfaces for users to issue missing but required treatment consents. See authors' paper "Consent-Based Workflow Control in EMRs" for more information (Yu, Wijesekera, & Costa, 2014).

Privacy Consent

Patient privacy is the second major concern in consents. In general medicine, informed privacy consent, provides the proper opportunity and knowledge for patients and/or research participants to understand and decide how the medical community can use and share their identifiable medical information. The Health Insurance Portability and Accountability Act (HIPAA) defines Protect Health Information (PHI) as "information that identifies the individual or for which there is a reasonable basis to believe can be used to identify the individual" (Federal Register, Vol. 78, No. 17, 2013, pp1689). HIPAA and other healthcare-related privacy laws mandate how patients' PHI may be used and disclosed. Every medical entity/provider must obtain a patient or guardian's informed consent before sharing and/or using patient PHI except for specified purposes of use and disclosure, such as treatment, for public health activities. In authors' previous work, the authors analyzed HIPAA in a great detail. However, HIPAA only governs covered entities.

Similar to treatment consent for genetic diseases, studies of, and methodologies for, protecting privacy of genetic information have lagged behind scientific advances. The harms of wrongly releasing or misusing genetic information are more than the physical harm, but so-called "psychosocial" harms (Strouse, 2005), which may cause societal discrimination (uninsurability, unemployability), even breakdown of family relationships. Prince et al. describe three practical genetic counseling cases that illustrate genetic discrimination (Prince, & Roche, 2014). The fundamental covenant of protecting patient privacy is embodied in patient-doctor privilege. Compromising genetic information privacy may stigmatize someone as carrying a genetic marker for a disorder or disease. Many researchers have suggested adopting traditional information protecting methodologies to protect patients' confidentiality. Yet, unlike other clinical datum, genetic information is unique and traceable to an individual or group of individuals who share a genetic inheritance (Mascalzoni, et al., 2008, & Gostin, Hodge, 1999). For example, certain genetic information of an individual may not only precisely identify him/her as high risk of certain hereditary disease(s), but also indicate that his/her relatives may have the same risks due to a hereditable gene. Consequently, traditional methodologies for privacy protection, such as de-identification, are not as well suited to the new area. Informed consent complied with proper privation laws tailored for genetic research and clinical usage constitutes a strong basis for ensuring appropriate genetic privacy.

In the past decade, consent management has received considerable attention from researchers, healthcare organizations, and publications proposing different ways to improve electronic consent management. Especially, most of those e-consent approaches focus mainly on sharing medical data, privacy, and security aspects (Grimson, Stephens, Jung, Grimson, Berry, & Pardon, 2001; Saranummi,

2005). For example, "eConsent: The Design and Implementation of Consumer Consent Mechanisms in an Electronic Environment," Coiera and Clark (2004) provided guidelines for designing an e-consent system. Another relevant work is by Ruan C. and Yeo S.S. (2009) that used a UML Model to design an e-consent system. They first identified various parts necessary to specify the e-Consent rules about patient record protection, then used UML to model the properties required by an e-consent system to make the associated patient record protection rules explicit and verifiable. That theoretical work was neither used to design nor implement an e-consent system that works with an EMR.

Rusello G. et al. (2008) proposed a consent-based healthcare management workflow where patients can control disclosing of their medical data based on workflows that are related to inter-institution transfers such as consults. Others have proposed e-consent management to be integrated with EMR or electronic health records systems (Bergmann, Bott, Pretschner, & Haux, 2007; O'Keefe, Greenfield, & Goodchild, 2005; Sheppard, Safavi-Naini, & Jafari, 2009; Win, & Fulcher, 2007). Win et al. (2002) in their paper "Implementing patients consent in electronic health record systems" expressed patient consent using an interface-based approach. Regarding enforcement of privacy consents in existing EMR systems, Bhatti, R. and Grandison, T. (2007) quoted several reports about healthcare privacy, concluding that IT system security mechanisms to enforce patients' consents for privacy were under-utilized and often bypassed. As mentioned in authors' previous works, privacy consent has a lot in common with treatment consent. Nevertheless, they are different in the following aspects:

1. **Issues/Objects are Dealt with Differently:** For privacy consent, patients decide how to use or disclose their identifiable medical information; by contrast, for treatment consent patients decide what should be done to their body.
2. **Who is Covered:** In privacy consent, HIPAA covers the medical information in what are known as covered entities. These are health providers/hospitals/health plans/healthcare clearing house and the like. Non-covered entities, such as private pharmaceutical factories have to abide by state privacy laws and organizational policies.
3. **The Type of Consent Affects the Government's Ability Override Patient Wishes:** The patient does not solely control consent regarding sharing of a patient's identifiable information. This type of consent also depends on the purposes of use and disclosure and a hierarchy of controls applies to the final decision. For example, HIPAA or state law can override a patient who rejects sharing his/her identifiable medical information that relates to a "Serious Threat to health or safety (OCR, 2003, pp 8)" Pursuant to an individual's right to be free of unwanted bodily invasion, patients have more power when deciding their treatment procedures. Consequently in normal care, providers must execute valid treatment consents.

The differences between the two categories of informed consents preclude using the same methodology to obtain informed consent for protecting privacy, especially because privacy rules that reflect public policy may override patient wishes. Thus, the additional factors of governmental override add complexity to protecting privacy for information sharing management in EMR systems. In HIPAA, the purpose of using and disclosing PHI provides a good example; it requires additional components for managing and enforcing this kind of consent in EMR systems in different levels. The traditional authentication strategy, like Role-based Access Control (RBAC), is insufficient (Al Faresi, Wijesekera, & Moidu, 2010). Authors' approach combines patient consents with the hierarchy privacy rules of regulation to determine the correct subsequent actions.

Participating Research Consent

Protecting and respecting participants of human subject research is the third major concern in healthcare domain. In most cases, informed consent for participating in human subjects research is a prerequisite. Participation in research allows researchers to generate and analyze new data or use their old data/samples. Traditional medical research may be well designed within a fixed time. The participants are informed with sufficient information about the study purpose, the procedures used in the study, and potential risks and benefits, etc. and the participants have the right to withdraw their consent at any time.

Contemporary medical research, especially biomedical research, provides many challenges to the currently accepted ethical standards of informed consent in both categories (Mascalzoni, et al. 2005; Knoppers, 2005; Petersen, 2007)

One challenge of designing consent for participating biomedical research and consent for performing a medical treatment is: in general medicine, clinicians seek patients' permission to perform planned procedures and/or to use their medical information for treatment. The patients are knowledgeable about the risks/benefits of performing procedures. Correspondingly, the benefits or risks of participating a genetic study may not be foreseen at the time of consent. As stated in (Strouse, 2005; The Presidential Commission for the Study of Bioethical Issues, 2013), obtaining informed consent in biomedical research settings present differences in required techniques and approaches when compared to clinical practice. In addition, informed consent is a process rather than an occurrence at the one-point action. Another challenge of consent for reusing sensitive medical data or samples in research is: in general medicine, patients reasonably consider that their medical information constitutes their own private information and, hence, are unwilling to either share or have divulged such information beyond participated study, as well as they, are easily able to withdraw such consent at any time. Conversely, the new genetic researches based on the enormous existing data or samples around the world, and may develop over time, which cause re-consent or completely strike out widely shared genetic data is impossible. The fundamental ethical principle of research consent may no longer be suitable. Irrespective of the purpose of research, methodologies for respecting participants and preventing them from both emotional distress and social risk have not, however, kept pace with rapid medicine and technique advances.

Hence, it is no surprise that some genetic medical practices and biomedical research are performed without obtaining appropriate informed consent. For example, researchers may entice participants to participate in a proposed study without providing them with the proper informed consent forms. To address this issue, some researchers advocate different methodologies such as using overly stringent policies to protect participants from harm, and to encourage trust in the research study itself. Obtaining written informed consent of testing to produce genetic data is such an example. But this approach potentially risks limiting scientific innovation (Hallinan, et al., 2015) Genetic research advances also benefit public health (Khoury, & Dorman, 1998). One of the evidences is breast cancer 1 (BRCA 1), where a gene mutation that can be used for general population to predict and prevent from disease (Struewing, & Abeliovich, 1995). Other researchers have proposed a new, open-consent model for medical and scientific genetic research (Lunshof, et al., 2008) or open-access policies for genetic data sharing (Kaye, et al., 2009) in order to achieve research goals quickly. Some researchers disagree on these proposed divergent methodologies and question if such policies may result in a new threat to research participants. Without the consensus of ethical and legal framework for biomedical research consent may result in a perceived breach of the patient's right to privacy and erosion of the ever-sacred principle of researcher/doctor-patient confidentiality (Petronio, 2012; McGuire & Secko, 2009; Beskow, 2010). The authors balance the power of research goads and individual interests by implementing and enforcing related laws and organizations guideline in authors' designed prototype consent management system, for example, by recommending the conditions to apply a waived research consent by the federal "common rule" in federally funded research; guidelines for broad consent given by the Council for International Organizations of Medical Sciences (CIOMS, 2006). Additionally, the nature of genetic research may not promise short-term benefits to the participants and considerable risks in the research must be as part of participating research consent forms.

Components of Consent Forms

Due to the absence of an agreed upon views on the components of medical consent forms, the contents of consent forms may vary greatly. Nonetheless, many studies explored this issue and proposed various recommendations on the essential content of informed consent. Carmen Ayuso et al. (2013) proposed ten minimum elements of information to be included in all informed consent forms for whole-genome sequencing (WGS) in the clinical setting. They did so after searching and reviewing applied documents from 554 documents in the Pubmed-Medline and Embase, such as Scope, Benefits, Risks, Voluntary, Alternative test, Future use, Incidental findings, etc. The authors also examined many paper-based consent forms and found that they include a large number of attributes. As shown in authors' previous work, the authors found 21 attributes in eight dialysis consent forms. Authors' examinations have led to categorizing the consents as follows:

1. **Informed Consent Giver:** The person with the legal right to make health care or participating decisions, such as parents or legal guardians of minors, healthcare proxies, healthcare providers or third parties.
2. **Disclosed Information:** At a minimum, includes procedure (treatment procedure for treatment consent, data usage for privacy consent, research procedure for research consent, and so on), benefits, risks and alternative procedures.
3. **Patient's Decision:** Includes the decision (deny or accept) by providing all required conditions and attributes such as signatures, date, etc.

Consequently, consents are based on all input variables, such as consent giver, treatment specification, related consent rules, and the like. Usually, they are represented in the physical forms in writing, electronic forms in the computer applications, or in some other legally acceptable manner. Hence a well-designed consent form should be obtained when activities require it. In authors' prototype system, electronic consent forms are automatically generated based on the collected attributes and regulations and enforced to obtained as practice workflow demands.

The various rules generated from laws, organization policies or sub-discipline medical guidelines affect each component of consent. Therefore, to be valid, informed consent must comply with state and federal laws and regulations applicable to medical sub-disciplines, as well as depend on some specific situations such as treatment type, research type, facility location and the purposes of use and disclosure of sensitive patient information for medical information sharing consent.

Consent Rules

As stated above, the relationship between consent components and governed rules are expounded below:

1. Informed consent giver component is governed by a competency rule; that is there to validate that the patient has sufficient maturity to grant informed consent;
2. Disclosed information component is governed by information or disclosure rules. An essential component is the concept of autonomy that allows competent adult persons and emancipated children to make their own decisions based on the understanding of given information. Nonetheless, the scope of the disclosure of required information is still debated, especially in genetic consents.
3. Patient's decisional component is governed by decisional capability rule, which is for evaluation of patient competency for understanding information about the procedure or using/sharing medical data and the ability to provide a rational, voluntary agree or deny decision. In (Fisher, 2002), authors described four psycho-legal standards of:
    a. Communicating a choice,
    b. Factual understanding,
    c. Appreciation of the situation, and
    d. Rational manipulation of information that is used to evaluate patient competence in granting consent.

However, no widespread consensus exists on how the decisional capacity of treatment consent should be measured.

Consent statutes and regulations are complex. Authors' previous work (Yu, Wijesekera, & Costa, 2014) showed the complexity of determining patient competency for treatment consent. One of the issues is that each state has its own laws defining minors, at times differing by treatment type. Various statutes and regulations and laws governing informed consents change over time. For example, a medical lawsuit that establishes precedent may trigger a new or amended statute or regulation or alter how a law is interpreted. Nevertheless, studies of consent laws are scarce, perhaps because ever changing laws would cause such studies to have a short shelf-life. Yet, no implementation method or modeling changes to consent laws are available that govern specific institutional practices (Beauchamp, & Childress, 1989). Consent is rendered unreliable without adhering to corresponding changes in laws. Even more, at times ambiguity adds to complexity (e.g., precedent changing interpretations of the law that, due to ambiguity, is subject to multiple interpretations). This causes breakdowns between concepts that people use and data that computers interpret. Thus, a methodology for acquiring proper consent based on evolving law must be dynamic.

Issuing proper medical consent demands to evaluate all consent rules and to determine the type of consent to be obtained from the appropriate consent provider as well as allowing exceptions to achieve the flexibility. For example, an incapacitated patient (perhaps temporarily due to injury or medication) may be considered not to possess a sound mind or may have been determined not to have the mental capacity (such as developmental disorders or clinically determined mental impediments) needed to provide legally binding informed consent. Similar exceptions exist with respect to children or young adults, who may not be considered mature to provide consent (Appelbaum, & Grisso, 1995).

Figure 3. High-level genetic services workflow

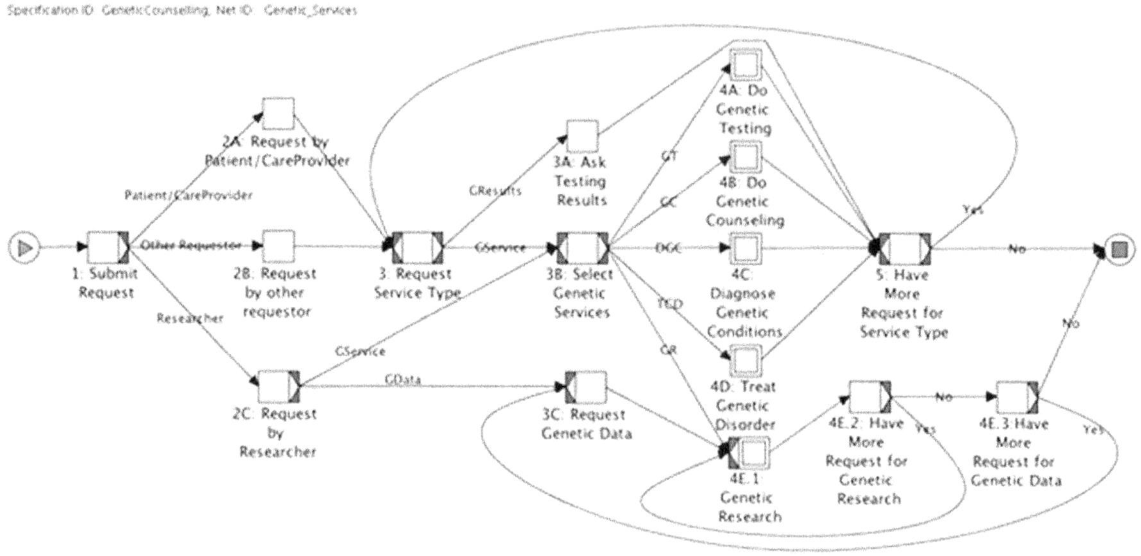

System Architecture

Authors' system architecture (shown in Figure 3) consists of the following components: (1) User Interface (UI) for EMR system users, (2) EMR's Runtime System, (3) WfMS — Workflow Management System - a runtime system that enforces medical treatment workflow, (4) CMS — Consent Management System, and (5) corresponding databases.

1. **UI:** Enables interactions between EMR systems and EMR system users (usually refer to people, such as members of the treatment team and quality care team that may want to review the logs, etc.)
2. **EMR System:** Provides clinical functions, including the display of patient demographic information, vital signs, medication, lab order/results, etc.
3. **Workflow Management System:** Designs and executes workflow models, consisting of a workflow editor, workflow runtime engine and other components such as a workflow task handler that enforce the completion of a specific task.
4. **Consent Management System:** Evaluates and obtains appropriate patient's consent form, if needed. It contains different consent services, such as Patient Privacy Consent Management Service (PPCMS) and Patient Treatment Consent Management Service (PTCMS).
5. **Related Databases:** WfMS' databases contain healthcare and medical research workflow specifications composed of tasks describing processes and WfMS' data; while EMR systems' databases contain patients' or research participants' medical records and other EMR systems' data.

As stated, previous work describes the details of the developed consent management and workflow-based EMR design. The enhanced Workflow-based EMR system includes:

A CMS connected to WfMS that contains different consent management services, such as treatment consent management service, privacy consent management service, participating research management service, and so forth. The authors describe two of main consent management services below:

1. A PTCMS that contains a Treatment Consent Management System (TCMS) and Treatment Consent Rule Management System (TCRMS), which ensure treatment consents comply with treatment consent laws and policies. TCMS generates the appropriate informed treatment consent forms automatically and obtains the consent before passing to the next task.
2. A PPCMS contains a Privacy Override Privilege Management System (PoPMS) and a Privacy Consent Rule Management System (PCRMS). When an entity requests using or disclosing protectable patient information through the EMR system, the sub-component, the PoPMS in the system will check the requester, which may be a government agency, patient, covered entity, business associate or a researcher. Then PoPMS retrieves the purpose of disclosure and use of sensitive medical information based on federal, state privacy rules or organization policies. For example, in HIPAA, without any stated purposes, a patient or his/her authorized representatives is allowed to require this patient's PHI. In this situation, the request is assigned as "required disclosure" by default. If the request is an "authorized use" and disclosures, the request will trigger PCRMS to obtain a patient's informed privacy consent, which when given by the patient can be used for disclosure. In this design, the Ontology Service (OS) plays a role in obtaining valid consent forms. OS includes an ontology editor (to edit terms and rules), a rule set that codifies treatment or privacy consent laws and a reasoner that derives components of the consents that are displayed as consent forms by the EMR system. PCMS returns the final decision made by privacy rules with the highest override privilege to the EMR system. For authorized uses and disclosures request, the decision is shown on a patient's valid privacy consent.

Similar in design to the TCMS, PoPMS can retrieve or generate the valid informed privacy consent forms automatically and passes the patient's decision of sharing his/her sensitive medical information. The Enhanced Workflow-based EMR System Architecture is shown in Figure 1.

Informed consent is managed by the combination of WfMS and CMS. Based on the kind of consent required, corresponding consent management service is triggered. Following, the authors use PPCMS as an example to show how does the system work. PCRMS must be able to ascertain the consents, if any, are missing, but are required for making the final decision; if so, they must be obtained prior to disclosure. See, Figure 2 for the interaction among the WfMS engine; the EMR systems; and PPCMS and OS.

Step 1 EMR System → WfMS: When a requestor starts to request an individual's sensitive medical information in an EMR system or the request is issued during other workflow tasks, a "launch case" event request with workflow specification I.D. or name is sent to WfMS engine; WfMS engine enables the work item(s) based on control flow defined in the workflow specification and input data. If the enabled work item(s) do not request consent service, then go to Step 8. Otherwise,

Step 2 WfMS → CMS: If a procedure/step needs to check patient's informed privacy consent, the CMS is triggered. Furthermore, base on requested consent type, a corresponding consent management service is triggered, PPCMS in this case.

Figure 1. Workflow-based EMR system with consent management architecture

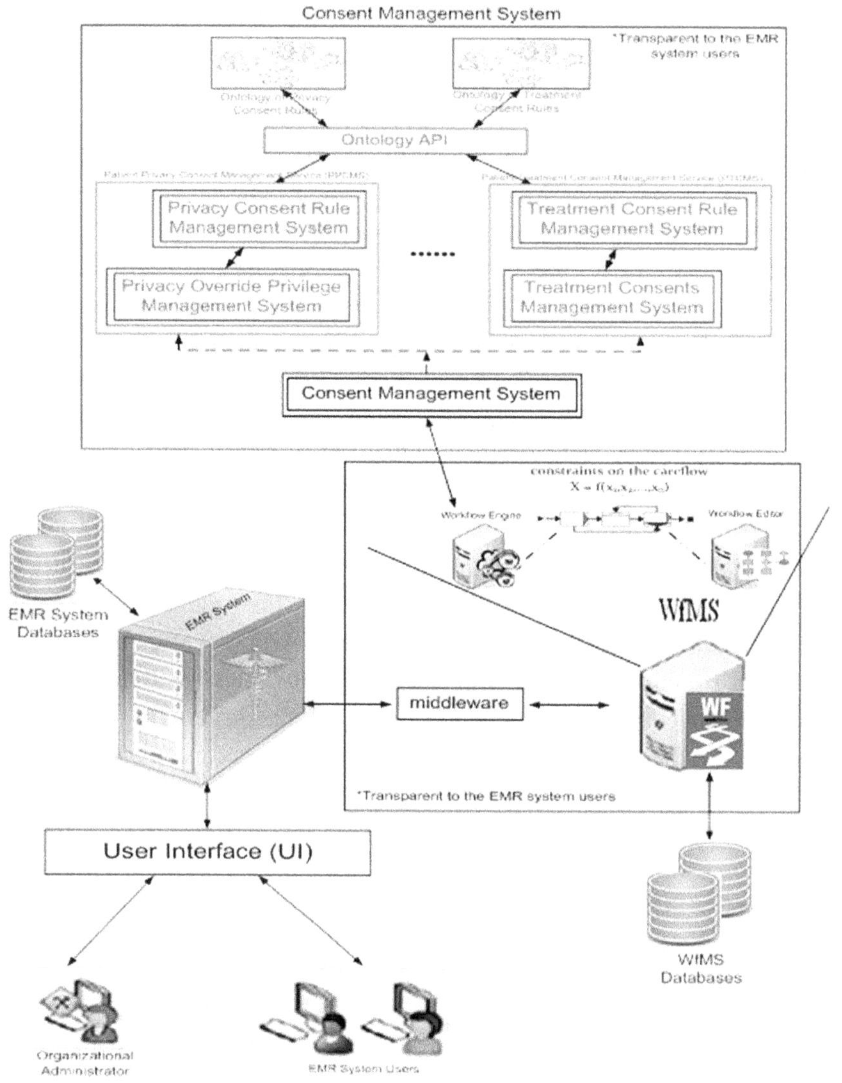

Step 3 PPCMS → OS: PPCMS uses OWL API to connect to the OS with patient's information and other required consent information.

Step 4 OS → PPCMS: OS retunes the results reasoned based on the rules to the PPCMS.

Step 5 EMR System → PPCMS: This additional step is triggered only when informed consent is required. EMR system requests the PPCMS to the kind of the privacy consents should be issued.

Step 6 PPCMS → EMR: System Similar to the previous step, except this step is triggered only if the consent service is called. PPCMS returns the answers to EMR System.

Step 7 PPCMS → WfMS: PPCMS passes results to CMS, then the CMS forwards results to WfMS, the WfMS decides if procedures should continue or be aborted based on the workflow specification.

Figure 2. Interactions between the WfMS; the EMR system; and PPCMS and OS per session

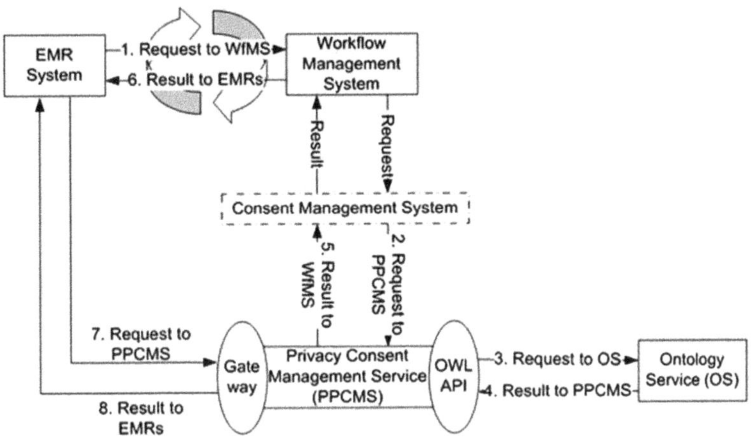

Step 8 WfMS → EMR System: WfMS sends a notification to EMR system. The available work item(s)/ step(s) will notify EMR system users via UI. Then, the interactions between WfMS and EMR system are repeated.

In the next section, the authors use informed consent for genetic services as a case study to show how genetic informed consents placed new challenges on the traditional ethical standards of informed consent. It also illustrates how appropriate consents can be electronically obtained and automatically enforced using a system that combines medical workflows and hierarchically, ontologically motivated rule enforcement.

CASE STUDY ON GENETIC SERVICES

In authors' previous works (Yu, Wijesekera, & Costa, 2014), the authors mainly address the consent for medical treatments, with a focus on informed consent for procedure-oriented treatment regimes. A preliminary study convened jointly by the National Institute of Health (NIH) and the Center for Disease Control (CDC) (Clayton, 1995) presents the risks and ethical issues involved in collecting and storing tissue samples for genetic tests in a research setting. Herein, the authors present a unique approach, which is based on the premise that acceptable genetic service regimes are captured in workflows to automatically obtain or generate (when needed) the deferent types of informed consent for clinical usage (collectively called *genetic services*) and genetic research. Moreover, the authors combine genetic privacy laws and policies relevant to informed consent with an encompassing and customizable genetic services workflow to show consent enforcement for ensuring appropriate genetic information privacy.

Background

Genetic studies comprehensively utilize genotypic and phenotypic data (Ritchie, et al., 2015). Studies have shown that preventive care, in which genetic services and researches play an important role, costs significantly less than treatment upon disease onset (Németh, et al., 2013). Examples include genetic mutations causing certain kinds of breast cancers (BRC-1 and BRC-2), ovarian cancer, sickle cell anemia, behavior disorder, β-thalassemia, left ventricular noncompaction cardiomyopathy and Alzheimer's disease, etc. Those genetic advances have encouraged some genetic services to become medically acceptable common practice to provide preventive and preemptive treatment for hereditary diseases. Concurrently, rapid advancement of genetic research continues to lengthen the list of predictable diseases (Rehm, et al., 2016). Many of those achievements are produced by researches using large sets of stored genetic information and samples. As stated in (Kerath, et al., 2013), the utilization of existing biobanks' stored information has become the cornerstone of human genomic and epigenomic studies. The concept of open access in the field of genomic research is expressed in the Bermuda Principles and the Fort Lauderdale Agreement, which have been widely applied in North America and the UK for funded genetic research. Sharing genetic data is vital for maximizing the use of such information to benefit patients and the general public. However, concern for ensuring genetic privacy is growing.

Genetic exceptionalism is defined in a paper (Gostin, & Hodge 1999) as "*the societal practice of treating genetic data as different from other types of health data for the purposes of assessing privacy and security protections*." The Federal Government and some states enacted several genetic-specific legislations to protect the genetic privacy and prevent discrimination. For example, HIPAA considers genetic information to be confidential medical information and regulates healthcare providers. In spite of Gostin & Hodge (1999) argued this definition is flawed in the light of two reasons:

1. Strict protection of genetic data threatens the accomplishment of public goods;
2. There is no clear demarcation separating genetic data from other medical data.

The majority of scholars agree that genetic information has its particular characteristics from other medical data. Some researchers say that *genetic information is essentially familial in nature and is referred to as the Genetic Information is Familial Thesis (GIFT)* (Liao, 2009), sharing such information will benefit related groups of individuals. Yet, others, who advocate the view of humans possessing the rights of *do not want to know* (Sherlock, 2009, & Liao, 2009), disagreed with the familial approach in their literatures. Sharing such data introduced new challenges. Inter alia, related regulations are many. For example, some countries have regulations to enforce sharing such information among family members (Lucassen, & Kaye, 2006, & American Society of Human Genetics Social Issues Subcommittee on Familial Disclosure, 1998) and others do not. Both research and clinical uses of genetic information pose ethical issues on medical consent:

- **Ethics:** Privacy involving genetic information differs from traditional medical informed consent. For example, protecting patients' private information is an important medical ethics and legal obligation. The key point is that the healthcare industry's current level of privacy and confidentiality is not yet entirely suitable for genetic privacy in both clinical medical practice and biomedical research. Genetic privacy consent has not been linked-up to applicable laws as part of an EMR workflow that enforces appropriate consent as a predicate to using genetic information in research and clinical practice. Protecting patient privacy in the context of genetic information leads to other equally unique types of challenges.
- **Legal Issues:** Requirements differ based on the usage. For example, generating data requires written informed consent that meets strict requirements, whereas sharing genetic data for research may have a less stringent opt-out consent. Genetic information can be traceable not only to individuals

but also identify data owner's relatives and makes family trees susceptible to stigma (Roach et al., 2010). Therefore, genetic privacy has been proposed as categorical privacy that differs from traditional individual-centered concepts of privacy in literature (Lunshof, 2008). Furthermore, genetic privacy laws vary from state-to-state and may be inconsistent with and be more or less stringent than federal law.

- **Social Implications:** Societal views are often reflected in law and/or organizations' policies, so societal implications are likely inextricably intertwined with laws and policy governing genetic privacy and what constitutes informed consent.

As a solution, the authors provide an encompassing framework consisting of workflow-enforced genetic privacy as well as biomedical consent management consistent with state and federal genetic privacy laws such as a statute, regulation, and precedent. These missing regulations presented issues for the authors' prototype implementation that have been resolved by having default rules.

Related Work in Context

EMRs play a vital role in sharing medical information among participating actors based on their usage scenarios. In addition, using EMRs for genetic services present a unique set of challenges (Mascalzoni, 2008). Belmont et al. (2009) highlighted the privacy, ethical and legal issues of handling genetic data in EMRs. Additional, Scheuner et al. (2009) conducted a case study to verify if existing EMR systems meet genetic information needs. This study, involved results, and conclusions gathered from discussing 56 patient's electronic medical records within10 EMR specialists, 16 medical geneticists, and 12 genetic counselors, shows an overall lack of support for functionality, structure, and tools for clinical genetic practice. A more recent study on the state of EMRs supporting genomics for personalized medicine again identifies the designing of the structure of data as a challenge (Ullman-Cullere, 2011). The authors also identified genetic services workflow management as a priority area that needs further research, development, and testing. The authors, too, observed that current EMR systems for genetic services still cannot support the ability to obtain/generate informed privacy consents and enforce them in EMRs (Yu et al., 2015).

Some researchers suggested that the proper legislation on generating and using genetic information is pivotal to improving genetic privacy (Gymrek et al., 2013). In 2013, HIPAA (45 C.F.R. §160.103) Omnibus Rule included genetic information as PHI to be regulated under the privacy portion of HIPAA. Nonetheless, states may have different definitions of genetic information. The combination of Federal privacy laws and state laws from many states form a fragmented regulatory and statutory landscape for permissible information sharing and consent management. Indeed, significant regulatory gaps create additional burdens in providing automated ways to obtain and generate information consent in EMRs.

As mentioned, an informed consent management system in genetics is needed. To the best of authors' knowledge, to date, there is no such system implemented in EMR systems that can accommodate the rapid advancements of genetics research and the evolving nature of the genetic privacy landscape. To comply with different genetic privacy laws under various circumstances in clinical practice and genetic research is challenging. EMR systems evolved with differing architectures to satisfy different requirements at different stages of technology development. Many treatises (Locatelli, Restifo, Gastaldi & Corso, 2012; Shortliffe, & Cimino, 2006; Wickramasinghe, & Geisler, 2008) have detailed EMR system evolution. Today, EMR systems are indispensable. Because medical organizations have over two decades adopted costly EMR systems ($25M-$45M per large hospital and $8B for the Defense Health Agency), medical organizations are understandably reluctant to switch to new systems. Consequently, a strategy of integrating a genetic consent management with existing EMR systems may provide a solution that the authors advocate.

Proposed Approach

Authors' solution to the issue is to enhance an existing EMR system with a workflow management system to choreograph predefined procedures, as the authors have prototyped using open source solutions. Although there will be other components that drive the EMR systems, EMR users will not notice a difference in interaction by using authors' solution.

During the time that genetic services have been around sub-disciplines or education papers have also defined de-facto workflows for some genetic services. For example, The Genetic Counseling Definition Task Force defines Genetic counseling as "The process of helping people understand and adapt to medical, psychological, and familial implications of genetic contributions to disease." However, the authors were unable to find a documented and modeled comprehensive workflow. Therefore, the authors need to create a genetic services workflow model. The authors describe a genetic services workflow specification in the next section.

High-Level Genetic Services Workflow

The methodology used to generate a genetic services workflow involves the following steps:

1. The authors interviewed genetic researchers to get their individual practice workflows.
2. The authors collected the paper-based documents used to record events and data that are associated with the workflows.

Finally, the authors combined (1) and (2) to generate a more comprehensive workflow. The authors describe the high-level workflow process first; then describe its one of sub-processes genetic counseling with the requesters involved in the processes separately and show an embedded consent management system.

The high-level genetic services, modeled using a workflow editor is shown in Figure 3. The shown workflow covers the high-level view of the genetic services consisting of multiple requested genetic services, as shown in Figure 1, the leftmost node with a right-pointing green arrow inside a circle is the starting point of the workflow, and the rightmost circle with a filled red square ends the workflow. Atomic Task (using a single box in Figure 3, as (1: Submit Request) denotes "a single task to be performed by a human participant or an external application"; Composite Task (using a double box in Figure 1, as (4B: Do Genetic Counseling) represents "A container for another workflow process (also called a sub Net)"; The starting point is the process of receiving different request for a genetic service by different requestors, such as care providers, researcher, etc. When genetic service or genetic information using/ sharing, the consent management system is triggered automatically in authors' design. Details follow.

"Do Genetic Counseling" Sub-Workflow

The continuous workflow that the authors call "do genetic counseling," named *4B: Do Genetic Counseling,* has two composite tasks in *Do Genetic Counseling* sub-workflow, *Pre-test Genetic Counseling,* and *Post-test Genetic Counseling,* as shown in Figure 4 and Figure 5. This sub-workflow is based on a presentation on clinical genetic counseling from Stanford University's Clinical Genomics program (Merker, 2014). In addition to the previous presentation, the authors used another presentation by O'Daniel et al. (2012) on Genomic Medicine for additional details. Here the authors provide a detailed documentation and overview of the Genetic Counseling workflow. The following list provides the details of the individual tasks involved in the process of providing genetic counseling to a patient or care provider.

1. Collection of Medical Records, Family History, and Social History:
    a. **Require Genetic Counseling:** A case originates with a physician's referral for genetic counseling. Alternatively, a patient self-requests genetic counseling after learning of a manifestation of a genetic disorder in a family member.
    b. **Patient Walk-ins:** Upon arriving at the genetic counselor's office, a self-requests patient is asked to provide social and family history. Concurrently, the Genetic Privacy Consent is obtained. Additionally, if copies of medical records are provided, they are recorded in the system. In authors' workflow model, the patient is presented with a detailed family and social

Figure 4. Pre-test genetic counseling

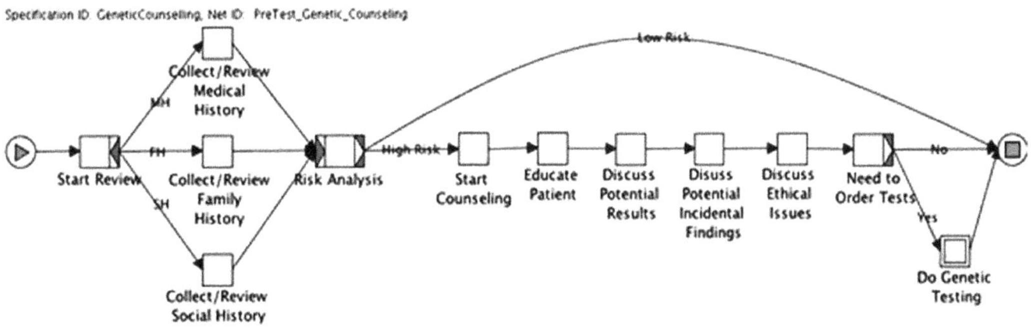

Figure 5. Post-test genetic counseling

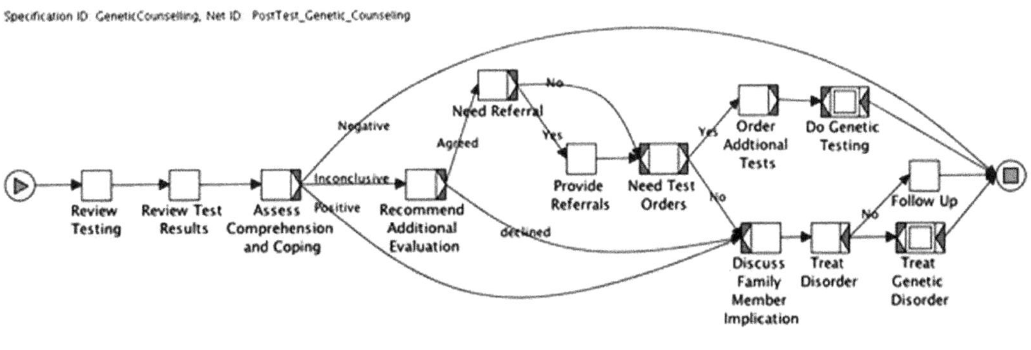

history questionnaire to assess the risk of a suspected hereditary disease. Authors' workflow produces a questionnaire on suspected Hereditary Cancer Syndrome based on forms developed by the Virginia Women's Center (Virginia women's center website).

   c. **Physician's Referrals:** When a physician refers a patient for genetic counseling, the patient is asked to sign release forms for medical records (Genetic Privacy Consent) from the referring physician (if not already provided). If not, and the patient brings in copies of medical records, they are recorded in the system.
   d. **Review Requirements:** Information collected from the patient is reviewed for completeness. If any, missing information is collected from the patient, patient's primary care physician or public sources of ancestry information. This is shown in the "*Collect More Information*" task in the modeled workflow (Figure 4). When all of the information (to the best of patient's knowledge) is collected, one or more of following people review the collected information: Genetic Counselor, Molecular Pathologist, and/or Medical Geneticist. Next, check for the ami-ability of genetic test to answer the questions posed by the patient or the referring physician.
2. **Pre-Test Counseling:** Once an insurance or payment authorization is obtained, the patient meets with a genetic counselor for pre-test counseling. The genetic counselor performs the following sub-tasks for pre-test counseling:
   a. An informed consent is obtained for counseling, i.e., Genetic Counseling Treatment Consent. As a part of this informed treatment consent, the counselor provides the patient with information about the expected risks and benefits of this process.
   b. The family, social, and medical history provided by the patient is reviewed.
   c. The counselor discusses the expected range of results and their impact on the patient and his/her relatives. Additionally, the counselor discusses other potential incidental findings that may be in the report. Incidental findings are those findings in the test results that are not associated with the primary reason for conducting the test, but indicative of other recognizable genetic disorders. The counselor also discusses ethical issues that could arise from conducting or disclosing these test results. Before ordering the tests, any questions or clarifications from the patient are answered. At this moment, the counselor will obtain a doing lab consent, which belongs to the Medical Treatment Consent.
   d. If applicable, consent for sharing information or using their samples for current or future possible research purposes (Participating Genetic Research Consent) is collected.
3. **Lab Work:** Blood or tissue samples are collected from the patient for genome sequencing. Generally, one tube of blood is collected for sequencing. An additional tube may be collected for confirmatory studies. Another tube of blood may be collected from the patient with appropriate consent for research purposes. The blood and tissue samples are then sent to a laboratory for sequencing, and the sequenced genetic information is returned to the genetic counseling team. The authors do not model the workflow for genome sequencing in the laboratory in this chapter.
4. **Post-Test Counseling:** Once the sequencing results are reported back to the genetic counseling team, a draft report is prepared. This draft report is reviewed by a review team consisting of Genetic Counselors and/or Medical Geneticists, Physicians, and/or content experts. Once reviewed, the final report is uploaded into the EMR and is ready for the patient. Ideally, this report should be delivered electronically to the EMR. When the patient meets the counselor to discuss the test results, the following sub-tasks are performed:

a. The counselor reviews the test results with the patient. Once the review is complete, the counselor assesses the comprehension and coping skills of the patient.
b. If the additional evaluation or referral for treatment (e.g. prophylactic mastectomy) is warranted, referrals or orders are placed by the genetic counselors. Alternatively, the patient may decline the recommendations of the genetic counselor. If the recommendations are declined, it is recorded in the EMR and if needed, a second opinion is scheduled.
c. The counselor finally discusses implications of the findings on related family members. At this point, the genetic counselor may recommend the patient to inform related family members personally about the test results and treatment options by providing templates. Alternatively, they may obtain consent (Genetic Privacy Consent) to disclose test results to affected family members.
d. Lastly, if required, the counselor may schedule follow-up appointments.

5. **Disclosure and Other Consents:** At the end of the genetic counseling process, the care provider may be required to obtain consent to retain samples and/or genetic information (sequencing results) and genetic test reports based on state and federal regulation. Additionally, the care provider may require additional disclosure consents to share information with other individuals or entities as required by law. If consent to retain genetic samples and test information is denied, they must be destroyed and/or purged from the EMR records. Once these housekeeping tasks are complete, the genetic counseling workflow comes to an end.

Consent Management in the Genetic Counseling Workflow

As discussed earlier, there are various types of informed consent required for Genetic Counseling, which mainly include treatment consent; genetic information use/disclosure consent, so-called genetic privacy consent; genetic research consent; and retention consent. If a proper workflow in not enforced for genetic counseling in the EMRs, it may leave healthcare providers and/or health-care organizations open to lawsuits. Existing laws limiting genetic information disclosures do not generally consider ethical issues involved during the disclosure process. Ethical issues present an abstract concept that needs to be carefully considered by genetic counselors on a case-by-case basis. Additionally, an organization's ethical guidelines may regulate disclosure of genetic information, which upon disclosure may tangibly affect a third party.

In this section, the authors describe how the authors enforce all of the required consents in the genetic counseling workflow. The authors describe the enforcement of disclosure consent in this work. Other types of consent may be enforced in the workflow very similar to the disclosure consent.

When a task requires consent in the genetic counseling workflow, the consent management system is invoked to manage the consent requirements. The authors also adopted workflow technologies to model the consent management processes as a workflow specification, shown in Figure 6. In the case of information disclosure consent, the consent must comply with federal and state laws, as well as organization policies.

In developing authors' prototype, the authors studied genetic-related privacy laws in great detail. At first, the authors examined the papers and publications (Rothstein, 2014; & American Health Information Management Association, 2013), which focused on the federal genetic privacy laws. There are four major federal laws for genetic information sharing as shown below:

Figure 6. Genetic consent management workflow

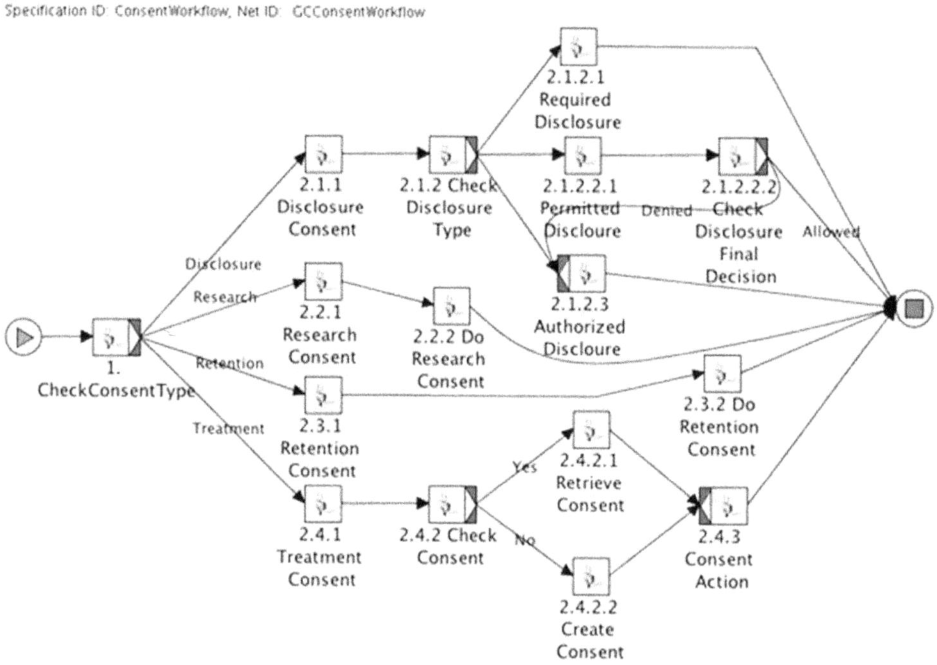

1. Genetic Information Nondiscrimination Act of 2008 (GINA) (2008). GINA regulates employers and health insurance companies but not healthcare providers who use genetic information. GINA protects individuals from discrimination based on genetic conditions. However, GINA does not apply to federal government employees or employers with fewer than 15 employees.
2. HIPPA (45 C.F.R. §160.103). The 2013 Omnibus Rule included genetic information as PHI to be regulated under the privacy portion of HIPAA. However, HIPAA only mandates a portion of genetic information requestors such as covered entities.
3. The Common Rule applies only to institutions that perform federally funded research on human subjects; private research institutions may voluntarily agree to comply with federal standards. Among other issues, the Common Rule sets out explicit standards for informed consent by research subjects, although an ethics board may waive these requirements.

Although these laws guide establishing policies for genetic information sharing, none of them absolutely protects genetic privacy. In addition to federal laws, many state laws and institutional polices add to the informed consent management.

Now the authors are reviewing genetic privacy laws from states that apply to genetic privacy in published literature (Mulholland, 1998; & National Conference of State Legislatures, 2008) and online resources. Many states have their own genetic privacy laws with different levels of requirements to protect genetic privacy.

For example, California has a more strict genetic privacy law while some states such as Alabama do not have any regulations specific to genetic data. Furthermore, the genetic information use and sharing of genetic services will vary based on the types of the requestor (such as genetic counselors, researchers), and the purpose (such as diagnosis, research, payment). Without an understanding of informed consent, it is problematic to make consent information semantics explicit and hence discoverable automatically in a software system.

Computer science defines "Ontology" as "the explicit specification of a conceptualization" (Gruber, 1995) or "explicit formal specifications of the terms in the domain and relations among them (Noy, & McGuinness, 2001)." Consequently, ontologies can be used to model a domain of discourse as a set of representative primitives, such as classes, object properties, data properties and relationships between them. Many papers present reasons to use ontologies to formulate shared vocabulary (knowledge) of a given healthcare domain of interest (Gruber, 1993), to ensure interoperability within the various healthcare domains (by ontology matching). Ontologies have been used to represent actionable knowledge in biomedicine (Dang, Hedayati, Hampel, & Toklu, 2008; Garde, Knaup, Hovenga, & Heard, 2007; Matos, Campos, Braga, Palazzi, 2010; Rosse, & Mejino Jr, 2003; Yu, 2006) due to their ability to capture domain knowledge in a formal yet simple and incremental manner, as well as their easy and powerful application in reasoning processes (Valls, Gibert, Sánchez, & Batet, 2010). Other healthcare fields include decision support and information integration. Thus, the authors developed a medical treatment consent ontology as a preliminary notation to formalize the predicates used in creating consent rules.

The rules used to model treatment consents are of the form "$predicate_1(x_{11},x_{12},..,x_{1n}),\ldots \ldots,$ $predicate_m(x_{m1},x_{m2},,,x_{mk}) \rightarrow predicate(y_1,\ldots y_p)$" where the predicate instances stated left of the arrow symbol → are taken as the body of the rule and read as a conjunction of $predicate_1(_{x11},x_{12},,,x_{1n})\wedge,\ldots,\wedge$ $predicate_i(x_{i1},x_{i2},,,x_{ij})\wedge,\ldots,\ \wedge predicate_m(x_{m1},x_{m2},,,x_{mk})$ and the consequent is $predicate(y_1,\ldots,y_p)$. The intended meaning is that if the conditions specified in the antecedent hold, then the conditions specified in the consequent also hold. The authors show patient maturity evaluation rules for each state based on its consent laws as a case study in authors' published paper (Yu, Wijesekera, & Costa, 2014). In (Yu, Wijesekera, & Costa, 2014), the authors used open source software for implementing authors' framework YAWL Management System as the workflow management system and OpenMRS as authors' EMR system, Ontology Web Language (OWL) to describe authors' consent ontology, implemented using Protégé and applied Pellet as tour ontology reasoner. Similar techniques are used to obtain valid genetic privacy consents in addition to the privacy disclosure decision made by the highest override privilege as shown in Figure 7. As a result, additional task, which applied checking disclosure decision privilege rules, is added to genetic privacy consent service workflow.

Implementation

The authors developed a functioning prototype that addresses many aspects to develop an automated and integrated informed genetic information consent system. The prototype collages the data gathered during interactions with the medical provider with the application laws, regulations and policies to address the privacy issues specific to genetic information. The first component of implementing the genetic privacy enforcement gathers the required information from an EMR system. This foundation allows the rules to be seamlessly integrated with the operations of the medical facility and maximizes the use of existing data to reduce additional data entry. The authors extended an open-sourced EMR by adding a tab to launch the consent workflow management system for an EMR system user. The workflow gathers additional information regarding aspects of the tasks being performed and then executes the path based on the purpose for accessing the genetic information (Disclosure, research, or treatment).

Figure 7. Structure of the hierarchy overrides privilege to override the privacy disclosure decision

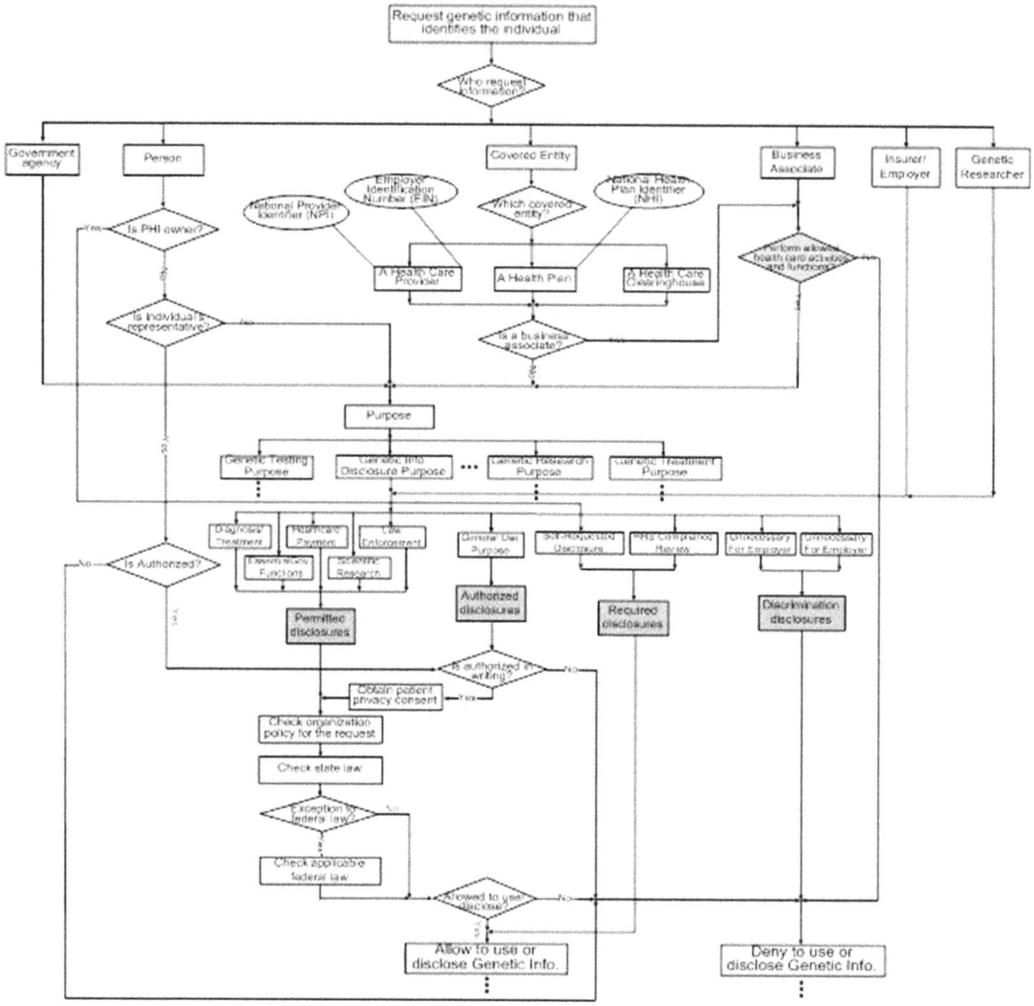

Once all the required information has been gathered from either the EMR database or from the users by invoking workflow-based prompts, the workflow management engine calls consent management system whenever an informed genetic consent is required. When a corresponding consent service is triggered, it implements an ontology described below to reason if the requested access is permitted or if not a consent form is required to generate. The access evaluation is done at each level in the hierarchy that is applicable to state, federal genetic privacy laws, and organization policies. By definition, federal laws are at the top of the hierarchy followed by state laws, local laws and then organizational policies. The hierarchical structure dictates how conflicts between laws and policies can be resolved based on the decisions made at each level. (For example, Federal Laws set a number of restrictions on the use of genetic data in research. Unless explicitly allowed in the Law, an organization cannot write conflicting policies.) The workflow engine evaluates the results from each level to return an overall decision as to whether access is allowed along with incorporating any other requirements that must be enforced (such as retention periods, written consent, de-identification, etc.)

In order to support the consent service, the authors developed an ontology to capture the various aspects of enforcing privacy laws and policies. As shown in Figure 8, the ontology has four major entities:

- **Requester:** The person making the request to access the medical information including their role, associations with a specific organization, and information about this organization,
- **Resource:** The part of the electronic medical record being requested along with information about the subject (or patient)
- **Request:** Details on the purpose for requesting the information. The four specific purposes applicable to genetic information are disclosure, research, testing and treatment. The prototype currently implements the information disclosure component with the applicable specific instances for Self-Request by the Patient, Law Enforcement, etc.
- **Response:** The results of the reasoner applying the appropriate rules along with a list of any obligations that must be enforced by the EMR and specific consent clauses that are needed for the associated approvals. (A subclass for Federal Responses allows information about HIPAA-specific requirements to be gathered.)

The ontology diagram shown in Figure 8 contains some main properties and instances used in authors' work so far. The ontology is implemented using the Protégé platform with the laws (Federal and State), and the organizational policies are enforced using DLQuery and the Pellet reasoner. The predicate used in each rule uses the Request instance with the associated properties to gather additional information

Figure 8. The ontology diagram

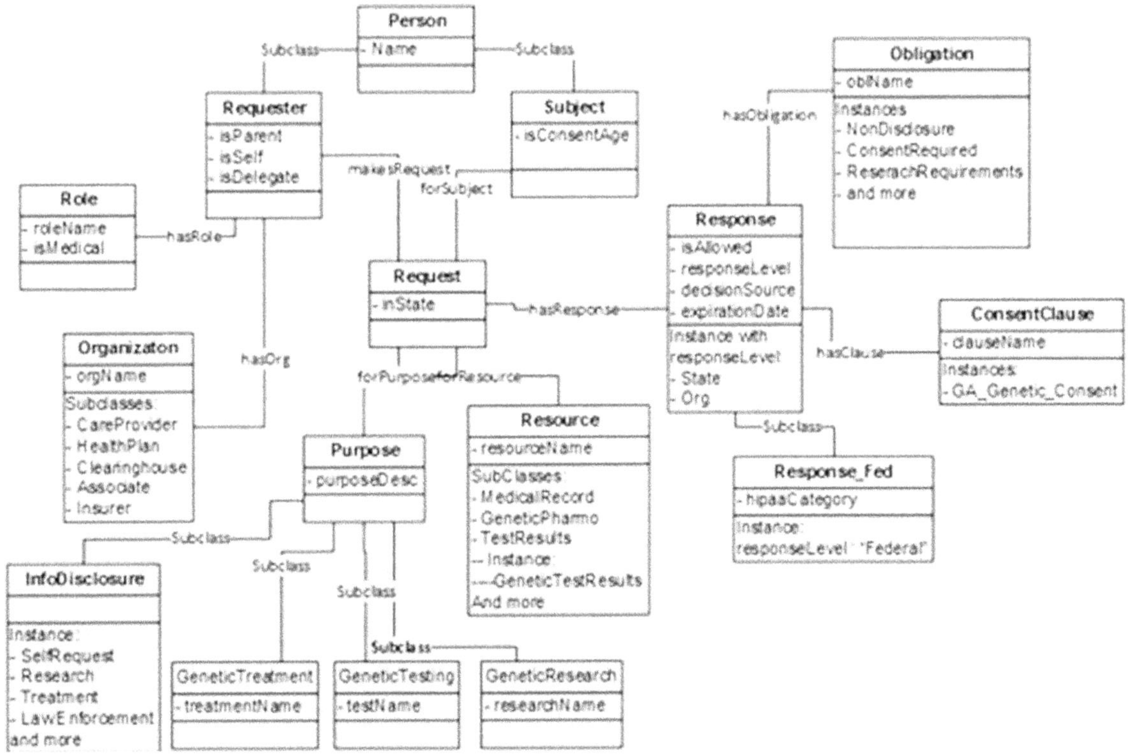

on the Requester and the Resource. The appropriate Response instance (Federal, State or Organization) receives the outcome of the rule regarding whether access is permitted or denied the specific law or policy that generated the result, and the appropriate obligations and clauses.

The Override property implements the hierarchy of Federal/State laws and organizational policies described above. The override property is set as a meat-rule implementing a more strict law being evaluated that permits a looser law or policy to provide a different answer or supplemental information. So, if a Federal law permits access but has a clause where a state or organization can set a different policy to deny access, the override property in the Federal response is set to "True." Alternatively, the organizational policy might still permit access but add more clauses to the consent agreement that must be signed.

For example, HIPAA permits access to medical records even genetic data for treatment. In Georgia, there are additional obligations and consent requirements when the resource being accessed is from genetic testing. The Response structure allows both sets of answers to be passed back to the workflow engine for further evaluation and execution.

As an example of the implementation of obligations and overrides, the first DLQuery checks for the Federal law for access to the genetic Test Results for Treatment. The response is set to provide the corresponding information for the associated HIPAA category for Permitted, and therefore other laws can override the decision.

makesRequest(?r, ?req), forPurpose(?req, ?pur), purposeDesc(?pur, "Treatment"), hasResponse(?req, ?res), responseLevel(?res, "Federal") -> isAllowed(?res, true), canOverride(?res, true), hipaaCategory(?res, "Permitted"), decisionSource(?res, "HIPAA"), hasRule(?res, 4)

The next part of the example below shows the DL Query for the related request which sets the location in Georgia and that the rule can be executed if the Federal response allows an Override. The State response then allows access but with an additional obligation for a Consent Agreement and the agreement must have text specific to Georgia.

isSelf(?r, false), makesRequest(?r, ?req), inState(?req, "GA"), forResource(?req, ?resource), forPurpose(?req, ?pur), purposeDesc(?pur, "Treatment"), resourceName(?resource, "GeneticTestResults"),

Figure 9. Outcome of the decision of accessing genetic data using Pellet reasoner

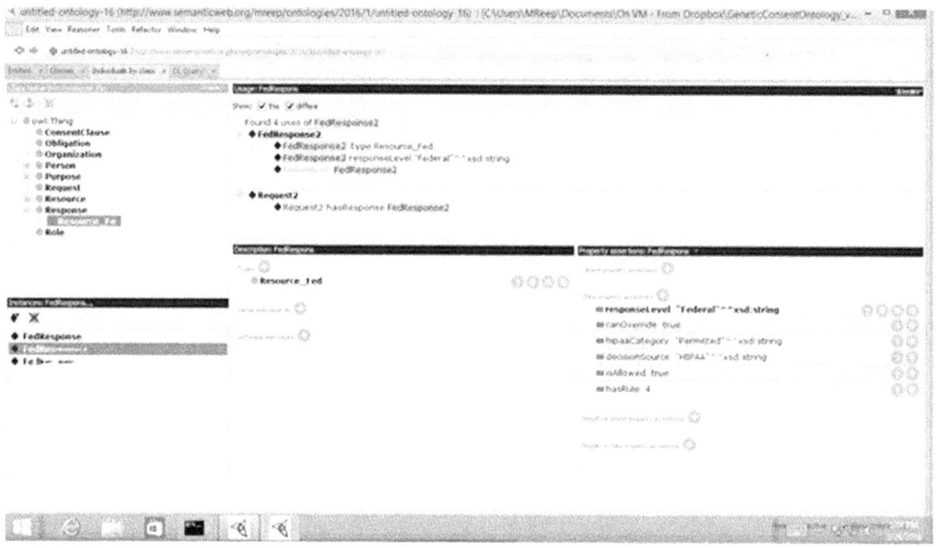

Figure 10. Outcome of the decision of accessing genetic data using Pellet reasoner

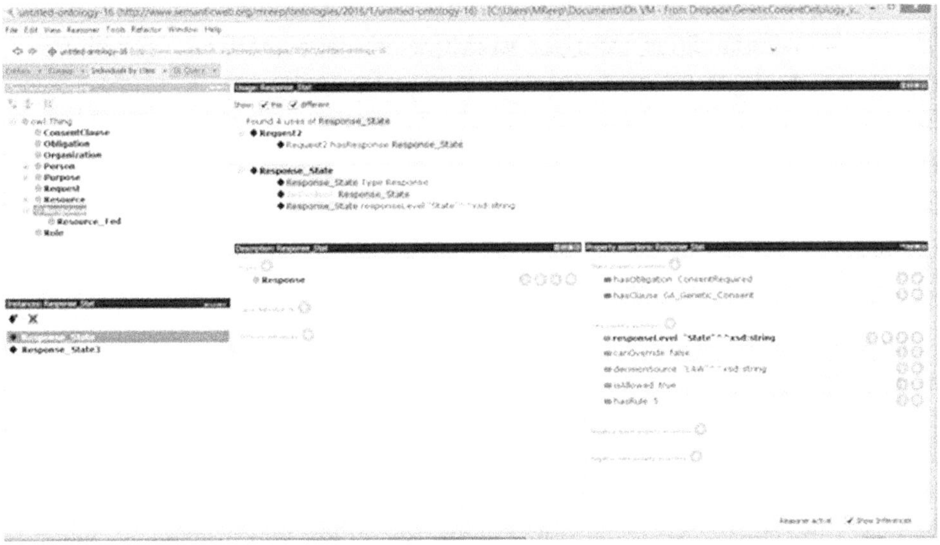

hasResponse(?req, ?res), responseLevel(?res, "Federal"), canOverride(?res, true), hasResponse(?req, ?resst), responseLevel(?resst, "State"), oblName(?obl, "ConsentRequired"), clauseName(?clause, "GAGeneticConsent") -> isAllowed(?resst, true), canOverride(?resst, false), decisionSource(?resst, "GA_LAW"), hasObligation(?resst, ?obl), hasClause(?resst, ?clause)

Once the reasoner has evaluated the rules, the workflow engine will retrieve the Response, Obligation and Clauses instances through Java API calls to Protégé in order to enforce the results. The first part of the enforcement determines if access to the requested resource is allowed or denied. In order to consolidate the responses into one answer, first the Federal response is checked and, if an override is permitted, the state level is evaluated followed by the organizational level. If the consolidated response is determined to be a denial, then the EMR workflow ends with a message and information on the law or policy that generated the denial is provided. If the consolidated response is to allow the requested access, the workflow displays information on the required obligations and requests acceptance to these conditions for data access. If consent is required, the applicable genetic privacy consent form will be retrieved for granting consent by legal consent giver. The workflow ends with access decision being provided to the requested genetic data.

Finally, the authors describe security issues, which are important considerations for any EMRs:

- **Access Control:** The medical team as a whole provides the required services to a patient who visits the medical center, from acceptance of a patient to the end of the treatment at the facility. Each team member plays a designated role in providing care with a set of assigned duties that are choreographed with each other, forming workflows. The team together provides the care planned for the patient. The authors used a role-based access control model to provide confidentiality.

Furthermore, enforced informed treatment consent and privacy consent can be viewed as more complex access controls with more complex rules.

- **Accountability:** To monitor the quality of care and be consistent with continuous improvements, an EMR system must enable auditing capabilities. HIPAA requires logging all PHI requests and the system actions for auditing. Authors' workflow-enforced EMR system with consent management allows the quality care team to review both procedures and outcomes from workflow logs and EMR system logs and consent logs, which provide an audit trail that satisfies accountability requirements.

CONCLUSION

Adding an executable consent-enforced service into workflow-based EMR systems to manage informed consent at runtime includes not only all benefits provided by workflow enforced EMR systems (Yu, & Wijesekera, 2013), but also provides significant benefits to medical practitioners and patients by reducing medical malpractice and potential medical treatment errors caused by missing informed consents (Yu, Wijesekera, & Costa, 2014). This work also improves the patient-caregiver relationship, risk management, decreases malpractice costs, enhances audit capabilities and fosters continuous care process improvement. Another advantage of authors' approach is the protection of patients' privacy by authors' EMR system. Additionally, this system can accommodate changes to policies and standards.

Solving the new consent management challenges in the area of genetic service, authors' approach allowed a single consent management system to handle different consent services based on the procedures' purposes. Authors' approach stores all genetic consents in the EMR system. Gaining consents and dealing with exceptions are recorded in the workflow management system. Thus, these records are readily available for quality of care audits and reviews.

Finally, using ontological techniques in a consent management system and creating a consent ontology enable keeping current of each State's evolving consent laws. Failure to track consent law changes closely and in near-real time is a sure recipe for failure.

Authors' work introduces an inspiring framework to extend existing EMR systems to avoid treatment errors caused by deviation from standardized treatment workflow and potential breach of privacy, or "psychosocial" harms to the individuals, as well, the many serious negatives that flow from lack of proper, informed consent.

Authors' ongoing work will expand this EMR system to automatically generate required consent rules from revised or newly enacted laws so that the operational EMR quickly reflect these changes, to allow patients to revoke consents and to appoint or re-appoint consent holders. This research path also includes further developing the evaluation rule repository to cover other more specific treatment scenarios.

REFERENCES

Faresi, A. L. A., Wijesekera, D., & Moidu, K. (2010). A comprehensive privacy-aware authorization framework founded on HIPAA privacy rules. In *Proceedings of the 1st ACM International Health Informatics Symposium*. ACM.

American Health Information Management Association. (2013). *Analysis of Modifications to the HIPAA Privacy, Security, Enforcement, and Breach Notification Rules under the Health Information Technology for Economic and Clinical Health Act and the Genetic Information Nondiscrimination Act; Other Modifications to the HIPAA Rules*. Retrieved August 16, 2014, from http://library.ahima.org/PdfView?oid=106127

American Society of Human Genetics Social Issues Subcommittee on Familial Disclosure. (1998). ASHG STATEMENT Professional Disclosure of Familial Genetic Information. *American Journal of Human Genetics*, *62*(2), 474–483. doi:10.1086/301707 PMID:9537923

Anonymous. (2007). *Healthcare's most expensive piece of paper*. DialogMEDICAL. Retrieved May 10, 2013, from http://www.dialogmedical.com/wp- content/uploads/2010/04/ROI%20White%20Paper%20 05-07.pdf

Appelbaum, P. S., & Thomas, G. (1995). The MacArthur Treatment Competence Study. I: Mental illness and competence to consent to treatment. *Law and Human Behavior*, *19*(2), 105–126. doi:10.1007/BF01499321 PMID:11660290

Ayuso, C., Millán, J. M., Mancheño, M., & Dal-Ré, R. (2013). Informed consent for whole-genome sequencing studies in the clinical setting. Proposed recommendations on essential content and process. *European Journal of Human Genetics*, *21*(10), 1054–1059. doi:10.1038/ejhg.2012.297 PMID:23321621

Beauchamp, T. L., & Childress, J. F. (1989). *Principles of Biomedical Ethics* (3rd ed.). New York: Oxford University Press.

Belmont, J., & McGuire, A. L. (2009). The futility of genomic counseling: Essential role of electronic health records. *Genome Medicine*, *1*(5), 1. doi:10.1186/gm48 PMID:19439060

Bergmann, J., Bott, O. J., Pretschner, D. P., & Haux, R. (2007). An econsent-based shared EHR system architecture for integrated healthcare networks. *International Journal of Medical Informatics*, *76*(2-3), 130–136. doi:10.1016/j.ijmedinf.2006.07.013 PMID:16971171

Bhatti, R., & Grandison, T. (2007). *Towards improved privacy policy coverage in healthcare using policy refinement*. Berlin: Springer. doi:10.1007/978-3-540-75248-6_11

Boonstra, H., & Nash, E. (2000). Minors and the right to consent to health care. *The Guttmacher Report on Public Policy*, *3*(4), 4–8. PMID:12134879

Bourgeois, F. C., Taylor, P. L., Emans, S. J., Nigrin, D. J., & Mandl, K. D. (2008). Whose personal control? Creating private, personally controlled health records for pediatric and adolescent patients. *Journal of the American Medical Informatics Association*, *15*(6), 737–743.

Buchanan, A. (2004). Mental capacity, legal competence and consent to treatment. *Journal of the Royal Society of Medicine*, *97*(9), 415–420.

Clayton, E. W., Steinberg, K. K., Khoury, M. J., Thomson, E., Andrews, L., Kahn, M. J. E., & Weiss, J. O. et al. (1995). Informed consent for genetic research on stored tissue samples. *Journal of the American Medical Association*, *274*(22), 1786–1792. doi:10.1001/jama.1995.03530220052033 PMID:7500511

Coiera, E., & Clark, R. (2004, March/April). e-Consent: The design and Implementation of consumer consent mechanisms in an electronic environment. *Journal of the American Informatics Association, 11*(2). PMID:14662803

Compbell, D. (June, 2004). Case and Commentary – Listen to the family. *Morbidity & Mortality Rounds on the Web. AHRQ.* Retrieved August 8, 2013, from http://webmm.ahrq.gov/case.aspx?caseID=62

Dang, J., Hedayati, A., Hampel, K., & Toklu, C. (2008). An ontological knowledge framework for adaptive medical workflow. *Journal of Biomedical Informatics, 41*(5), 829–836. doi:10.1016/j.jbi.2008.05.012 PMID:18602872

Del Carmen, M. G., & Joffe, S. (2005). Informed consent for medical treatment and research: A review. *The Oncologist, 10*(8), 636–641. doi:10.1634/theoncologist.10-8-636 PMID:16177288

Health insurance portability and accountability act. U.S. department of health and human services. (2013). Retrieved February 20, 2014, from http://www.gpo.gov/fdsys/pkg/FR-2013-01-25/pdf/2013-01073.pdf

Fisher, C. B. (2002). Goodness-of-Fit Ethic for Informed Consent. *A. Fordham Urb. LJ, 30*, 159. PMID:15868667

Garde, S., Knaup, P., Hovenga, E. J., & Heard, S. (2007). Towards Semantic Interoperability for Electronic Health Records--Domain Knowledge Governance for open EHR Archetypes. *Methods of Information in Medicine, 46*(3), 332–343. PMID:17492120

Genetic Information Non-discrimination Act of 2008 (GINA). *Pub. L. 110-233*, 122 Stat. 883, codified as amended in scattered sections of 26, 29, and 42 U.S.C.

Gostin, L. O., & Hodge, J. G. Jr. (1999). Genetic privacy and the law: An end to genetics exceptionalism. *Jurimetrics*, 21–58. PMID:12465649

Grimson, J., Stephens, G., Jung, B., Grimson, W., Berry, D., & Pardon, S. (2001). Sharing health- care records over the internet. *IEEE Internet Computing, 5*(3), 49–58. doi:10.1109/4236.935177

Grisso, T., & Appelbaum, P. S. (1998). *Assessing competence to consent to treatment: A guide for physicians and other health professionals*. Oxford University Press.

Hall, D. E., Prochazka, A. V., & Fink, A. S. (2012). Informed consent for clinical treatment. *Canadian Medical Association Journal, 184*(5), 533–540. doi:10.1503/cmaj.112120 PMID:22392947

Gruber, T. R. (1993). A translation approach to portable ontology specifications. *Knowledge Acquisition, 5*(2), 199–220. doi:10.1006/knac.1993.1008

Hallinan, D., & Friedewald, M. (2015). Open consent, biobanking and data protection law: can open consent be 'informed'under the forthcoming data protection regulation?. *Life Sciences, Society and Policy, 11*(1), 1.

Gruber, T. R. (1995). Toward principles for the design of ontologies used for knowledge sharing? *International Journal of Human-Computer Studies, 43*(5), 907–928. doi:10.1006/ijhc.1995.1081

Gymrek, M., McGuire, A. L., Golan, D., Halperin, E., & Erlich, Y. (2013). Identifying personal genomes by surname inference. *Science, 339*(6117), 321–324. doi:10.1126/science.1229566 PMID:23329047

HIPAA Compliance Assistance. (2003). *Summary of the HIPAA privacy rule*. Office for Civil Rights. Retrieved February 20, 2014, from http://www.hhs.gov/ocr/privacy/hipaa/understanding/summary/privacysummary.pdf

Holder, A. R. (1987). Minors' rights to consent to medical care. *Journal of the American Medical Association*, *257*(24), 3400–3402. doi:10.1001/jama.1987.03390240106033 PMID:3586272

Kaye, J., Heeney, C., Hawkins, N., De Vries, J., & Boddington, P. (2009). Data sharing in genomics—re-shaping scientific practice. *Nature Reviews. Genetics*, *10*(5), 331–335. doi:10.1038/nrg2573 PMID:19308065

Kerath, S. M., Klein, G., Kern, M., Shapira, I., Witthuhn, J., Norohna, N., & Taioli, E. et al. (2013). Beliefs and attitudes towards participating in genetic research–a population based cross-sectional study. *BMC Public Health*, *13*(1), 1. doi:10.1186/1471-2458-13-114 PMID:23388465

Khoury, M. J., & Dorman, J. S. (1998). The human genome epidemiology network. *American Journal of Epidemiology*, *148*(1), 1–3. doi:10.1093/aje/148.1.1 PMID:9663396

Knoppers, B. M. (2005). Consent revisited: Points to consider. *Health Law Review*, *13*(2-3), 33–38. PMID:16459412

Liao, S. M. (2009). Is there a duty to share genetic information? *Journal of Medical Ethics*, *35*(5), 306–309. doi:10.1136/jme.2008.027029 PMID:19407036

Locatelli, P., Restifo, N., Gastaldi, L., & Corso, M. (2012). Health Care Information Systems: Architectural Models and Governance. In C. Kalloniatis (Ed.), *Innovative Information Systems Modelling and Techniques* (pp. 71–96). Rijeka, Croatia: InTech. doi:10.5772/38212

Lunshof, J. E., Chadwick, R., Vorhaus, D. B., & Church, G. M. (2008). From genetic privacy to open consent. *Nature Reviews. Genetics*, *9*(5), 406–411. doi:10.1038/nrg2360 PMID:18379574

Mascalzoni, D., Hicks, A., Pramstaller, P., & Wjst, M. (2008). Informed consent in the genomics era. *PLoS Medicine*, *5*(9), e192. doi:10.1371/journal.pmed.0050192 PMID:18798689

Matos, E. E., Campos, F., Braga, R., & Palazzi, D. (2010). CelOWS: An ontology based framework for the provision of semantic web services related to biological models. *Journal of Biomedical Informatics*, *43*(1), 125–136. doi:10.1016/j.jbi.2009.08.008 PMID:19695346

Merker, J. (2014). *Establishing a clinical genomics program at an academic medical center.* Regional APC/PDAS Meeting, Kauuai.

McGuire, A. L., & Beskow, L. M. (2010). Informed consent in genomics and genetic research. *Annual Review of Genomics and Human Genetics*, *11*(1), 361–381. doi:10.1146/annurev-genom-082509-141711 PMID:20477535

Mulholland, W. F. (1998). Genetic privacy and discrimination: A survey of state legislation. *Jurimetrics*, *39*, 317. PMID:11762444

National Conference of State Legislatures. (2008). *Genetic privacy laws.* Congressional Research Service. Retrieved March 2008 from http://www.ncsl.org/research/health/genetic-privacy-laws.aspx

Németh, A. H., Kwasniewska, A. C., Lise, S., Schnekenberg, R. P., Becker, E. B., Bera, K. D., & Talbot, K. et al. (2013). Next generation sequencing for molecular diagnosis of neurological disorders using ataxias as a model. *Brain*, awt236. PMID:24030952

Noy, N. F., & McGuinness, D. L. (2001). *Ontology development 101: A guide to creating your first ontology*. Retrieved February 20, 2014, from http://protege.stanford.edu/publications/ontology_development/ontology101.pdf

O'Daniel, J., Scott, J., Varga, E., Speights, V., & Gordon, E. (2012). Lecture iv: Genomic medicine: Communicating with the patient. *TRiG Curriculum: Lecture 4.*

O'Keefe, C. M., Greenfield, P., & Goodchild, A. (2005). A decentralized approach to electronic consent and health information access control. *Journal of Research and Practice in Information Technology*, *37*(2), 161–178.

O'Leary, C. (2010). Informed consent-principles and practice. *ASA Newsletter*, *74*(2), 20–21.

Petersen, A. (2007). 'Biobanks'" engagements": Engendering trust or engineering consent?'. *Genomics. Social Policy*, *3*(1), 1–13.

Petronio, S. (2012). *Boundaries of privacy: Dialectics of disclosure*. Suny Press.

Presidential Commission for the Study of Bioethical Issues. (2013). Retrieved March 23, 2015, from http://www.bioethics.gov/sites/default/files/Informed%20Consent%20Background%20090413.pdf

Prince, A. E., & Roche, M. I. (2014). Genetic information, non-discrimination, and privacy protections in genetic counseling practice. *Journal of Genetic Counseling*, *23*(6), 891–902. doi:10.1007/s10897-014-9743-2 PMID:25063358

Rehm, H. L., Hynes, E., & Funke, B. H. (2016). The changing landscape of molecular diagnostic testing: Implications for Academic Medical Centers. *Journal of Personalized Medicine*, *6*(1), 8.

Riaño, D., Real, F., López-Vallverdú, J. A., Campana, F., Ercolani, S., Mecocci, P., & Caltagirone, C. (2012). An ontology-based personalization of health-care knowledge to support clinical decisions for chronically ill patients. *Journal of Biomedical Informatics*, *45*(3), 429–446. doi:10.1016/j.jbi.2011.12.008 PMID:22269224

Ritchie, M. D., Holzinger, E. R., Li, R., Pendergrass, S. A., & Kim, D. (2015). Methods of integrating data to uncover genotype-phenotype interactions. *Nature Reviews. Genetics*, *16*(2), 85–97. doi:10.1038/nrg3868 PMID:25582081

Roach, J. C., Glusman, G., Smit, A. F., Huff, C. D., Hubley, R., Shannon, P. T., & Shendure, J. et al. (2010). Analysis of genetic inheritance in a family quartet by whole-genome sequencing. *Science*, *328*(5978), 636–639. doi:10.1126/science.1186802 PMID:20220176

Rosse, C., & Mejino, J. L. Jr. (2003). A reference ontology for biomedical informatics: The Foundational Model of Anatomy. *Journal of Biomedical Informatics*, *36*(6), 478–500. doi:10.1016/j.jbi.2003.11.007 PMID:14759820

Rothstein, M. A. (2014). Privacy and Confidentiality. Routledge Handbook of Medical Law and Ethics, 52.

Ruan, C., & Yeo, S. S. (2009). Modeling of an Intelligent e-Consent System in a Healthcare Domain. *J. UCS*, *15*(12), 2429–2444.

Russello, G., Dong, C., & Dulay, N. (2008). Consent-based workflows for healthcare management. In *Policies for Distributed Systems and Networks, POLICY. IEEE Workshop on* (pp. 153-161). doi:10.1109/POLICY.2008.22

Salgo v. Leland Stanford, Jr., Univ. Bd. of Trustees, 317 P. 2d 170, 181 (Cal. App. Ct. 1957).

Saranummi, N. (2005). PICNIC architecture. *Studies in Health Technology and Informatics*, *115*, 37–60.

Scheuner, M. T., de Vries, H., Kim, B., Meili, R. C., Olmstead, S. H., & Teleki, S. (2009). Are electronic health records ready for genomic medicine? *Genetics in Medicine*, *11*(7), 510–517. doi:10.1097/GIM.0b013e3181a53331 PMID:19478682

Secko, D. M., Preto, N., Niemeyer, S., & Burgess, M. M. (2009). Informed consent in biobank research: A deliberative approach to the debate. *Social Science & Medicine*, *68*(4), 781–789. doi:10.1016/j.socscimed.2008.11.020 PMID:19095337

Sheppard, N. P., Safavi-Naini, R., & Jafari, M. (2009). A digital rights management model for healthcare. In Policies for Distributed Systems and Networks. *POLICY 2009.IEEE International Symposium* (pp. 106-109). doi:10.1109/POLICY.2009.8

Sherlock, E. (2009). *Disclosure of patient's genetic information without their consent- Is the "public interset" really a Sufficient Justification?* Genomics Law Report. retrieved March 2, 2015, from http://www.genomicslawreport.com/index.php/2009/11/10/disclosure-of-patients-genetic-information-without-their-consent-is-the-public-interest-really-a-sufficient-justification/

Shortliffe, E. H., & Cimino, J. J. (2006). *Biomedical informatics*. Springer Science + Business Media, LLC.

Strouse, D. S. (2005). Informed consent to genetic research on banked human tissue. *Jurimetrics*, 135–152.

Struewingl, J. P., & Abeliovich, D. (1995). The carrier frequency of the BRCA1 185delAG mutation. *Nature Genetics*, 11.

Studdert, D. M., Mello, M. M., Levy, M. K., Gruen, R. L., Dunn, E. J., Orav, E. J., & Brennan, T. A. (2007). Geographic variation in informed consent law: Two standards for disclosure of treatment risks. *Journal of Empirical Legal Studies*, *4*(1), 103–124. doi:10.1111/j.1740-1461.2007.00083.x

Ullman-Cullere, M. H., & Mathew, J. P. (2011). Emerging landscape of genomics in the electronic health record for personalized medicine. *Human Mutation*, *32*(5), 512–516. doi:10.1002/humu.21456 PMID:21309042

Valls, A., Gibert, K., Sánchez, D., & Batet, M. (2010). Using ontologies for structuring organizational knowledge in Home Care assistance. *International Journal of Medical Informatics*, *79*(5), 370–387. doi:10.1016/j.ijmedinf.2010.01.012 PMID:20185360

VHA HANDBOOK 1004.05, Transmittal Sheet. (2005). *IMEDCONSENT™*. Retrieved August 17, 2013, from http://www.va.gov/vhapublications/ViewPublication.asp?pub_ID=1857

Virginia women's center - cancer family history questionnaire. (n.d.). Retrieved May 22, 2015, from https://www.virginiawomenscenter.com/assets/HEREDITARY_CANCER_RISK_ASSESSMENT_FORM.pdf

Wickramasinghe, N., & Geisler, E. (Eds.). (2008). *Encyclopedia of Healthcare Information Systems*. Hershey, PA: Medical Information Science Reference. doi:10.4018/978-1-59904-889-5

Wirth, T., Parker, N., & Ylä-Herttuala, S. (2013). History of gene therapy. *Gene*, *525*(2), 162–169. doi:10.1016/j.gene.2013.03.137 PMID:23618815

Win, K., Song, H., Croll, P., & Cooper, J. (2002). Implementing patients consent in electronic health record systems. *Proceedings of CollECTeR*.

Win, K. T., & Fulcher, J. A. (2007). Consent mechanisms for electronic health record systems: A simple yet unresolved issue. *Journal of Medical Systems*, *31*(2), 91–96. doi:10.1007/s10916-006-9030-3 PMID:17489500

Yu, A. C. (2006). Methods in biomedical ontology. *Journal of Biomedical Informatics*, *39*(3), 252–266. doi:10.1016/j.jbi.2005.11.006 PMID:16387553

Yu, B., & Wijesekera, D. (2013). Building Dialysis Workflows into EMRs. *Procedia Technology, 9*, 985-995.

Yu, B., Wijesekera, D., & Costa, P. (2014). Consent-Based Workflow Control in EMRs. *HCIST- International Conference on Health and Social Care Information Systems and Technologies*, 72-79.

Yu, B., Wijesekera, D., & Costa, P. (2014). An Ontology for Medical Treatment Consent. *The 9th International Conference on. Semantic Technologies for Intelligence, Defense, and Security - STIDS 2014*.

Yu, B., Wijesekera, D., Costa, P., & Hiremagalore, S. (2015). Genetic Counseling Using Workflow-based EMRs. *The 10th International Conference on. Semantic Technologies for Intelligence, Defense, and Security - STIDS2015*.

KEY TERMS AND DEFINITIONS

Consent Ontology: An ontology of consent.

Electronic Medical Record (EMR) System: An electronic system that manages medical data.

Genetic Counseling: Counseling related to genetic issues.

Genetic Services: A set of services that generates or uses genetic data.

Medical Informed Consent: A decision and permission to perform a procedure in medicine.

Participating Research Consent: A decision and permission to participate in medical research.

Privacy Consent: A decision and permission to use and disclose information.

The Health Insurance Portability and Accountability Act (HIPAA): The federal laws to protect patients' PHI for covered entities.

Treatment Consent: A decision and permission to treat medically.

Workflow Management: A management system for executing workflows.

Chapter 14
Improving Quality Improvement Collaboratives:
Mixing Communication Media to Attain Multiple Measures of Success

Priscilla A. Arling
Butler University, USA

Edward J. Miech
Regenstrief Institute, USA

Greg W. Arling
Purdue University School of Nursing, USA

ABSTRACT

For several decades, researchers have studied the comparative effects of face-to-face and electronic communication. Some have claimed that electronic communication is detrimental to outcomes while others have emphasized its advantages. For members of healthcare quality improvement (QI) collaboratives, a mix of both of types of communication is often used, due to geographical dispersion. This chapter examines the outcomes of a specific QI collaborative, the Empira Falls Prevention project in Minnesota, USA. Levels of electronic communication between collaborative members were found to be associated with a positive patient outcome, specifically a reduction in falls. Electronic and face-to-face communication differed in their association with success measures for the collaborative. The findings suggest that the two modes of communication can be leverage to attain maximum benefits from participating in a quality improvement collaborative.

DOI: 10.4018/978-1-5225-1724-5.ch014

INTRODUCTION

Despite the prevalence of electronic communication in the workplace researchers continue to debate the effectiveness of electronic media for getting work done in teams. Some have stated that electronic interaction is a poor replacement for face-to-face and can lead to misunderstandings and damaged personal relationships (Hinds & Bailey, 2003; Nardi & Whittaker, 2002). Others argue that despite the drawbacks, electronic communication is essential, particularly when work involves group members that are physically or temporally dispersed (Olson & Olson, 2000). Recently research has begun to suggest that the use a mix of communication modes enhances outcomes (Caughlin & Sharabis, 2013; Malhotra & Majchrzak, 2014). In health care settings using both electronic and face-to-face communication is commonplace. Shift work and multi-disciplinary patient care mean that caregivers are at times together at the same place at the same time, but also often work physically and temporally apart. In addition the increasing complexity of and drive to improve the quality of healthcare has given rise to one type of healthcare group, comprised of members from dispersed organizations, the *quality improvement collaborative*.

Members of quality improvement (QI) collaboratives share knowledge and act as resources for each other, with the goal of improving implementations of evidence-based practices (Newton, Davidson, Halcomb, Denniss, & Westgarth, 2006). A key purpose of a collaborative is to provide a formal structure that can be used by individuals to build networks of support and gain access to expertise in implementation areas. Many collaboratives hold scheduled conferences where members learn about problem-solving techniques and evidence-based practices, and individuals have the opportunity to meet in person. Members also share experiences during collaborative meetings. Other tools used in collaboratives can include site visits, written reports and sharing of data via electronic methods (Nembhard, 2009). Multiple studies have reported collaborative successes in improving processes, including studies in the areas of colorectal, perinatal, and diabetes care (Gould, 2010; Hicks et al., 2010; Jackson et al., 2010). Others, however, have suggested that collaboratives have only modest effects on outcomes and have concluded that little is known about the specific components that affect a collaborative's effectiveness (Schouten, Hulscher, van Everdingen, Huijsman, & Grol, 2008). In addition few studies have assessed or found a positive effect on patient outcomes (Nadeem, Olin, Hill, Hoagwood, & Horwitz, 2013). Therefore there is a need for research on the behaviors of collaborative participants and the effect on outcomes (Lindenauer, 2008; Nadeem et al, 2013).

This chapter seeks to better understand how a mix of electronic and face-to-face communication employed by individual participants in a collaborative can affect measurable, objective outcomes in health care. To do so, the authors present a study of a fall prevention project carried out by Empira, a quality improvement collaborative of Minnesota nursing homes.

BACKGROUND

Quality Improvement Collaboratives and Communication

In quality improvement collaboratives, members from multiple organizations work together to share information on effective interventions and ways to overcome barriers to implementations (Cretin, Shortell, & Keeler, 2004; Kilo, 1998). A central premise underlying success for collaboratives is that members learn and benefit from each other. The collaborative also offers access to experts via a variety of communication methods. Inter-organizational communication is a key differentiator in terms of whether or not collaborative participation benefits specific members (Nembhard, 2009).

Inter-organizational communication between collaborative members is likely to occur both face-to-face and electronically, since participants typically come from geographically dispersed locations. Both collaborative organizers and members have a choice as to the mode by which they communicate and the extent to which they communicate via that mode. In addition to hosting face-to-face learning sessions, collaboratives often provide participants with a mix of methods by which to communicate including collaborative-specific websites (extranets), phone calls, and written reports (Kilo, 1998; Nembhard, 2009; Nadeem et al, 2013). While studies have reported the benefits of in-person learning sessions and meetings (e.g. Nembhard, 2009; Ovretveit, 2002; Schouten et al., 2010), relatively little is known about the extent to which face-to-face or electronic communication between members, outside of regularly scheduled meetings, influences outcomes.

Face-to-Face vs. Electronic Communication in Dispersed Groups

In any group, physical and temporal dispersion of members influences who is contacted, how often and by what mode of communication, either face-to-face or electronic. Face-to-face access is limited to proximal others while electronic access is possible regardless of physical distance from team members. Even when people are just 30 feet away from each other, face-to-face contact drops significantly (Allen, 1977).

Even when face-to-face communication is limited, research suggests that the level and quality of face-to-face communication may be higher than electronic. Face-to-face communication is synchronous and the physical context shared by communicators makes the repair of misunderstandings faster and easier, which reduces conflict between individuals and increases the frequency of communication (Hinds & Bailey, 2003). Face-to-face interaction engenders social bonding through the involvement of the human body that is not easily replicated electronically (Nardi & Whittaker, 2002). Face-to-face interaction also enhances individual commitment to the relationship, which encourages further future interaction (Kraut, Galegher, & Egido, 1987; Nardi, 2005). In groups, the social bonding and shared physical context associated with face-to-face interaction are critical to developing mutual knowledge, and in particular learning what knowledge others possess (Cramton, 2001; Monge & Contractor, 2003). Many believe therefore that face-to-face communication, as compared to electronic communication, provides the highest quality knowledge exchange and the most benefits.

However electronic communication is frequently used to span physical and temporal gaps that may otherwise restrict group member contact (Griffith, Sawyer, & Neale, 2003). Since electronic communication is asynchronous it can also improve the timeliness of information exchange (Ramirez, Walther, Burgoon, & Sunnafrank, 2002). Electronic communication expands the range and diversity of an individual's contacts in a network, which can increase overall communication (Monge & Eisenberg, 1990). Group members do not have to wait for individuals to be physically present to send them an email or to leave a voice or text message, nor does a group member have to get another's immediate attention. Information can be shared electronically when it is convenient for the sender, even if the receiver is unavailable, which can improve the timing of the information.

Increasingly research has found that leveraging a mix of face-to-face and electronic communication can improve outcomes. Caughlin and Sharabis (2013) studied the relationships of over 300 undergraduate students and found that interpersonal satisfaction was higher when individuals used both mediated and face-to-face communication. Geissler and colleagues (Geissler, Hasenbein, Kanatouri, & Wegener,

2014) compared electronic-based and face-to-face coaching sessions. They suggest that while electronic communication has specific advantages, a blended approach using both modalities for coaching reaps the most rewards. Indeed research has begun to suggest that 'virtuality', the mix of electronic and face-to-face communication used, should be measured both at the individual and task level (Dennis et al, 2008, Orhan, 2014). That is, depending upon the goal, each mode of communication has advantages and disadvantages.

EMPIRA FALLS PREVENTION COLLABORATIVE STUDY

To investigate the impact of electronic and face-to-face communication the authors studied a single QI collaborative, the Empira Falls Prevention project. The project ran from October 2008 through September 2011 in the state of Minnesota. The goal of the project was to reduce the prevalence of falls among nursing home residents. Empira assisted with the development and implementation of fall prevention strategies through facility-based project coordinators (PCs). The PCs established fall prevention teams or committees in their facilities. The collaborative held regularly scheduled meetings at once a month. Empira leaders and members also communicated by email, phone, or texting outside of meetings. The collaborative facilitated the project by searching for and presenting information on evidence-based practices for falls prevention, training members, consulting and problem solving with PCs, and collecting and reporting project data. On average the 15 project facilities reduced the rate of falls for their residents by 31% between 2007 (the year before the project began) and 2010.

Communication Data: Collection and Analysis

Both quantitative and qualitative data were collected and analyzed. Quantitative data regarding collaborative members' communication were collected at the August 2011 meeting of the collaborative. Members were asked to complete a survey regarding their communication patterns and opinions related to the collaborative and their facility's project. Thirty-four survey responses were received from nineteen project coordinators and fifteen therapeutic recreation directors participating in the collaborative. Five of the survey respondents were from Empira or from a corporate headquarters, and did not have associated facility fall reduction data. These responses were excluded from the analyses. The number of respondents per facility ranged from 1 to 3. The final dataset analyzed included 29 individual survey responses, representing 15 facilities. Due to exploratory nature of the study and the small sample size, the analysis was limited to observed correlations between factors.

Two measures of communication outside of regularly scheduled meetings were captured via the survey. The communication question asked: "Thinking about all of your communication with other collaborative members (outside of your facility), how often do you send or receive information about falls prevention via the following methods?" Six methods were listed: in-person (outside of collaborative meetings), voice telephone, texting telephone, email, website, other. For each method, respondents were asked to choose from the following frequencies, with the weighted value of each in parentheses: every day (5), several times a week (4), once or twice a week (3), at least monthly (2), less than once a month (1) or do not contact (0). From these responses two variables were constructed: "In-Person Communication," the level of face-to-face communication conducted with collaborative members outside of scheduled meetings; and "Electronic Communication," the sum of all technology-based communication outside of scheduled meetings.

Respondents were asked to provide subjective assessments of collaborative outcomes by rating both the effectiveness and success of the Empira Falls Prevention Collaborative when it came to helping them carry out falls prevention project in their facilities in the following areas:

- Effectiveness in helping to figure out how to sustain the project in the facility;
- Effectiveness in helping to obtain staff buy-in in the facility for the project;
- Effectiveness in keeping everyone in the collaborative informed;
- Success in stimulating new quality improvement ideas;
- Success in figuring out how to measure other areas of quality;
- Success in creating a better organizational climate for quality.

The variables were measured on a four point Likert scale with '1' being not effective or not successful, to '4' being highly effective or highly successful.

Qualitative data were collected from two group interviews conducted at project meetings and inform the quantitative findings. Demographic, descriptive data about respondents were also collected and are discussed in the results section.

Fall Reduction Data: Collection and Analysis

Each facility's percentage change in the prevalence of residents experiencing new falls was based on a quality indicator that is part of the Minnesota Nursing Home Report Card. The rate of new falls is calculated quarterly based on standardized resident assessment data collected and reported to the state by all the state's 370 nursing facilities. For the purposes of this study, the authors compared the change in the rate of falls between 2007, the year before the project began, and 2010, the most current year for which falls data were available for all facilities. Each facility's decrease or increase in fall reduction percentage was captured as the Fall Reduction Percentage. The Fall Reduction Percentage for the collaborative facilities ranged from a 10% increase to a 55% decrease, establishing that there was considerable variation in outcomes across the 15 sites. Two facilities experienced an increase in falls in the year reported, one with a 10% increase and the other with a 4% increase. The range for facilities whose falls decreased was from 14% to 55%.

STUDY FINDINGS

Survey Respondent Descriptions

Of the 29 individual respondents, 24 (83%) were female. The majority (19, 65%) had a bachelor's degree or equivalent, while 31% (9) had some college and 1 (3%) have a master's degree or higher. Twelve of the respondents (41%) were licensed RN's, 3 (10%) were licensed recreational therapists, and the 14 others had various licenses or certificates including LPN, Nursing Home Administrator, Activity Director, CTRS, social worker and CPI instructor. Most of the respondents (20, 69%) were between 45 and 64 years of age. Eight (28%) respondents were between 26 and 44 years old and one (3%) was between

18 and 25. The average length of time in job for respondents was 8.42 years, while the average length of time in the facility for each was 10.17 years. The average respondent had spent 20.92 years in long term care and had been with the collaborative for 2.77 years.

Impact of Communication on Fall Reduction Percentage

Electronic communication was significantly and positively correlated to improvement in fall reduction ($r=0.532$, $p<0.05$). In-person communication, by contrast, was not significantly related to changes in facility fall rates.

To investigate the communication variables further, the authors looked at the correlations between those variables and perceptions of the collaborative's effectiveness and success. Electronic communication was correlated to the perceived effectiveness of the collaborative in keeping members informed ($r=0.761$, $p<0.01$), effectiveness in helping members sustain projects ($r=0.605$, $p<0.05$) and effectiveness in obtaining staff buy-in at the facility for the project ($r=0.713$, $p<0.01$). In-person communication was positively correlated to success in creating a better organizational climate for quality ($r=0.531$, $p<0.05$), success in stimulating new ideas ($r=0.692$, $p<0.01$), and success figuring out how to measure other areas of quality ($r=0.518$, $p<0.05$). The findings above support research that has found that a mix of electronic and face-to-face communication should be used, each selected based on the task to be executed (Dennis et al, 2008; Geissler, et al, 2014; Orhan, 2014).

IMPLICATIONS

An important finding from this study is that electronic communication between collaborative members has a positive effect on patient outcomes, in this case, fall reduction. Respondents who experienced the highest level of electronic communication with collaborative members were based in facilities with the highest fall reduction percentages. The findings also suggest that different modes and levels of communication used by collaborative members outside of meetings influence the benefits reaped from participation. Electronic communication was related to perceived collaborative effectiveness. In-person communication, although not directly related to fall reduction improvement, was related to perceived success in other areas.

Electronic Communication's Contribution to Effective Change

The results highlight the importance of the electronic communication in today's work environment, where groups are geographically dispersed and timely access to information is critical to being effective in a job. The relationship between electronic communication and fall reduction improvement suggests that an important advantage of participating in a collaborative is conveying knowledge outside of face-to-face scheduled meetings. Through electronic communication members received information when it was most needed and most effective. This in turn had a positive impact on patient care and individual patients. Members with the highest electronic communication levels outside of meetings also felt that the collaborative kept them informed, assisted with obtaining staff buy-in, and assisted in figuring out how to sustain their project.

Qualitative data from the focus group interviews provided additional insights as to how and why electronic communication in the collaborative was associated with fall reduction and perceptions of collaborative effectiveness.

In the interviews several respondents reflected upon their use of email outside of meetings, including the quality and purpose of that contact. One respondent discussed how she assessed the value and quality of email communication, both for sending questions and receiving answers:

For me, high quality is, did I get the answer? (laughing) How many of you have sent me, 'Is this a fall?' Yes. No. But that's it...did we get an answer, did we solve the problem?

For the respondent above, email was used to get answers quickly and help define ambiguous situations, such as what is considered a fall and how to solve a unique problem. Another member referred to how email was used to get more general information related to learning:

Another example, if I needed a Power Point or something to do some education.

A third individual noted how electronic communication was used to efficiently set up face-to-face interaction and extend communication network contacts. Emails could be sent to coordinators who could direct the collaborative participant to others who had the needed information.

And sending an email out to (name here) and say can I have a contact meeting and getting it back timely.... it was a very valuable contact to get the information that I needed to help at a facility.

And when the interviewer asked:

Do you just pick up the phone or fire off an email between meetings to get charged up?

Several members answered simultaneously 'Emails', emphasizing the effectiveness and efficiency of the asynchronous, text based mode of communication.

The comments reflect how electronic communication was leveraged to acquire information quickly, whether it was structured, educational content such as in PowerPoint slides or more informal, expert feedback on a specific fall situation. The high use of email communication also highlights how asynchronous communication was used by members to make the best of use of their time, while still quickly obtaining information. As one member noted above, a key attribute of the communication is getting the information in a timely manner, when it is needed and from someone they know can offer support. Malhotra and Marjchak (2014) found when tasks are not routine, the use of electronic media has a positive relationship with outcomes in distributed groups. For members of this collaborative, email was used to get quick answers to unique situations.

Another member, who joined the group later in the project, noted that he would have appreciated having more information electronically recorded from the group, so he could quickly access and pick up on what had already been learned:

..it would have been nice to have something that was, well, this is what my predecessor did before me. You now, they worked on this and this and have all this stuff recorded that I could just kind of come and pick it up instead of, OK, what do I do? .. It just would have been smoother I think if something had been recorded exactly what was done and exactly what I need to be doing moving forward.

These results support prior work by Dennis and colleagues (Dennis, Fuller, & Valacich, 2008) that notes that asynchronous communication modes such as email, are well suited for when individuals need to acquire large amounts of diverse information quickly, and need time to make sense of the information individually. More synchronous modes such as face-to-face, however, are more suited to discussion of each individual's interpretation of a situation, agreeing on the meaning of information and reaching a common understanding. Many of the comments highlighted the ways in which face-to-face communication benefited collaborative members.

Face-to-Face Communication Benefits

The differences in the benefits accrued from face-to-face communication suggest what topics required in-person interaction for successful communication as well as the areas of collaborative success that relied more on in-person communication. One member noted how he waited until he saw a collaborative member in-person before talking about some topics:

I think for a lot of times with me if there was something that I had a question on or something that I would want to know I would save that and wait until ...everyone was there or bring it up or maybe if like let's say if [NAME] drove with me that day I would ask her in the car ... on the way to the meeting.

The quantitative results suggest that respondents found face-to-face interaction important for stimulating new quality improvement ideas, figuring out how to measure other areas of quality improvement and for creating a better organizational climate for quality.

One member noted how in-person interaction helped her particularly when she ran out of ideas:

You run out of ideas so I think the biggest thing for me is being able to share the experience ... We kind of have things in our tool kit to move forward

The quantitative findings suggest that the 'tool kit' the member mentions above contains more than information on how to address falls. The in-person interaction helps members figure out how to measure other quality improvement areas and how to improve the climate for QI in her facility. The ability to take learning and apply it to other areas in the facility was echoed by another respondent:

I think one of the most profound things that I noticed was the root cause analysis that we applied to other areas of our operation... We have (grown) in so many other areas besides falls.

In-person communication facilitated acquiring and applying knowledge to new areas. Through face-to-face communication, individuals could easily and quickly repair any misunderstandings about a new application of information. In addition the social bonding that occurs encouraged members to share both their successes and failures with the group, the trial and error that goes along with addressing new areas.

The social bonding and commitment to relationships that occurs during face-to-face communication was highlighted by another member, who was relatively new to the group:

... people bring suggestions so there was a lot of communication and you felt comfortable. .... I've been in nursing for a long time but you felt very open and you're eager to learn and felt very accepted.

One member remarked on watching others in the group communicate face-to-face on how to address a problem and how the interaction facilitated more than just conveying information; the group came away with a shared understanding:

..the background would be presented and .. the discussion would just take off and they'd arrive at some conclusion, so there was time for both, so it was very valuable.

FUTURE RESEARCH AND DIRECTIONS

Several next steps for research are recommended based on this study. It would be useful for additional research to look at the differences between electronic and face-to-face communication in QI collaboratives. Specifically, the link found here between electronic communication and patient outcomes needs to be studied in different health care contexts and patient outcomes. Particularly as new types of electronic communication become available and embedded in every day use, the impact of leveraging those modes should be considered. In addition, a study with a larger sample that compared several collaboratives with similar objectives would help to refine these findings.

CONCLUSION

This study is one of only a handful of studies to find a positive effect of a collaborative on patient outcomes, in this case, fall reduction. It supports earlier work that has found positive effects of QI collaboratives in health care settings. The research also was unique in that it identified a specific component of the collaborative associated with that outcome, electronic communication among members. Finally, the findings suggest that different modes and levels of communication used by collaborative members outside of meetings influence the benefits reaped from participation. This work is among the first to examine the differences between the face-to-face and electronic communication in QI collaboratives and the association between communication modes and outcome measures. The authors found that face-to-face and electronic modes of communication differed in their association with improved outcomes in reducing falls as well as with self-reported measures of success.

For practitioners, this study suggests that collaborative leaders and participants should try to take full advantage of multiple modes of electronic communication available today. Websites, blogs, chat capabilities, and video conferencing are just a few of the electronic modes by which shared knowledge and networks of contacts cultivated in face-to-face meetings can be extended and leveraged outside of meetings when participants return to their geographically disparate locations. By using both face-to-face and electronic modes of communication, collaborative participants can construct new networks of contacts and then use those networks to effectively implement ideas in a timely manner to achieve measurable quality improvement in target areas.

REFERENCES

Allen, T. J. (1977). *Managing the Flow of Technology*. Cambridge, MA: MIT Press.

Caughlin, J. P., & Sharabis, L. L. (2013). A Communicative Interdependence Perspective of Close Relationships: The Connections Between Mediated and Unmediated Interactions Matter. *Journal of Communication*, *63*, 873–893.

Cramton, C. (2001). The Mutual Knowledge Problem and Its Consequences for Dispersed Collaborations. *Organization Science*, *12*(3), 346–371. doi:10.1287/orsc.12.3.346.10098

Cretin, S., Shortell, S. M., & Keeler, E. B. (2004). An Evaluation of Collaborative Interventions to Improve Chronic Illness Care. *Evaluation Review*, *28*(1), 28–51. doi:10.1177/0193841X03256298 PMID:14750290

Dennis, A. R., Fuller, R. M., & Valacich, J. S. (2008). Media, Tasks and Communication Processes: A Theory of Media Synchronicity. *Management Information Systems Quarterly*, *32*(3), 575–600.

Geissler, H., Hasenbein, M., Kanatouri, S., & Wegener, R. (2014). E-Coaching: Conceptual and Empircal Findings of a Virtual Coaching Programme. *International Journal of Evidence Based Coaching and Mentoring*, *12*(2), 165–187.

Gould, J. (2010). The role of regional collaboratives: The California Perinatal Quality Care Collaborative model. *Clinics in Perinatology*, *37*(1), 71–86. doi:10.1016/j.clp.2010.01.004 PMID:20363448

Griffith, T. L., Sawyer, J. E., & Neale, M. A. (2003). Virtualness and Knowledge in Teams: Managing the Love Triangle of Organizations, Individuals, and Information Technology. *Management Information Systems Quarterly*, *27*(2), 265–287.

Hicks, L., O'Malley, A., Lieu, T., Keegan, T., McNeil, B., Guadagnoli, E., & Landon, B. (2010). Impact of health disparities collaboratives on racial/ethnic and insurance disparities in US community health centers. *Archives of Internal Medicine*, *170*(3), 279–286. doi:10.1001/archinternmed.2010.493 PMID:20142575

Hinds, P., & Bailey, D. (2003). Out of Sight, Out of Sync: Understanding Conflict in Distributed Teams. *Organization Science*, *14*(6), 615–632. doi:10.1287/orsc.14.6.615.24872

Jackson, G., Powell, A., Ordin, D., Schlosser, J., Murawsky, J., Hersh, J., & Members, V. C. C. C. P. C. et al. (2010). Developing and sustaining quality improvement partnerships in the VA. *Journal of General Internal Medicine*, *25*(1), 38–43. doi:10.1007/s11606-009-1155-x PMID:20077150

Kilo, C. M. (1998). A Framework for Collaborative Improvement: Lessons from the Institute for Healthcare Imrpovements Breakthrough Series. *Quality Management in Health Care*, *6*(4), 1–13. doi:10.1097/00019514-199806040-00001 PMID:10339040

Kraut, R., Galegher, J., & Egido, C. (1987). Relationships and Tasks in Scientific Research Collaboration. *Human-Computer Interaction*, *3*(1), 31–58. doi:10.1207/s15327051hci0301_3

Lindenauer, P. K. (2008). Effects of quality improvement collaboratives. *British Medical Journal*, *336*(7659), 1448–1449. doi:10.1136/bmj.a216 PMID:18577558

Malhotra, A., & Majchrzak, A. (2014). Enhancing Performance of Geographically Distributed Teams Through Targeted Use of Information and Communication Technologies. *Human Relations*, *67*(4), 398–411. doi:10.1177/0018726713495284

Monge, P., & Contractor, N. (2003). *Theories of Communication Networks*. New York, NY: Oxford Univ.

Monge, P., & Eisenberg, E. (1990). Communication Networks and New Media in Organizations. In J. Fulk & C. Steinfield (Eds.), *Organizations and Communication Technology* (pp. 143–172). Thousand Oaks, CA: Sage.

Nadeem, E., Olin, S., Hill, L., Hoagwood, K., & Horwitz, S.Understanding the Components of Quality Improvement Collaboratives. (2013, June). A Systematic Literature Review. *The Milbank Quarterly*, *91*(2), 354–394. doi:10.1111/milq.12016 PMID:23758514

Nardi, B. (2005). Beyond Bandwidth: Dimensions of Connection in Interpersonal Communication. *Computer Supported Cooperative Work*, *14*(2), 91–130. doi:10.1007/s10606-004-8127-9

Nardi, B., & Whittaker, S. (2002). The Place of Face-to-Face Communication in Distributed Work. In P. Hinds & S. Kiesler (Eds.), *Distributed Work* (pp. 83–110). Cambridge, MA: MIT Press.

Nembhard, I. M. (2009). Learning and Improving in Quality Improvement Collaboratives: Which Collaborative Features Do Participants Value Most? *Health Services Research, 44*(2), 358-378.

Newton, P. J., Davidson, P. M., Halcomb, E. J., Denniss, A. R., & Westgarth, F. (2006). A Introduction to the Collaborative Methodology and Its Potential Use for Management of Heart Failure. *The Journal of Cardiovascular Nursing*, *21*(3), 161–168. doi:10.1097/00005082-200605000-00002 PMID:16699354

Olson, G., & Olson, J. (2000). Distance Matters. *Human-Computer Interaction*, *15*(2), 139–178. doi:10.1207/S15327051HCI1523_4

Orhan, M. (2014). Extending the Individual Level of Virtuality: Implications of Task Virtuality in Virtual and Traditonal Settings. *American Scientist*, *4*, 400–412.

Ovretveit, J. (2002). How to run an effective improvement collaborative. *International Journal of Health Care Quality Assurance*, *15*(4/5), 192–196. doi:10.1108/09526860210437403

Ramirez, A., Walther, J. B., Burgoon, J. K., & Sunnafrank, M. (2002). Information-Seeking Strategies, Uncertainty, and Computer-Mediated Communication: Toward a Conceptual Model. *Human Communication Research*, *28*(2), 213–228.

Schouten, L. M. T., Hulscher, M. E., van Everdingen, J. J., Huijsman, R., & Grol, R. P. (2008). Evidence for the impact of quality improvement collaboratives: Systematic review. *BMJ (Clinical Research Ed.)*, *336*(7659), 1491–1494. doi:10.1136/bmj.39570.749884.BE PMID:18577559

Schouten, L. M. T., Hulscher, M. E. J. L., van Everdingen, J. J. E., Huijsman, R., Niessen, L. W., & Grol, R. P. T. M. (2010). Short- and long-term effects of a quality improvement collaborative on diabetes management. *Implementation Science; IS*, *5*(1), 94. doi:10.1186/1748-5908-5-94 PMID:21110898

KEY TERMS AND DEFINITIONS

Asynchronous: Not occurring at the same time; occurring at different points in time.

Electronic Communication: Interaction between two or more individuals that is carried out via technological assistance, regardless of the physical proximity of the individuals.

Face-to-Face Communication: Interaction between two or more individuals that is carried out without any technological assistance, typically in close physical proximity.

Synchronous: Occurring at the same time.

Virtuality: A measure of the level of the mix of electronic and face-to-face communication used by an individual or group.

Chapter 15
We Can Trust without Data, But We Are Accountable Only through Measurement

Vahé A. Kazandjian
The Johns Hopkins University, USA

ABSTRACT

Traditional expectations about healthcare continue to be challenged by the umbrella concerns about accountability and trust. The core of this challenge is two-fold: healthcare providers have seen the absolute trust placed into their intentions and practices erode through the quantification of quality and safety of care, and, the recipients of care have been empowered with timely and specific data to demand accountability rather than unquestionably trust providers. The purpose of this chapter is to review the key dimensions of the operationalization of performance measurement and the translation of its findings to statements about quality and safety of care. The past four decades have seen the continuous discovery and refining of analytical tools to quantify what once was taken for granted: that patients always receive the best care possible. These tools have uncovered the probabilistic nature of medicine and the resulting nature of the relationships outcomes have to processes. Hence the expectations of patients, payers of care and policy makers require being continuously modified to reflect the limitations of medicine and healthcare. The education of various audiences as to what the measures mean not only is a necessary requisite for sound project design but also will determine how the accountability model is shaped in each environment based on the generic measurement tools results, local traditions of care and caring, and expectations about outcomes.

INTRODUCTION

There is, as it should be, ongoing debate in health services research about the best tools for measuring health care performance. Yet, and in parallel with the search for the best tools, external requirements for data reporting and accountability about quality and safety of care are shaping the focus of inquiry, the nature of the measurement strategies, and the models of accountability. The central themes for the debate could be summarized under the following categories:

DOI: 10.4018/978-1-5225-1724-5.ch015

- The focus of the inquiry;
- The adoption of state of the art measurement science; and,
- The promises about how the healthcare system would increase appropriateness, enhance its safety, and demonstrate these changes in a systematic and ongoing way;
- The communication with and education of those responsible for policy.

This chapter addresses the topic of quality through the measurement of performance specifically in hospitals. It is not the purpose of this chapter to review performance measurement systems, but to discuss the above three categories as fundamental to all performance measurement and evaluation systems. As an illustration, voluntary data reporting about medication safety is discussed addressing the three themes of this paper: focus of inquiry, measurement, and the promises for increasingly appropriate and safe health care services.

THE FOCUS OF THE INQUIRY

"*Where to look?*" is the first question during an inquiry, and one would assume that there is sufficient and progressive guidance to professionals to initiate this inquiry. Unfortunately, that is not the case. "Traditional" aspects of care and caring have been evaluated ad nauseam in the past fourty years with variable outcomes. The focus on the area of inquiry not only varies by the health care system's traditional beliefs on how services should be delivered (Cylus et al, 2015; Ladhani, et al., 2014; Hyppönen, et al., 2014; Moses, et al., 2103; Merlino & Raman, 2013), but also by the expectations of the recipients of care (Health Affairs, 2016; Danforth et al, 2013; Carvalho, 2013; Marcieca et al, 2013). The introduction of recipient expectations regarding access to quality care, empathy by the caregivers, and affordability of the services is a relatively new paradigm even in health care systems with a tradition of accountability. The novelty of the paradigm is in its departure from the purely "professional model" (Jha et al, 2014; Parchman & Burge, 2004; Firth-Cozens et al, 2004; Snyderman & Williams, 2003; Redman & Lynn, 2004) where expectations are defined à priori by those who deliver the care and caring. The dissonance between the professionals' opinions about appropriateness and the recipients' expectations of good outcomes becomes apparent when performance measurement systems are also used towards accountability (Kazandjian, 2002; Kazandjian et al, 2005). Challenging the professional model of beliefs is a departure from the central concept of trust inherent in a few true professions. Perhaps the most apparent parallel in challenging the concept of trust is one between the profession of medicine and that of clergy (Kazandjian, 1999). Indeed, if a profession is based on peer-review, such as medicine and clergy, than the exclusive ownership of the knowledge they own and keep are for the well-being of the people they serve and therefore of late, clergy and medicine have been challenged to demonstrate accountability through quantitative, periodic, and measured demonstration of how their social mission is being accomplished. This request by communities is a significant departure from the traditional relationship of "*don't ask, just trust*" whereby the outcomes of services provided were not directly linked to the belief in the appropriateness of the process. This is of significant importance as quantification of performance naturally links processes to outcomes and eliminates all subjective feelings of trust that cannot be substantiated. In other words, the concept of trust is built on the belief that, in all situations, the professional will be providing the most appropriate service to those in need of those services. And that such an appropriate service would be delivered in the most adequate and efficient way within the context of knowledge and resources. Therefore, within the context of trust, it is the process that matters not the outcome.

The parallel between clergy and medicine can be taken a step further to encompass the issue of safety that is now central to many health care environments. That appropriate services were provided in the most adequate and efficient manner is not enough. Rather, the environment is expected to be of minimal harm to the recipients and even in some situations harm free (Pronovost & Kazandjian, 1999; Phelps & Barach, 2014; Wachter, 2004). Further, the trust in the provider of the services is being challenged by questioning if, in all situations, all precautions have been taken to minimize or eliminate actual and potential harm to patients. Thus, health care in particular, and the concept of trust in general have new meanings in today's societies as the safety of care is analysed from its undesirable perspective – that of harm. Indeed, it is rare that quantification methods of performance report on what has been done "safely" but rather report on what has caused harm, or at least predisposed to potential harm.

THE ADOPTION OF STATE OF THE ART MEASUREMENT SCIENCE

Epidemiological sciences have established a solid method of inquiry dealing with diseases and environmental factors, health care systems (especially hospitals) have rarely adapted epidemiological techniques for performance measurement. It is, therefore, worthwhile exploring relationships between epidemiological investigative techniques and the understanding of what happened to whom and why within a health care setting.

The starting point of any epidemiological inquiry is the outcome. The observation of an effect on a group of people leads the investigators to look back and understand, under what circumstances and eventually why, that observed effect had resulted. Thus, the traditional method of investigation is always retrospective. Further, once the retrospective analysis has identified possible candidates that may have "caused" the observed outcome, a certain predictive model can be developed to anticipate these effects when those factors exist individually or through the interaction, leading to the outcome. Finally, the forecasting model that results from synthesizing the knowledge gleaned from investigations would result in specific activities, such as education and prevention to eliminate or minimize the happening of these often undesirable outcomes. Therefore, the generic dimensions of epidemiological investigation are:

- Retrospective analysis to understand the reasons for the observed outcome;
- The synthesis of relationships among the possible causative factors;
- The design of a predictive forecasting model to be used in the future as an anticipatory strategy; and,
- The establishment of a series of activities towards eradication or prevention of the factors possibly causing the observed outcomes.

Not only do epidemiological investigative methods have a generic and highly portable method of inquiry, the statistical and mathematical tools that support each of the above four steps are well established and widely used. The systematic, scientific, and replicative steps of inquiry, therefore, should have a benefit to health care settings when performance measurement is undertaken. Epidemiological methods add an anticipated acceptability to the investigative methods by drawing their examples from health and disease in various social environments. Given those existing scientific methods, one would expect that performance measurement in health care would also result in a science that would be acceptable to various health care settings and methods of health care provision (Elwyn et al, 2015)

The ongoing challenges that the field of performance measurement in health care faces and the still unachieved consensus about best methods seem to indicate that such "scientification" of performance measurement is not yet reached (To et al, 2003; Kazandjian & Lied, 1999; McCarthy, Schoen & Radley, 2014; Rosen et al, 2014; Caughey, Kalisch Ellett & Wong, 2014). Previously, I had introduced the analogy between epidemiology and the study of performance in health care organizations as "epidemiology versus epinosocomiology" (Kazandjian, 2014). Indeed, if epidemiology is the study of what happens to populations, then epinosocomiology would be the study of what happens to hospitals. Is there merit to such a parallel concept when studying the question of performance and eventually translating that performance into quality of care? I believe there is. And the reasons for the usefulness of such an analogy can be found in the following similarities between the two approaches.

MEASUREMENT IS GLOBAL BUT EVALUATION IS LOCAL

The variability across health care systems to systematize the relationship between measuring performance, interpretation / evaluation, and accountability defines the pillars to a model that, curiously enough, is portable across health care systems (McKinney, (2013, Veillard et al, 2012, Drösler et al, 2009). Specifically, the first pillar centers the quantification of performance which is increasingly placed within the context of indicators that follow either epidemiological or econometric scientific methods. By definition, since these methods are scientific, they are generic to all environments – one does not measure an aspect of performance differently in different contexts. Rather, it is the interpretation of what the measurement has resulted in that will vary by social context and cultural sets of beliefs. The second pillar of this model, namely the interpretation/evaluation of the findings is a reflection of norms and principles. It is at this level that the customization to local environments evaluating health care becomes crucial. If it is "destiny" (Kazandjian, 1997; Yen, 2013) that a patient dies, then the interpretation of the outcome has little influence on how the provider's dedication to saving a patient's life is evaluated. When oncogenes become well-known culprits in certain inherited types of cancers, in cultures believing in destiny oncogenes seemed to override patient's lifestyles or risk-taking behaviors. Further, in such a culture, it may be believed that medicine could do little to change the course of destiny. Finally, in a culture that believes that science can fix anything, the slightest deviation from perfect outcomes will become fair game for litigious behavior and enhanced mistrust between providers and communities (Nicol, Mohanna & Cowpe, 2014). The third and final pillar is that of accountability, which encompasses trust. In the accountability context, and as noted previously, trust is not a dichotomous concept, i.e., there is no 100 percent versus zero percent trust. Rather, trust is a continuous concept. The level of trust is a function of the type and amount of knowledge the recipients have about the process and the anticipated outcome. In a situation like that, the concept of trust will influence different services variably at different points in time during the health care encounters and interactions. The continuous nature of the concept of trust in this model makes the understanding of performance evaluation more complex, because the "value" to be placed upon the performance (hence "evaluation") will be affected by the levels of trust, leading to anticipation, satisfaction, and acceptance.

THE VALIDITY OF THE TOOLS IN MEASURING QUALITY

Studying the Appropriateness of Health Care Delivery

Doing the right thing to the right person at the right time has often been used to describe a good performance. It is a complex three-dimensional proposition which often results in additional dimensions given the interaction between each of those three. For example, doing the right thing is predicated upon the knowledge individual providers or even organizations have about the latest relationships between methods of care and outcomes. In today's lexicon, this dimension of good care is often described as "evidence-based." Evidence should, therefore, be there between what is done and what is expected to happen in order to assist in and justify doing the right thing. But the mere presence of such evidence is not enough. Indeed that knowledge should be available to providers in a timely and complete manner (Ioannidis, 2016)

The second dimension of "doing the right thing to the right person at the right time" is that of the proper application of the evidence-based care to the right patient. Clearly, there is increasing evidence in health care that the wrong patients may be receiving treatment which in absentia of the patient itself may be evidence-based to treat a well-defined condition (Sackett, 1997). Thus, looking at doing the right thing to the right patient has to be dissociated from doing the right thing as a separate performance dimension. If the care were provided to the wrong patient, it is superfluous and unnecessary to explore if the right care was provided for the right condition. Indeed, it becomes almost experimentation and goes beyond the realm of safety and accountability. No matter how unacceptable it is to provide the care to the wrong patient, it may be useful in the abstract to have a parallel evaluation system that tries to link the diagnosis to the treatment. "Doing the right thing to the right patient at the right time" an organization or individual can, therefore, learn much about the practice of matching the right care for a given diagnosis. Although this suggestion may seem controversial, it is part of the systematic uncovering of the relationships between what is done, why it is done, and what impact it has had upon the individual patients or the organizational profile in total.

The third and final dimension is that of the right time. This concept could be expanded beyond the terminology of time or timing to connote the efficiency during the production of the services. However, efficiency does not supercede appropriateness. In other words, producing the wrong service in an efficient way does not make it appropriate. However, in situations (and these are most of the situations) where the appropriate care is decided upon and appropriately provided to the right patient, the production efficiency dimension becomes important. Understanding the efficiency in the production, and specifically the timeliness of it is a task often repeated in understanding any industry's mode of production and hence, the residual capability to be enhanced. While many models exist on how to produce services more efficiently, the discussion of efficiency has direct linkages to appropriateness but also to expectations of both recipients and providers. Figure 1 provides a set of relationships between the concept of appropriateness and production efficiency. This schematic builds upon the distinction provided by Donabedian between efficiency of the production and services and the appropriateness of that service (Donabedian, 1976). The expanded model as provided in this section takes those concepts into the operational setting and places them within the actual reality of ever growing demands by actual and potential recipients upon the health care system. The expectation of individuals, groups, or even larger geopolitical entities (cantons, states, even countries) may be influencing clinical practice in ways that are new and worth understanding. In the 1980's, "defensive medicine" was one of the explications

Figure 1.

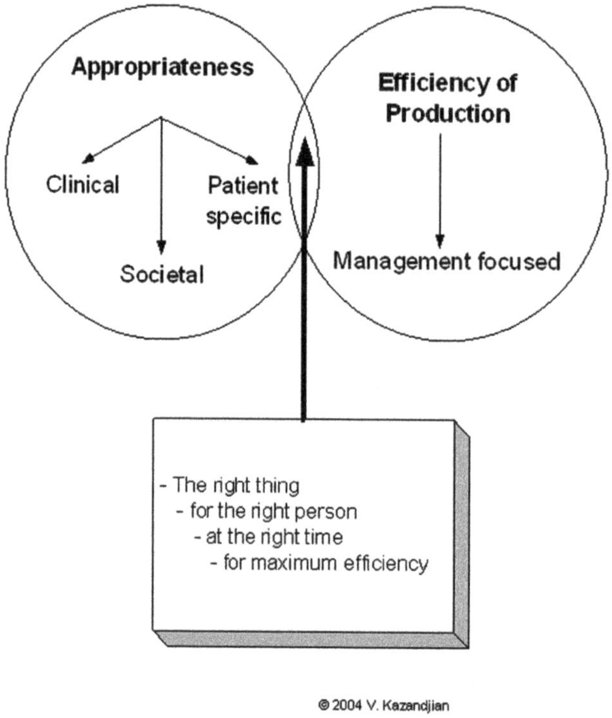

given to variation in rates of surgery (Brachfeld, 2002). Today, Cesarean section rates, as they continue to escalate again (Betrán et al, 2016), may see defensive medicine (Schifrin & Cohen, 2013; Minkoff, 2012) and patient expectations identified as underlying confounders. It is certainly beyond the scope of this chapter to explore these questions in much detail yet they cannot be ignored. Understanding variation may uncover factors beyond the realm of statistics, such as organization of the health care system, reimbursement methods, and support of professionals to improve their performance.

VARIATION IN THE DEFINITION OF VALIDITY

Performance measurement tools, no matter in what health care environment they are being used, are expected to at least demonstrate their validity. Although the statement seems a truism, often the validity of the tools may be confused with the intentions of the users. For example, in health care environment where the physician is the ultimate judge of the quality of care, any tools that would be used to measure performance and eventually translate it to quality would clash with the opinion of the physicians no matter how valid are the tools. Such a situation is often seen in health care environments where the physician is not only the deliverer of the care but also the keeper of the science. With increasing amount and specificity of data, the definition of the "keeper of the science" has changed. It is practically a recipe for disaster to believe and expect that a physician can keep up and understand all the new knowledge derived from data about quality, appropriateness, efficiency and safety of various better practices. Curiously, the same tools, epidemiological and clinical in nature, are also seen as incomplete and even predisposing to inappropriate care. Therefore, it is the validity of the tool that is questioned at the outset by various health care providers and also groups advocating different interests (Wong et al, 2016). For example, when inpatient mortality analysis was first conducted in the United States in the mid-1980s by the then-called Health Care Financing Administration (HCFA), clinicians, health care researchers, politicians, various payers of care, and even pharmaceutical companies all questioned the validity of the tool. Few, in fact, questioned the appropriateness of looking at mortality, as mortality in hospitals or soon after discharge has been and remains a central indicator for health care (Goodacre, Campbell & Carter, 2013).. The validity of the tool, therefore, has consequences beyond its narrow definition from a statistical vantage point. Clearly, the tool should measure what it is intended to measure as the most fundamental statistical requirement proposes. But the validity of the tool for purposes of this article is more germane to how a group accepts validity versus trust. It is worthwhile elaborating on this issue further.

A VALID MEASURE VERSUS A TRUSTWORTHY INTERPRETER

The discussion of evidence-based approaches brought forth the importance of dissociating subjective, opinion-based assessments from those that are based in facts and replicable across time and space. The evidence, when existent about the relationship between process and outcome, for example, eliminates the need for guesswork and experimentation minimizing the odds of error and harm. Further, it eliminates the need for the individual providers' art of matching the right process to a diagnosis in anticipation of a good outcome. Similarly, the validity of the tool when established through replication eliminates the skepticism among users regarding the relevance of the tool toward performance measurement.

There is a caveat, however, and a large one. When performance measurement systems are based on rates, thus follow epidemiological methodologies of designs aimed at quantifying events out of the possible occurrence of those events (numerator and denominator constructs) they provide a set of tools that should remain unaffected by the ambient situation. For example, a bacteremia rate of five percent will be calculated the same way no matter where in the hospital the infection occurs. However, it is relatively rare to have a "standard" for a "good" or "desirable" outcome rate in health care. What is the right rate for bacteremia in the intensive care unit? What is the right rate for Cesarean sections? Further, what is the right rate for patient satisfaction? The multi-factorial reality underlying every health care outcome makes it a formidable challenge not only to design the right rates but to identify their magnitude and usefulness of the signal given by an indicator. That is why the relationship between validity of the tool and the opinion of the experts is often found in challenging or even antagonistic postures. It is true that increasing discoveries of evidence-based relationships between processes and outcomes would enhance our ability to identify magnitudes and directions that over time could connote validity (content validity) to the tool. Until then, the challenge of the measurement tool versus the opinion of the users would remain.

A PARTIAL SOLUTION TO LACK OF EVIDENCE AND QUESTIONS ABOUT VALIDITY

The solution to placing an observed performance profile (i.e., rate) within the context of quality is to conduct comparisons with similar performers. Indeed, the health services research literature of the past 35 years is ripe with examples on how comparative analysis was able to convince providers in further understanding their performance profiles even when no untoward outcomes were observed. The first milestone in this strategic approach to performance review and evaluation could be related to Small Area Variation Analysis (SAVA) methodology (Kazandjian, Durance & Schork, 1989). The methods of looking at the rates of surgical procedures by geographical area (hence the name Small Area Variation Analysis) goes back to a short article published in the SCIENCE journal back in 1973 (Wennberg & Gittelsohn, 1973). The attraction of that article's message – that there were many-fold variations across geographical regions for seemingly the same procedures – prompted massive involvement by local and federal governments into the field of health care delivery and indirect judgment about quality. For example, the National Center for Health Services Research (HCHSR) was transformed as the Agency for Health Care Quality and Research (AHCQR) with significant amounts of funding to primarily minimize variation in health care delivery. The underlying rationale for such an approach was that the variation is bad and minimizing variation would increase the quality and minimize cost. Over time, the understanding of the factors leading to variation has lessened the initial attraction of the simplicity of the pursuit to minimize variation. Today, we realize that the variation will exist to a large extent due to variables that may be unknown or due to variables that locally could justify the observed performance profile (Curtis et al, 2016)

If comparative analysis did not succeed in providing an easy and direct effect on understanding and improving quality, the concept of comparison analysis promoted a fundamental method of inquiry. The attraction of comparison analysis is that it takes away the questions about the *golden standard* regarding how good quality would translate into a rate. Comparative analysis immediately proposed that while the ultimate rates may not be known, learning from each other, and improving processes in the delivery of the care was the first step towards improving performance. Providers who did not believe that they were performing differently than their peers suddenly were faced with quantitative profiles of their peer's performance and realized that they may be outliers. Finally, hospital trustees and management were provided with tools to ask questions about "Why are we different?" to their clinicians whereas before they were able only to question performance when an undesirable and tragic outcome was observed. Even then, the explications were often rooted into clinical and biological variables and not readily understood by non-clinicians (Kazandjian, 1996)

Comparative analysis, therefore, is a partial solution for the lack of evidence regarding the relationship between process and outcome. Further, the establishment and ongoing conduct of comparative analysis provides also insights into the validity of the tools used in this process. For example, when rates are calculated and applied to various health care settings to measure the same aspect of care, it is expected that the rates' statistics will not be affected by the local norms and method of care delivery. In other words, the numerator and denominator should be able to be captured with the same exactitude and fidelity to the structure of the data elements that went into the construct of the rate. If, therefore, the tool is portable across different health care settings and can be populated with data elements that would allow the rates to measure what it is intended to measure, over time it will satisfy the skepticism of users regarding the validity of the tool. In the initial phase of comparative analysis, the tool may be seen as having a different type of validity, namely the validity of its ability to induce dialogue and even improvement in performance. And dialogue, as opposed to defensive posture leading to rejection of any method of quantification, is at the heart of trusting. Providers not trusting comparative analysis would not collaborate with researchers and policy makers rendering even the most valid tool and approach moot and futile pursuits. Perhaps that distinction between "construct validity" and "operational validity" is important when dealing with incomplete knowledge about the associations between performance and outcomes. Therefore, the lack of evidence regarding the processes and outcomes coupled with the reproducibility of the tools mechanics (type of data elements to be captured, the time limits of the information, the way the data can be identified and audited, etc.) will help the establishment of a systematic inquiry within that health care system. Eventually, that inquiry would transform itself into a systematic set of questions about appropriateness of the care, the proper selection of patients, the communication level between patients and providers, and ultimately, internal measurement of outcomes. Until then, the road will be serpentine and bumpy, and many of the issues related to the tool itself will be raised every time there is a dissonance between the message of the performance measurement outcomes and the clinical application of existing knowledge. With persistence, the tool will be seen more as an enabler and facilitator than a direct measurement tool for quality of care. When that realization is achieved, a health care system would have demonstrated its maturity in the use of performance measurement tools and its willingness to go to the next level which is the translation of the tools message into aspects of quality and accountability. Until then, the process of inquiry and dialogue facilitated by the measurement tool may weigh more in the balance of its statistical validity contrasted to its usefulness toward performance amelioration

The validity of the tools as was discussed at the outset could be along two major categories. First is the validity associated with the construct primarily dealing with the statistical validity of indicators and second, is the validity defined through the usefulness of the tool itself towards performance improvement by initiating trust and dialogue among providers, researchers and policy makers.

THE CONSTRUCT VALIDITY OF THE PERFORMANCE MEASUREMENT TOOL

The construct validity is relatively easy to evaluate. Indeed, if the tool is measuring what it is supposed to be measuring, then the building of the tool and its sub-dimensions (e.g., the type of indicators, the sources of data it will be using, and the ability of the tool to show variability and change in the rates direction over time) can be addressed through standard construct validation methods. The validation of this dimension for a tool aiming at measuring performance would require two types of focus: one, a "bench evaluation," and the second, a field evaluation. The bench evaluation is similar to testing of any two focusing only on its physical characteristics (i.e., construct) and the results it yields under the controlled environment of the bench testing. The field testing, in contrast, requires an ongoing and systematic assessment of how the tool is used in the field and what results it yields. In this situation, the environment is not well-controlled, and the inter-, as well as intra- user variability in the use of the tool, is often unpredictable. The two types of tests result in the evaluation of the construct validity of the tool. A simple example is that of testing photographic equipment. Bench testing of lenses could yield much detail about the validity of the construct and its prowess. Indices have been developed to assess the extent to which a lens shows flare, aberrations, distortions, and contrast. Yet, a good lens in itself would never yield a good picture. The intervening factor is certainly the photographer who follows the recommendations of the manufacturer for optimal performance of the lens. Yet, a good photo goes beyond the appropriate use of the lens. It involves the expectations and the creativity of the user, but also the ability of the user to place the photo within a context that other viewers would identify with and appreciate. At the end of the day, many great photos could be taken with less than perfect lenses if the creativity and keen eye of the photographer have found the right angle to capture the moment.

Usefulness of the Tool Toward Performance Improvement

The second type of validity associated with the performance tool is that of content validity or the usefulness of the tool itself. This aspect is more fundamental when discussing performance improvement in health care than construct validity. Indeed, health care providers are known for their acceptance of approaches, technology, and overall mode of practice when examples of the relationship between processes and outcomes are provided by other health care providers. In other words, comparative analysis and recommendations by professional brethren often count more than the recommendations of experts. In fact, the whole concept of evidence-based medicine which is now struggling to find its place in better performance strategies could be said to represent the type of feedback from the field as mentioned above. Evidence-based practice in its most generic meaning depicts a persistent, replicable, and measurable relationship between what is done and what results. As mentioned, variation analysis of the mid-1980s has made more health care providers believe in learning from others and emulating successful practices than perhaps all the protocols published in medical journals have promoted. Therefore, when discussing content validity, the usefulness of the tool in different environments and the testimonials often in the shape of case studies from fellow organizations and direct care providers would count heavy in the decision of an organization to adopt a performance measurement tool or reject another.

How Do We Approach Policy Makers with Our Message to Improve the Existing System?

Leaders are Negotiators

While measurement and accountability initiatives are necessary for ameliorating any healthcare system, the ultimate difference is made when those involved in policy understand and support such efforts. This phase of performance improvement, I propose, is also the domain and responsibility of healthcare professionals, primarily those involved in the research aspects of quality and safety of care.

Why? Because we often preach to the choir by continuously refining the tools for measurement and reporting. As an academic and researcher in this field for more than 30 years, I have come to believe that many of our efforts have marginal benefits at this point. The harvest has been done – we know how to measure, evaluate, and to a large extent report while realizing the limitations and caveats of our epidemiological and quantitative methods. What the next generation of "quality and safety" professionals is entrusted to achieve is the education and support of policy makers to adopt, implement and require monitoring of measurement to build healthcare systems that keep up with the times of new knowledge, more demanding expectations, and social responsibility.

My experience in numerous countries and governments has also made me realize that the key requirement for successful communication with policy makers is our ability to speak the language of negotiation. This is not always a natural characteristic of a researcher who is trained to be an "absolutist" when it comes to theories or even field findings. Indeed, the finding is either statistically significant or not; a case study is duplicable in other settings or is not; and a theory is supported when our peers say so.

Policy makers are often not our peers. That is why successful healthcare actions, based on the translation of theory and field findings to policy, are contingent on negotiating the operationalization of an idea while keeping its validity intact. Is it possible to systematize the steps of these negotiations?

I propose a step-wise framework to negotiating which parallels that of the epidemiological inquiry, often known as the "W"s. These are:

What happened?

- *How* did it happen?
- *When* did it happen?
- *Who* was affected?
- *Why* did it happen?

The framework I propose could be called the "*Ws of Negotiating*" as follows:

- *What*: Is the idea clearly defined?
- *How*: Is the message adjusted to the audience?
- *When*: Is the timing conducive to the adoption of new ideas?
- *Who*: Is the audience a partner in the process?
- *Why*: Is there a common cause among all involved?

The "*Why*" is a common dimension and can be used in each step of the framework.

- **The *What*:** Within the context of this chapter, the "*What*" is the need for improving the quality and safety of care through measurement. Is that stated as a clear benefit to patients and a responsibility of the government? Or is it seen by the medical profession as an intrusion into the historically cherished autonomy? And why is the system in need of improvement? Does the measurement of its efficacy, effectiveness, appropriateness and responsiveness to population needs make the case that improvement is necessary?
- **The *How*:** There are often a myriad of entities one has to consider having a conflict of interest with any proposal for changing the status quo (it is safe to assume that patients are not such an entity). So how is the message i.e. that the system needs to ameliorate, adjusted to the audience (s)? If the goal is to propose new policies or regulations regarding adherence to evidence about efficacy and effectiveness of care (e.g., through Evidence-Based Medicine knowledge), can it be demonstrated that the system as is now does not apply this knowledge systematically? How will the clinical decision-making of individual physician's be addressed when dealing with the "art" of medicine argument? Will pharmaceutical companies see any benefit in supporting medication safety initiatives? Will hospitals see any decrease in readmissions as a direct threat to their revenues?

And again, why would any of these groups accept a proposal for change if there are no political, professional or financial incentives for them?

- **The *When*:** No matter how convincing and valid we think is our message, communicating it at the right time is critical. As in the horticultural adage, one cannot plant seeds in winter, no matter how great the seeds are. There seems to be an art and science in determining the appropriate timing for communication. Sometimes a new Minister of Health and a restructuring of the government is the time to promote ideas for improvement; sometimes it is when an epidemic is recognized, and sadly, other times when a wide-scale incompetency is documented such as was with the 1990

Institute of Medicine report in medical errors (Kohn, Corrigan, & Donaldson, 2000) No matter the impetus, the timing for the communication may require a "burning platform", a social cause when the appropriateness, efficiency or cost-effectiveness of health care services are under new focus.

- **The "*Who*":** As in any communication, what you say, how you say it and when, would not translate into action if the audience is not one that can act upon it. In healthcare, the stakeholders of the status quo are numerous and powerful – clinicians, pharmaceutical companies, device manufacturers, hospitals, and policy makers who may be influenced by each of these stakeholders. Promoting, implementing and continuously supporting change require two things: leadership or a tragedy!

I have a simple definition of leadership: it is doing it before you have to do it. I have followed this definition as a guide because it also builds into it the second requirement for change: a tragedy. Indeed, *having* to take action means that something significant has happened already and all action is reactive. Leadership, as I know it, can only be proactive as it is based on the concept of leading

CONCLUSION

Two words are at the core of this article's title. While *accountability* requires a demonstrated willingness and action toward responsibility and transparency, *trust* in healthcare has deeper historical roots. When sick, vulnerable and unaware of the consequences of our lessened health, we have learned to trust those and the systems to which we have given the social status of healers. In the past few decades that trust has been challenged through our ability to measure, quantify and compare the performances of our healers and healing organizations. In many instances, the quantification has led to changes in policy, to questioning if the trust is justified and if our social systems of providing health care and caring for patients' safety was cherished by leaders who were well informed about the healthcare system they oversaw. After all, an uninformed or ill-informed leader cannot be blamed for leading in the wrong direction.

Perhaps all boils down to measuring the right things, the best way, for the right reasons and communicating these to decision makers at the right time and in a language that is significantly separate from statistical and clinical terminology. Eventually, our collective goal is to make healthcare accessible, affordable, compassionate, safe and effective. Policy makers have the crucial responsibility to facilitate the implementation, support and continuously promote better practices not only in clinical and public health services but as a social good for all to benefit from. And it is the responsibility of healthcare professionals to collaborate with policy makers as colleagues and educators.

REFERENCES

Aff, H. (2016, Aprill). (Millwood). Patients' and Consumers'. *Use of Evidence.*, *35*(4), 564–565. doi:10.1377/hlthaff.2016.0171

Betrán, A. P., Ye, J., Moller, A. B., Zhang, J., Gülmezoglu, A. M., & Torloni, M. R. (2016). The Increasing Trend in Caesarean Section Rates: Global, Regional and National Estimates: 1990-2014. *PLoS ONE*, *11*(2), e0148343. doi:10.1371/journal.pone.0148343 PMID:26849801

Brachfeld, J. (2002). "Defensive Medicine" and malpractice suits. *Archives of Internal Medicine*, *162*(22), 2631. doi:10.1001/archinte.162.22.2631 PMID:12456244

Carvalho, D., & Biswas, D. (2013). Health care social media: Expectations of users in a developing country. *Med 2.0, 9*(2), e4. doi: 10.2196/med20.2720

Caughey, G. E., Kalisch Ellett, L. M., & Wong, T. Y. (2014). Development of evidence-based Australian medication-related indicators of potentially preventable hospitalisations: A modified RAND appropriateness method. *BMJ Open*, *4*(4), e004625. doi:10.1136/bmjopen-2013-004625 PMID:24776711

Curtis, E. M., van der Velde, R., Moon, R. J., van den Bergh, J. P., Geusens, P., de Vries, F., & Harvey, N. C. et al. (2016). Epidemiology of Fractures in the United Kingdom 1988-2012: Variation with Age, Sex, Geography, Ethnicity and Socioeconomic Status. *Bone*, *9*(87), 19–26. doi:10.1016/j.bone.2016.03.006 PMID:26968752

Cylus, J., Richardson, E., Findlay, L., Longley, M., O'Neill, C., & Steel, D. (2015). United Kingdom: Health System review. *Health Syst Transit.*, *17*(5), 1–126. PMID:27049966

Danforth, R.M., Pitt, H.A., Flanagan, M.E., Brewster, B.D., Brand, E.W., & Frankel, R.M. (2014). Surgical inpatient satisfaction: What are the real drivers? *Surgery, 56*(2), 328-35.

Donabedian, A. (1976). *Benefits in medical care programs*. Cambridge, MA: Harvard University Press.

Drösler, S. E., Klazinga, N. S., Romano, P. S., Tancredi, D. J., Gogorcena Aoiz, M. A., Hewitt, M. C., & Kelley, E. et al. (2009). Application of patient safety indicators internationally: A pilot study among seven countries. *International Journal for Quality in Health Care*, *21*(4), 272–278. doi:10.1093/intqhc/mzp018 PMID:19395469

Elwyn, G., Quinlan, C., Mulley, A., Agoritsas, T., Vandvik, P. O., & Guyatt, G. (2015). Trustworthy Guidelines – Excellent; Customized Care Tools – Even Better. *BMC Medicine*, *1*(13), 199. doi:10.1186/s12916-015-0436-y PMID:26324120

Firth-Cozens, J. (2004). Organisational trust: The keystone to patient safety. *Quality & Safety in Health Care*, *13*(1), 56–61. doi:10.1136/qshc.2003.007971 PMID:14757801

Goodacre, S., Campbell, M., & Carter, A. (2013). What do hospital mortality rates tell us about quality of care? *Emergency Medicine Journal*, *2013*(Sep), 23. doi:10.1136/emermed-2013-203022 PMID:24064042

Hyppönen, H., Reponen, J., Lääveri, T., & Kaipio, J. (2014). User experiences with different regional health information exchange systems in Finland. *International Journal of Medical Informatics*, *83*(1), 1–18. doi:10.1016/j.ijmedinf.2013.10.002 PMID:24200753

Ioannidis, J. P. (2016). Evidence-Based Medicine Has Been Hijacked: A Report to David Sackett. *Journal of Clinical Epidemiology*, *73*, 82–86. doi:10.1016/j.jclinepi.2016.02.012 PMID:26934549

Jha, V., Mclean, M., Gibbs, T. J., & Sandars, J. (2014). Medical professionalism across cultures: A challenge for medicine and medical education. *Medical Teacher*, *30*, 1–7. PMID:25073712

Kazandjian, V. A. (1996). The contribution of epidemiology to CQI: A commentary. *International Journal for Quality in Health Care*, *8*(4), 351–357. doi:10.1093/intqhc/8.4.351 PMID:8938496

Kazandjian, V. A. (1997). Genetic polymorphisms and breast cancer risk. *Journal of the American Medical Association, 277*(7), 533. doi:10.1001/jama.1997.03540310031027 PMID:9032157

Kazandjian, V. A. (1999). Power to the people: Taking the assessment of physician performance outside the profession. *Canadian Medical Association Journal, 161*(1), 44–45. PMID:10420865

Kazandjian, V. A. (2002). *Accountability through measurement: A global healthcare imperative*. Milwaukee, WI: ASQ Quality Press.

Kazandjian, V. A. (2014). Not Just Meaningful Data but Coordinated Data! Can Cloud Computing Promote Down-to-Earth E-Valuation of Disease and Healthcare? In Cloud Computing Applications for Quality Health Care Delivery. Hershey, PA: IGI Global. doi:10.4018/978-1-4666-6118-9.ch002

Kazandjian, V. A., Durance, P. W., & Schork, M. A. (1989). The extremal quotient in small-area variation analysis. *Health Services Research, 124*(5), 665–684. PMID:2584039

Kazandjian, V. A., & Lied, T. R. (1999). *Healthcare Performance Measurement: Systems Design and Evaluation*. Milwaukee, WI: ASQ Quality Press.

Kazandjian, V. A., Wicker, K., Ogunbo, S., & Silverman, N. (2005). Understanding safer practices in health care: A prologue for the role of indicators. *Journal of Evaluation in Clinical Practice, 11*(2), 161–170. doi:10.1111/j.1365-2753.2005.00516.x PMID:15813713

Kohn, L. T., Corrigan, J. M., & Donaldaon, M. S. (2000). *To err is human: building a safer health system*. Washington, DC: National Academy Press.

Ladhani, Z., Stevens, F. J., & Scherpbier, A. J. (2014). Does community health care require different competencies from physicians and nurses? *BMC Medical Education, 14*(1), 1. doi:10.1186/1472-6920-14-1 PMID:24387322

McCarthy, D., Schoen, C., & Radley, D. (2014). State health system performance: A scorecard. *Journal of the American Medical Association, 312*(2), 131–132. doi:10.1001/jama.2014.5374 PMID:24788783

McKinney, M. (2013). Partway across the quality chasm: Providers improve performance, but good measurement still lacking. *Mod Healthc, 43*(22), 6-7.

Mercieca, C., Cassar, S., & Borg, A. A. (2014). Listening to patients: Improving the outpatient service. *International Journal of Health Care Quality Assurance, 27*(1), 44–53. doi:10.1108/IJHCQA-03-2012-0033 PMID:24660517

Merlino, J. I., & Raman, A. (2013). Health care's service fanatics. *Harvard Business Review, 91*(5), 108–116, 150. PMID:23898737

Minkoff, H. (2012). Fear of litigation and cesarean section rates. *Seminars in Perinatology, 36*(5), 390–394. doi:10.1053/j.semperi.2012.04.025 PMID:23009974

Moses, H., Matheson, D. H., Dorsey, E. R., George, B. P., Sadoff, D., & Yoshimura, S. (2013). The anatomy of health care in the United States. *Journal of the American Medical Association, 310*(18), 1947–1963. doi:10.1001/jama.2013.281425 PMID:24219951

Nicol, E. D., Mohanna, K., & Cowpe, J. (2014). Perspectives on clinical leadership: A qualitative study exploring the views of senior healthcare leaders in the UK. *Journal of the Royal Society of Medicine*, *107*(7), 277–286. doi:10.1177/0141076814527274 PMID:25013095

Parchman, M. L., & Burge, S. K. (2004). The patient-physician relationship, primary care attributes, and preventive services. *Family Medicine*, *36*(1), 22–27. PMID:14710325

Phelps, G., & Barach, P. (2014). Why has the safety and quality movement been slow to improve care? *International Journal of Clinical Practice*, *68*(8), 932–935. doi:10.1111/ijcp.12413 PMID:25074334

Pronovost, P. J., & Kazandjian, V. A. (1999). A new learning environment: Combining clinical research with quality improvement. *Journal of Evaluation in Clinical Practice*, *5*(1), 33–40. doi:10.1046/j.1365-2753.1999.00160.x PMID:10468382

Redman, R. W., & Lynn, M. R. (2004). Advancing patient-centred care through knowledge development. *Canadian Journal of Nursing Research*, *36*(3), 116–129. PMID:15551666

Rosen, A. K., Chen, Q., Borzecki, A. M., Shin, M., Itani, K. M., & Shwartz, M. (2014). Using Estimated True Safety Event Rates versus Flagged Safety Event Rates: Does It Change Hospital Profiling and Payment? *Health Services Research*, *49*(5), 1426–1445. doi:10.1111/1475-6773.12180 PMID:24779721

Sackett, D. L. (1997). Evidence-based medicine. *Seminars in Perinatology*, *21*(1), 3–5. doi:10.1016/S0146-0005(97)80013-4 PMID:9190027

Schifrin, B. S., & Cohen, W. R. (2013). The effect of malpractice claims on the use of caesarean section. *Best Practice & Research. Clinical Obstetrics & Gynaecology*, *27*(2), 269–283. doi:10.1016/j.bpobgyn.2012.10.004 PMID:23206669

Snyderman, R., & Williams, R. S. (2003). Prospective medicine: The next health care transformation. *Academic Medicine*, *78*(11), 1079–1084. doi:10.1097/00001888-200311000-00002 PMID:14604864

To, T., Williams, J. I., Wu, K., Theriault, M. E., & Goel, V. (2003). Comparison of methods to identify outliers observed in health services small area variation studies. *Statistical Methods in Medical Research*, *12*(6), 531–546. doi:10.1191/0962280203sm350oa PMID:14653355

Veillard, J., Gula, C., Huynh, T., & Klazinga, N. (2012). Measuring and reporting on quality of care and patient safety in Canada: Focusing on what matters. *Healthcare Papers*, *12*(1), 32–37, discussion 50–57. doi:10.12927/hcpap.2012.22863 PMID:22543328

Wachter, R.M. (2004). *The End of The Beginning: Patient Safety Five Years After 'To Err Is Human'*. Health Aff (Millwood).

Wennberg, J. E., & Gittelsohn, A. (1973). Small area variations in health care delivery. *Science*, *182*(117), 1102–1108. doi:10.1126/science.182.4117.1102 PMID:4750608

Wong, A. H., Gang, M., Szyld, D., & Mahoney, H. (2016). Making an "Attitude Adjustment": Using a Simulation-enhanced Interprofessional Education Strategy to Improve Teamwork and Communication. *Simulation in Healthcare*, *1*(2), 117–125. doi:10.1097/SIH.0000000000000133 PMID:27043097

Yen, C. L. (2013). It is our destiny to die: The effects of mortality salience and culture-priming on fatalism and karma belief. *International Journal of Psychology*, *48*(5), 818–828. doi:10.1080/00207594.2012.678363 PMID:22551301

KEY TERMS AND DEFINITIONS

Accountability: Derived from the French word "compter", or to count, accountability is used as a demonstrable action regarding performance. In this chapter accountability includes trust but is incomplete without measurement.

Better Practices: This chapter does not use the term "best" practices as the goal to continuously improve the practices rather than use a binary "best" or "worst" as the framework of evaluation.

Epidemiological Inquiry Methods: These are all retrospective methods of understanding the "Why" and "How" of performance. In the context of accountability and trust, healthcare researchers are expected to use the epidemiological inquiry methods to establish the link between processes of care and their outcomes, giving priority to the appropriateness of the processes and the desirability of the outcomes.

Performance: The demonstrable interplay between the efficiency and effectiveness of producing a service.

Quality: The value put by clients (such as patients) upon the measured performance of the healthcare system.

Trust: The subjective propensity to believe that what is promised is fully pursued. In the context of accountability in healthcare, trust is necessary regarding the expected care and caring. However, data and measurement are needed to verify if indeed the trust was appropriate.

Validity: While the validity of a measurement tool is defined as its ability to quantify what was intended to measure, in this chapter validity is extrapolated to concept of goodness – that the care and caring by the healthcare system was what patient expected and were provided using better practices. Therefore this chapter synthesizes between validity, trust and accountability to define an evaluation framework for the quality of care.

Chapter 16
How to Make Your Work Really Influence Future Healthcare:
From Projects through Policies to Integration into Health Systems

Aleš Bourek
Masaryk University Center for Healthcare Quality, Czech Republic

ABSTRACT

Future health systems, besides traditional areas defined and addressed since 1980, face the advent of Proactive, Predictive, Prospective, Preventive, Participative and Personalized health care (HC). Reliable e-health platforms can help us with these challenges. They should be designed and implemented in a way to help ordinary people achieve extraordinary results. Even the best projects addressing HC systems improvement are not automatically qualified for implementation unless adopted by policy makers. The introduction of strategies with a potential for healthcare systems improvement to policy makers is necessary but difficult because of the complexity of the addressed issue. Illustrated on four projects, selected from the 25 the author participated in, from 1993 to 2016, principles, processes and attitudes found beneficial for successful policy implementation in various healthcare environments, are presented, to help with the integration of reliable electronic healthcare platforms into coming healthcare systems.

INTRODUCTION

Since 1980 quality of care is a central issue of interest to HC systems (Donabedian, 1980). With the turn of the century the challenge of ensuring the quality of health care remains high on the public and political agenda internationally, as a result of published reports based on at that time already existing platforms of hospital electronic medical records. Existing deficiencies were exposed in NHS (Gray, 1996) and in USA (Kohn, et al., 1999), and developed healthcare systems realized, that they must become Safe, Effective, Patient-centered, Timely, Efficient, Equitable, according to the Institute of Medicine (IOM) defined health care (HC) criteria (Institute of Medicine, 2001). Even before identifying and implementing good policy solutions for the above-stated criteria we became faced with other emerging issues in our

DOI: 10.4018/978-1-5225-1724-5.ch016

quest to build robust and functional future HC systems. If we base the process of HC systems improvement on a deficient set of criteria, we will undisputably end in a situation best described by the former Russian Prime Minister Alexander Chernomyrdin in the 1990s - *We wanted the best, but it turned out like always.* (The Economist, 2010). Electronic Healthcare Platforms and use of digital healthcare data is one of the drivers leading to a paradigm change in HC services provision. This requests a shift from paternalistic, curative (industrial age medicine) into shared care services resulting from the collaboration of all HC stakeholders (information society medicine) and HC (Bourek, 2011).We must be aware of and take into account needs of future health systems. Apart from areas defined by IOM, we will have to assure proactive, predictive, prospective, preventive, participative and personalized HC. Improvement of functionality and outcomes of HC systems and the success of implemented strategies depends on the volatility of the environment where they are implemented and is extremely impacted by unexpected turning points. All HC projects (although this may not always be obvious) result in policies. The final difference of the impact lies only in the size of the stakeholder network that is affected and in the duration of such effect. The policy (learned and accepted code of attitudes, conduct and possibly of behavior) will initially affect only the population which formed a part of the policy setting activity (project, training). Discovery, acknowledgment, and adoption of principles, processes and attitudes found beneficial for successful policy implementation in various healthcare environments are what determines how our improvement efforts and the work we do will influence future HC.

Health care and health systems improvement require a good understanding of two issues, namely of the "difficult problem" and the "policy." Both influence the success of what we are doing. The main attributes of difficult problems (complex issues) as elucidated by Dietrich Dörner (Dörner, 1975), and later by Joachim Funke (Funke, 1991) are - Complexity (large numbers of items, interrelations and decisions) with their enumerability, heterogeneity, connectivity with hierarchy relations, communication relations, allocation relations, - Dynamics (time considerations) with temporal constraints, temporal sensitivity, phase effects, dynamic unpredictability, - Intransparency (lack of clarity on the situation) with commencement opacity, continuation opacity, and - Polytely (multiple goals) with inexpressiveness, opposition, transience. The successful resolution of complex problems requires balanced addressing of each of these characteristics encountered. All mentioned characteristics are identifiable in HC systems and need to be considered to achieve improvement. The difficulty of such task is often demonstrated by a very quick turn-over rate of Ministers of Health who are, unjustifiably, blamed if "things end up as always". The noun "policy" can be interpreted as a course or principle of action adopted or proposed by the government, party, business, or individual. Terms close to policy are plan, strategy, stratagem, approach, code, system, guideline. The policy is in principle a practical activity aimed at changing a certain situation. It is a verbalized intent, helps with making decisions and is implemented by means of procedures or protocols. Analyzing the impact of 25 policies oriented projects the author participated in years 1993-2016 it became apparent, that at least in some situations a policy may be regarded as a "code" imposed on the system to disrupt or disturb it with expectations of achieving system performance, behavior, and attitude improvement. Often, for reasons addressed in the paragraphs "Project related observations and remarks" these expectations are not fully achieved. This article uses examples of finished projects in order to comment on the level of impact produced in their respective environments. It collates steps found beneficial to reach successful policy implementation and to avoid as much as possible situations where "though we did all the best we could; it ended up as always." An important lesson learned was that favorable acceptance on behalf of policy-makers is strongly context-dependent. Success is an emergent phenomenon born from "catastrophes" (from the singularity), unexpectedly appearing in places where in extreme conditions flaws were successfully identified and corrected. At the same time, the author is aware of limited implications of historical lessons for predictions and would like to emphasize, that a retrospective approach cannot lead to the identification of the causes of success. Everyone is a general after the battle - and many paths lead to the same point. The selected case-projects will be described briefly. Their detailed description, with the exception of the European Reference Networks project, was published in (Bourek, 2014). The author provides his observations, comments on policy introduction and shares some views about his anticipation of the future evolvement in this area. Projects are not presented in order to identify patterns but to disclose some of the logic of the process of getting a policy across to policymakers and other stakeholders of HC systems and helping the policy implementation into everyday life possibly to the level of becoming incorporated as habits of system behavior.

CASE PROJECT 1: CEEQNET (CENTRAL AND EASTERN EUROPE QUALITY NETWORK) UNIFIED CENTRAL AND EASTERN EUROPEAN SURVEILLANCE/MONITORING SYSTEM FOR HEALTHCARE QUALITY AND EFFICIENCY INDICATORS

Key concepts: standardization, harmonization, performance measurement, HC quality

Project Objectives

This four-year project (in full supported through the Programme of Community action in the field of public health (2003-2008) of European Commission DG Health and Consumer Protection, Grant Agreement Number - 2003105) offered to provide a unification methodology for efforts of five Central European countries (Austria, Czech Republic, Hungary, Poland, Slovak Republic) in the quest for standardization and harmonization of measurement methods used for evaluation of healthcare performance. Collaborating countries had a certain volume of data collected for various reasons in the process of providing health care. The project focused on the proper use of these existing relevant data sources and tried to form a "community of excellence" of institutions using their data for quality performance improvement. The result we wanted was strengthening the role of the health care consumer (eHealth application for hospital performance measurement and reporting) facilitating the appropriate informed choice of health care service providers.

Project Description

What set this project apart from another quality indicator and performance management projects was the use of primary data as obtained in each participating hospital (no additional data collection was required from the collaborating institutions in 4 countries of the project). Our used data was processed and in some participating countries uploaded continuously and in real time. The identified indicator "candidates" were computed from factual real world data, not from gamed data (Thompson et al., 2003; Weingart et al., 2000). The CEEQNET collaborative still is (to our knowledge) the only functional real-time benchmarking platform with the ability of extracting comparable measures from diverse existing countries and hospital-specific information systems handling administrative data (meaning all data that is already administrated electronically including clinical data) from four different European countries (Powell et al., 2003). There exists reasonable evidence that the indicator "candidates" as identified by this project are extractable from currently electronically administered data sets of the majority of countries of the European Union and that they will have the same meaning although coming from different HC systems. The CEEQNET platform provided dynamic views of all collected multi-national transformed and uploaded data. Rather than providing just a comparison of numbers it allows active searching for underlying facts leading to the recorded differences (e.g. that a subset of patients accounts for a recorded deviation). In some healthcare systems, the system allows drill down to each case of hospitalization and its episodes (departmental stays). This functionality actively facilitates the reflection process necessary for quality and safety improvement of healthcare services (Bourek, 2011). The flexibility and analytical capabilities of the CEEQNET platform (http://ec.europa.eu/health/archive/ph_projects/2003/action1/docs/2003_1_24_inter_en.pdf) allowed experimenting in the area of proposing and constructing of new measures and their subsequent testing of their potential value for indicator purposes. The system is ready to handle "what-if" scenarios and to test situations impossible to test in real life (reality). For instance, it is possible (in the systems "virtual reality") to treat a group of Czech patients (or "typical" Czech patient with an ICD code defined status) in the collaborating Polish hospitals and compare such treatment outcomes with the outcomes of the same group (or patient) treated in the Czech hospitals. This approach holds potential for use in the comparison of the health status of different European populations (Bourek, 2002; Milne et al., 1990). The project focused on the proper use of available data in project phases: - Analysis of the conditions of data sources and their evaluation for use of performance measurement. - Design of an information system assuring a/ Collection and standardization of data and their import into a relational database (ETL process - extraction, transforming, loading), b/ Proposal of relational and multidimensional database, c/ Proposal of algorithms and computation for obtaining Performance Quality Indicators (PQI), d/ Proposal of reporting based on key performance indicators, e/ Proposal of the technological implementation of an information system. – The design of an information system enabling visualization of the results and reporting the application of key indicators. - Implementation of information systems in participating institutions and Data and Reference Center of the project. - Evaluation of the usefulness of the proposed solution for quality management. - Creation of a network of institutions from different countries focused on standardization and unification of performance measurement and HC quality and efficiency improvement. 21 HC quality related indicator candidates were identified: Volume Measures (Abdominal Aortic Aneurysm Repair Volume, Carotid Endarterectomy Volume, Coronary Artery Bypass Graft Volume, Esophageal Resection Volume, Pancreatic Resection Volume, Pediatric Heart Surgery Volume, Percutaneous Transluminal Coronary Angioplasty Volume). Provider-Level Utilization Measures (Cesarean Section Delivery Rate, Laparoscopic Cholecystectomy Rate). In-Hospital Mortality Measures (Acute Myocardial Infarction Mortality Rate (MR), Congestive Heart Failure MR, Gastrointestinal Hemorrhage MR, Hip Fracture MR, Pneumonia MR, Acute Stroke MR). Post-Procedural Mortality Measures (Abdominal Aortic Aneurysm Repair MR, Coronary Artery Bypass Graft MR, Craniotomy MR, Esophageal Resection MR, Hip Replacement MR, Pancreatic Resection MR). These measures have the same meaning in the collaborating HC systems and are extractable from primary data (HC information systems) already administered in 5 European countries and most likely available in most EU HC systems.

Project Outputs

The project allowed the formation of a team of experts from the domain of quality of care, data reporting, and extensive database applications production from several European countries. A platform for online collaboration based on share point services was used for teamwork throughout the project, way back in 2007. Quarterly newsletters focused on international developments in healthcare quality, and safety management and performance measurement were produced and circulated to the CEEQNET community during the project duration in order to strengthen the community identity (West, 2001). Survey and analysis (audit) of available electronically administered healthcare environment data from collaborating countries was performed for the first time. Vulnerable areas in healthcare-related datasets were identified in some countries (e.g. non-existing coding of co-morbidities, which finally led to their implementation into the Slovak healthcare environment and systemic changes in data collection in the Czech Republic and Slovakia. Data samples were tested to verify the accessibility and level of data content. Auxiliary national data models were produced and subsequently used for the construction of a unified data model for all collaborating countries. Sufficient knowledge was gained enabling the production (if needed) of a new unified model after the inclusion of yet another country into the collaboration (each new included healthcare system calls for the production of a new unified model). Centralized project databases (data repository) robust enough for handling large data volumes were produced. The re-mapping of dimensions (their amalgamation) for participant countries was performed. The "candidate" quality indicators were redefined with the aid of nationally specific classifications. Selected quality indicators were computed, and reports created enabling the orientation in all the data contained in the database leading to the possibility of modeling and testing other potential quality indicators. The database and reports were accessible online (using a secure Internet connection) to all participants of the project and other authorized healthcare systems experts on the servers of the Stapro LLC. (as of the year 2012 this online database is closed and archived since the flow of data from countries outside of the Czech Republic ceased). Reports from the analysis potentially usable for further dissemination of measurement and benchmarking methods cutting across the participating EU countries as addressed by Marshall (Marshall et al., 2003) and standardized dataset enabling measurement and result comparison were published. The software-hardware-network platform utilizable as a tool for institutional healthcare management, based on quality performance information, was produced. Overview of data stored in the Central CEEQNET Data Repository is in (Table 1).

Table 1. CEEQNET global statistics (basic overview of the content of the CEEQNET Central Repository - database as of 30.03.2007)

CEEQNET Central Data Repository - database (basic facts)					
Parameter	**All Cases**	**AT**	**CZ**	**PL**	**SK**
Number of Cases - Hospital Episodes	370208	136932	107844	39671	85761
Number of Cases - Departmental Episodes	409381	158153	119863	40841	90524
Number of Comorbidities and complications (Secondary Diagnosis)	478625	319832	122683	2195	33915
Number of Procedures	789140	155481	480637	153022	0

The National Reference Center (NRC) of the project subsequently became the National Reference Center of Czech Republic that at present time serves the needs of Czech healthcare insurance companies and was used in the process of implementation of DRG in the country.

Project Related Observations and Remarks

The CEEQNET produced a functional cross-border system for healthcare quality performance evaluation based on administrative healthcare data (Iezzoni, 1996) in four countries. For communication issues with the Hungarian National Coordinator data from Hungary was not available. Several other challenges were encountered: - Low motivation of the participating hospitals. Things started to have a meaning for hospitals only after populating the database with the volume of data and the production of a user manual. Feedback related to data analysis had to be assured, and the local country management had to be more thoroughly instructed about the real-time availability of data/system access by the participating hospitals (Kiefe et al., 2001). - Technology barriers. Each hospital had a different IT system and a different structure. Data received from hospitals required transformation, even statistical files that should have existed in a standardized format slightly differed. – The complexity of data sources and their existing intersection. The most important area of intersection of all collected data across involved countries came from the common use of International Statistical Classification of Diseases and Related Health Problems (ICD-10) list. Limitations resulted from the existing use of different country or hospital-specific dimension values. Such items required remapping to typical "higher level" values to assure comparability, detailed information was inherently lost. – The inconsistency of data sources. The main limitation was the absence of a standard typical list of procedures (methods) and also encountered difficulties with remapping country coded-lists. - Transformation of data for logical data model needs. The only country with transparent, logical and complex healthcare data model in the CEEQNET collaborating countries was Austria. Data from all other participating countries required broad transformation. This turned the automated extraction-transformation-loading (ETL) into a very difficult exercise. - Factors affecting benchmarking activities between participating countries. Namely - different ways of organizing inpatient acute care, various descriptions of hospital and care types, the absence of a common coded list of procedures, low level of reliability of procedures and diagnoses coding in some countries. Project added value came from cataloging and description of currently used systems of performance measurement. Quality administrative data were defined for this study as:

1. Available through explicitly defined data interfaces;
2. Electronically recoded and collected in conformity with a unified methodology, at least at the national level (i.e. for national statistics, health insurance, fiscal purposes) (Powell et al., 2003).

Performance came to be considered composed of three elements:

1. Clinical production (Volume & Product Portfolio);
2. Clinical productivity (Human & Financial Inputs / Outputs);
3. Quality of care.

Despite all the limitations identified, the authors of this study saw at least some of the tools and methods designed during this study providing help in data transformation into information useful in hospital internal benchmarking in Czech hospitals, greatly aiding regional healthcare policy makers in information-based decision-making. Although this project was initiated at the time when it was an evidence-supported fact that performance measurement and benchmarking exerts a positive effect on the overall behavior of healthcare systems, it never reached the stage of general implementation as a policy in more extensive geographical areas. The use of available healthcare administrative data based on the proposed indicators was after the end of the project subsequently applied only in 34 Czech regional hospitals and only for internal benchmarking. No further development of the system took place, and it was used mainly by a health care professional managers who formed part of the CEENET project from its start. Even these policymakers never used all the capabilities of the system, complaining that they would like to "play with constructing their specific quality indicators", but due to political pressure and time constraints, they have no time to do so. No single hospital manager, to our knowledge, used the system to devise his performance measures tailored to the situation he was supposed to manage. The uploaded data was without exception used to produce the existing project established quality measures and to track their variation over time in the respective facility. The failure to deploy the system broadly for everyday use, from today's point of view, was mainly due to the difficulty of turning collected data (remapping) into indicators to the extent that they would be giving the same sense in all the different and country specific environments. The validation of the CEEQNET proposed indicators would have required a continuous effort of collaboration and financing that was not available. The barriers working against a broader dissemination of the use of the system were based mainly in the incapability of the project team to explain the functionality and usefulness of data collected automatically (robust against possible gaming efforts happening in all healthcare systems to improve the "image") to the ever-changing cohorts of policymakers on each national level of the countries forming the CEEQNET team. Again seen from today's point of view, the introduction of this project was premature in 2006/2007 on the information technology infrastructure of each of the project collaborating countries. The term "big data" and "cloud computing" was at that time virtually unknown. Also at that time the management of quality in individual healthcare systems in Europe was not mandatory and not even harmonized to a certain degree. Still the results of the CEEQNET project may be of future use when negotiating new policies on national and supra-national levels in Europe. Furthermore, the existing collected data sets may eventually find their use in the time-wise demonstration of the improvement of function of European healthcare systems. The adopted Directive on the application of patients' rights in cross-border healthcare (Directive 2011/24/EU of the European Parliament and Council) may again revoke the need for country comparable quality measures. A positive signal that projects such as CEEQNET have an influence on adopted policy lies in the fact that a number of the CEEQNET project people have participated in DG SANCO official consultations. The possibility and capability to shed light on existing hardships encountered in different phases and stages of healthcare related data collection in various national healthcare systems to European healthcare policymakers are a success of projects like the one described. Also, the interaction of various stakeholders during the projects allows for clarification of confusing issues and builds a trustworthy pool of professionals capable of collaborating with policymakers. Not only in this project the author has seen, that with a certain time-lag (often in the scope of several years) results of systemic projects have the potential to influence policy-makers on their quest to improve the functionality of healthcare systems.

CASE PROJECT 2: JOINT DEVELOPMENT OF CLINICAL PRACTICE GUIDELINES AND QUALITY INDICATORS AS A TOOL FOR QUALITY OF CARE IMPROVEMENT

Key concepts: clinical practice guidelines, performance measurement, healthcare quality

Project Objectives

Structured process methodology for the joint development of clinical practice guidelines (CPG) and indicators of quality and efficiency of health care (QI) was the main target of this project. Based on previous work it was known, that both healthcare quality "tools" share certain components, processes, and stakeholders. Project was conceived during the golden times of support for quality projects by the Czech Republic in the Decree No. 458 (May 10, 2000) on National policy for quality support aiming to unify activities leading to the growth of quality in all areas of the society in compliance with policies for quality support of the European Union. Quality Supportive Projects of all ministries (resorts) were to be monitored by the Council of the Czech Republic for Quality. According to the innovated status in 2005, the Council became the main governing body for the development of the quality of health care and was to prepare the National Program of Healthcare Service Quality in compliance with quality programs of the EU, WHO and internationally recognized quality approaches by means of "Projects for Support of the Quality of Care". Annually more than 30 projects originating through the collaboration of regional policy makers, opinion makers, healthcare professionals of all levels, academicians, economists, managers and IT specialists were proposed to the Council and depending on the resources allocated, many of these projects came to life and produced results still apparent in today's Czech healthcare environment.

Project Description

During preparatory and design phase know-how of organizations (AHRQ, HAS, SIGN) were extensively used and applied to functional components of Czech healthcare system. Project participants used a proprietary methodology of Lifecycle Development, EBM, algorithm design, recommendations of clinical criteria and process indicators based on rigorous analysis of the shortcomings of Czech healthcare. Czech healthcare already used an extensive database of "administrative" (care reimbursement) and clinically distinct (clinical registries) data which was used for the design and testing of Quality Indicators (QI) in defined coordination with Clinical Practice Guidelines (CPG) development process. The project group had some previous experience both in the area of development of structured CPGs (based on projects of developing Standards of Efficient Medical Care SEMC in the years 2000-2004 as a joint action of the Czech Medical Chamber and the Czech Medical Society of J. E. Purkyně) and QI. The new project was set up to identify and codify information on systemic solutions and present concrete examples from oncology in order to show the benefits of a systematic approach to policymakers on the level of Ministry of Health. It was known that only a small number of CPG producing organizations have a formal procedure for simultaneous development of QI in place. The methodology was first presented at the ISHIMR conference (Suchý et al., 2011) and consisted of:

Phase One: Development cycle of CPG
Phase Two: Development cycle of QI, especially the process QI

These two development cycles form synchronized tools for the National Set of CPG (NSCPG) and National Healthcare Services Indicator Set development (NHSIS). The main reasons for joint development of both systems were: - Both standards and indicators must be based on EBM and professional consensus, - Both systems involve almost identical teams of experts, - There is a similar approach for implementation in practice and the verification of their effect (evaluating validity), - Indicators are essential tools for evaluating the degree of fulfillment of the recommendations in clinical practice.

NSCPG was developed in order to create a nationwide standardized tool for improving the quality of care based on scientifically proven clinical recommendations where the effect can be measured by use of specific QI. Its development was based on the experience of similar major international systems (AHRQ, SIGN). It collects all information about CPGs, proposed and developed by the National Reference Center (NRC) in their respective 'life cycle' of which the main phases were: - Drafting of the CPG, - Processing scientific literature and formulation of key recommendations, - Production of a document on the CPG in different versions (depending on the purpose of publication), - Inclusion of measurable criteria and indicators and produced economic parameters of the CPG, - Supplementing the CPG by a chapter dedicated to patients (healthcare service consumers), - Peer-review (professional and public), - Publication of reports in various standard formats, - Implementation of standards in practice, - Evaluation of the effectiveness of standard. CPGs passed through this cycle in order to comply with scientifically-based recommendations to comply with - Evidence Based Medicine (EBM), - to be measured, tested, professionally assessed and consensually accepted by main Czech healthcare professional authorities. NSCPG was synchronized with NHSIS, which collects similar process indicators of quality and efficiency of care. Many indicators were developed for the development of CPG and were tied to specific clinical recommendations and criteria. CPGs were published in different versions, - Full version containing all administrative data, QI, and economic aspects, - Enhanced professional version of CPG, - Lay version designed for patients, as a Brief summary of key recommendations to become a guide arranged for practical situations in daily practice. The list was officially published on the website of Ministry of Health as National Set of Healthcare Standards (NSHS) (accessible at: http://www.mzcr.cz/dokumenty/vyvoj-narodni-sady-ukazatelu-zdravotnich-sluzeb_3783_1841_15.html and links from this URL) in the form of a simple overview to facilitate CPG development and to serve the authors, consultants and reviewers who are involved in the development, to provide information on the development phase and the fields covered by the respective standard. The individual items are accompanied by CPG supporting documents, primarily from professional research of related topics from abroad. Items included in the individual standards are then connected with the corresponding indicators of National Healthcare Services Indicator Set (NHSIS). Indicators are different in nature, revealing different aspects of quality and performance and are, therefore, also used in different ways for different purposes. Following types were defined and produced: - Indicators of coverage by preventive programs, - Indicators of centralization of cancer care, - Volume indicators, - Outcome indicators, - Productivity outcome indicators, - Utilization indicators, - Process Indicators. Their description, specification, and scope of use, is addressed in (Bourek, A., 2014). A simplified scheme of sequential CPG and process indicator development is presented in (Figure 1).

Figure 1. Design process for indicators

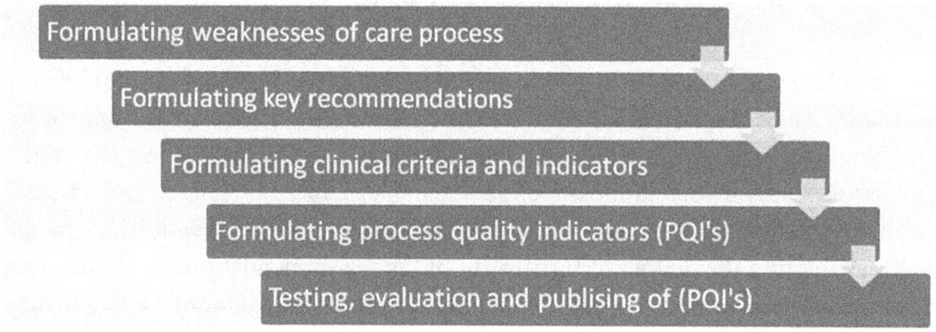

The produced Clinical recommendation is in text format formulated and recorded opinion voiced by experts aimed at improving quality and efficiency of care, based on evidence-based medicine (and rated according to the level of scientific evidence). It addresses only one single, clearly defined aspect of care, to which at least one clinical criterion may be allocated. The Clinical criterion is the most accurate textual formulation of a parameter evaluating some aspect (quality or effectiveness) of care. It does not necessarily contain information on how to measure or standardize or the form of statistical publishing of this parameter. Several relevant clinical criteria may relate to one key recommendation, but usually, one key recommendation is represented by one clinical criterion. The Indicator is a logically and mathematically precisely defined relation expressing the outcome measurement in the framework of the appropriate clinical criterion. It is possible to suggest more than one indicator for a single clinical criterion. The indicator contains comprehensive information on the manner and conditions of measurement, standardization and the format of statistical publication of this parameter. In the framework of the written CPG, the indicator is referenced to a particular indicator registry in the NHSIS, where the indicator is published with all the technical details. We required the authors of CPG, from the beginning of CPG development, to formulate the most important deficiencies in the respective care process in the existing national framework that the CPG implementation should ameliorate. Based on these deficiencies principal recommendations were defined so that it is possible to derive from them clear clinical criteria and subsequently produce relevant process indicators. These then represent the measure of the effective fulfillment of the recommendation issued in real daily care practice.

Project Related Observations and Remarks

In the course of the development of both sets (CPG and QI), we could already, to some extent, monitor and assess their benefits. The potential of quality indicators focusing on the health system (prevention in oncology, degree of centralization of care) was demonstrated as undisputable; yet during the project duration remained untapped because the first published results of our analysis were not too flattering to the Czech HC system. The best-recommended way of use for most indicators remains in the area of internal monitoring and quality improvement. During the last 15 years, we have found out that internal monitoring and self-benchmarking is much more readily accepted in the Czech healthcare environment then external evaluation and benchmarking. This, to a certain extent, seems to be a legacy of previous socialistic "centralized care" model, based on the fact that not only healthcare professional providers themselves, but also several active players on the healthcare policy playground (Ministry of Health, Czech Medical Chamber, Czech Medical Association, healthcare payers / sickness funds) tend to have a negative bias towards monitoring and evaluation, especially as the existing legislation does nothing to assure the "no-shame, no-blame" environment. Rather slow implementation of the presented work relates to the need of building trust and accountability of professional bodies handling datasets considered as proprietary and confidential and demonstrating the will of incorporating the voices of all interested parties involved in improving the quality of health care. A major drawback may also be a lack of representative patient organizations in the Czech healthcare arena as well as the fact that there is limited competition in the healthcare market since the majority of healthcare procedures are fully reimbursed by sickness funds. Patients are not involved in the process so put a little pressure on improving the efficiency of the system. Unfavorable (poor) results identified through the use of our system will best serve the workers of the respective healthcare institution to which they relate because they are equipped with local knowledge of organizational and clinical context and are in the best position to analyze and identify the causes of poor indicator values. As for process indicators, their development is an important task for improving the quality of care based on innovation and creation of a systematic basis of "clinical intelligence" exploiting available data generated in the healthcare system and readily available due to the level of added information and communication technologies and infrastructure of the Czech healthcare environment. Strengths of this project team were in 13 years of experience in the production of Czech hospital information systems and structured CPGs. Team member organizations were regarded by the professional public as trusted in relation to sensitive healthcare data handling and known for the confidential presentation of processed data only to involved healthcare stakeholders. By processing the primary data provided by participating institutions (data transformation), the project was able to achieve a high level of standardization of all collected datasets. Further development in the area of CPG and QI production in Czech Republic is possible not only by formulating new criteria and indicators for other clinical areas, but also in the gradual introduction and use of other existing and in the future introduced data sources as is planned in all systems strengthening their e-Health concepts (Bourek, A., 2011). Two major policy decisions and their practical implementation into everyday life have happened in the year 2013-2014, namely in the nationwide screening (cervical cancer, mammography, colorectal cancer) awareness program now in process and the performed centralization of child oncology care into seven National Centers. A very pleasant and unexpected side effect of this project was also the spontaneous adoption of the formal structure and process of producing CPGs by various Czech professional healthcare organizations.

CASE PROJECT 3: STRENGTHENING SEXUAL AND REPRODUCTIVE IN-SERVICE TRAINING CAPACITY OF THE MINISTRY OF HEALTH IN TURKEY

Key concepts: training cascade, monitoring, evaluation

Project Objectives

The main aim of this project was to begin collecting and sharing data on Sexual, and Reproductive Health (SRH) training outputs with an eye toward shared learning among involved centers. Questions addressed were: Are we doing the right things? Are we doing them well? Will the outputs of SRH convince the

Ministry of Health (MoH) policy makers of the usefulness of our approach? The illustrated work was undertaken in the years 2004-2007 (EUROPEAID/119528/C/SV/TR). The project was to provide one of the building blocks for a broad activity through which the government of Turkey aimed to increase the quality, availability, and accessibility of sexual and reproductive health services throughout the country. The strategy for this task was outlined in Woman's Health and Family Planning NSPHW/FP document, integrating woman's health and family planning into the primary health care system. The project was to improve the woman's health indicators on the national base and to reduce the existing discrepancies among regions and between urban and rural areas (long-term goal). The goal of the presented SRH sub-project was the creation of a training cascade for the provision of in-service training and to provide a set of tools enabling the monitoring and evaluation of the in-service training for use by the professionals of the MoH.

Project Description

Services related to Sexual and Reproductive Health (SRH) are provided in Health Centers by teams of physicians, nurses and midwives. The In-service Training Project was implemented by the Program Unit, which consisted of staff from the MoH and of the Technical Assistance Team providing technical advice to MoH throughout the SRH project implementation. The implementation of the SRH project "Strengthening SRH in-service training capacity" was operated within the framework of the Reproductive Health Program. The MoH established 12 regional training centers to cover all regions and to ensure sustainability through the implementation of training cascades for the entire provinces and establishing / strengthening a functional follow-up and monitoring system. Before the start of this SRH project, the implementation of SRH practices continuously relied on external projects for funding of in-service training. This was due to absent training policies, lack of coordination and lack of evaluation. As seen from daily activity reports, some directors continued to monitor in-service training in quantitative terms. Overall numbers trained were low relative to the size of the workforce and staff involved. Most in-service training for nurses and midwives had not been certified or accredited and had not contributed to significant professional development or advancement. In contrast, trainers attending the courses provided by the SRH project received formal recognition (Certificate of Attendance). Areas that were addressed (and co-financed by the World Bank) were defined as "improving the quality of care, the distribution of care, and cost-effectiveness of care". Specific objectives were to revise training materials on the basis of the performed pilot testing: - To strengthen SHR training capacity in selected areas (safe motherhood, emergency obstetric care, family planning, STI's, HIV/AIDS and SRH services for young people), - To establish/strengthen the monitoring and evaluation system for SHR in-service training, - To ensure dissemination of the in-service training results to policymakers and planners. Monitoring and evaluation (M&E) and dissemination activities included the following: - To provide a functional SRH training follow-up, M&E system (including software and manual), - To develop necessary forms and mechanisms for the establishment / strengthening of the M&E system, - To customize the system and oversee its functioning, - To perform follow-up M&E visits to each of the 12 regional training centers, -To train trainers of trainers (ToT) and M&E the total of 60 advanced trainers, - To produce the M&E report with the results of the assessment of the effectiveness of the trainers training, - To create an electronic database for 249 trainers, - To revise / streamline / improve robustness, selectivity and specificity of the M&E system based on the pilot survey (follow-up visits) of the 12 regional training centers assessed by members of the project and the representatives of the MoH. Performance measurement (PM) helped to eliminate much of the subjective impact by means of using the advantages of simple information technologies (IT). The application of the PM methodology served as a base for benchmarking and best practice identification. The main objective of measurement was to change (improve) the behavior of the system (people included) based on the data it produced. Key Indicators had to be identified and tested for selectivity, sensitivity, and specificity in order to demonstrate accountability for achieving the stated objectives. PM implementation was essential since: - If you do not measure results, you cannot tell success from failure, - If you cannot see success, you cannot reward it, - If you cannot reward success, you are probably rewarding failure, - If you cannot see success, you cannot learn from it, - If you cannot recognize failure, you cannot correct it, - If you can demonstrate results, you can win support. To bring the above principles into practice we devised an indicator list using the SMART framework of WHO for indicator production (WHO, 2004) intended for policymakers of MoH to monitor & evaluate the sustainability of the SHR Training Program in the following areas: - Educational materials, - Educational participation, - Local consensus process / involvement of stakeholders (trainer and trainees), - Audit and feedback. Even though the abovementioned indicators could have been constructed from the data collected by the SRH Project, after discussions with MoH representatives and senior project trainers, it was decided to perform the M&E using a simplified Basic Indicator Set. The basic set of M&E indicators of the in-service SRH training project was constructed to be as simple as possible and with the ability to address quantitative as well as qualitative issues. Main project quantitative indicators used were: - Number of training activities, - Number of training service providers (separate categories for OB/GYN, MDs, GPs, midwives, nurses), - Number of training centers active in SRH training, - Number of training modules (produced and distributed), - Number of CD-ROMs (produced and distributed). Three tools were produced by the process of M&E: - The in-service training and visits evaluation tool, - The Rapid Assessment tool (of the in-service training), - The Self-Assessment tool (for the evaluation of skills for conducting the course). The Manual on Monitoring and Evaluation of Sexual and Reproductive Health In-service Training was prepared in compliance with the project objectives and goals and providing a sound basis for data collection on all the necessary levels for the purpose of monitoring and evaluation of all the dimensions of the project and based on previously described experience (Haycock-Stuart et al., 2005; Johnston et al., 2000; Lawrence et al., 1996). It introduced and described three sets of tools and formed a sound basis for assuring sustainability and potential for subsequent PDSA improvement cycles. The manual was regarded as a starting point and continued to be developed according to identified needs. As the project team experience and understanding improved, additional information techniques and tips were added. The team invited any ideas and request from the trainees and directed them to the head of the SRH in-service training project. For policy makers of the MoH, the end-product of M&E electronic tools of the SRH Project was a reporting dashboard, enabling simple visualization of relevant information from data collected during the monitoring process in order to facilitate the evaluation phase of the project and for subsequent training cascades customized according to the requests of all the three main levels of decision-making identified (MoH, Training Center, Trainer / Trainee). The information contained in the data was made clearly visible and time evolution (trends) were visible where appropriate (Figure 2).

The "dashboard" provided the option of "pre-defined" views/reports requested by MoH. It formed an integral part of Plan Do Study Act (PDSA) managing for results process. To assure follow-up, the M&E system was devised and used to help allocate limited resources on the basis of objective quality determinations. Collected data was used to identify service training centers where outcomes of activities were superior. This served to direct trainees, research/improvement funding and advanced technology to these centers. These centers often provided a greater volume of training episodes in a given area and

Figure 2. Dashboard representation of the trainers benchmarking

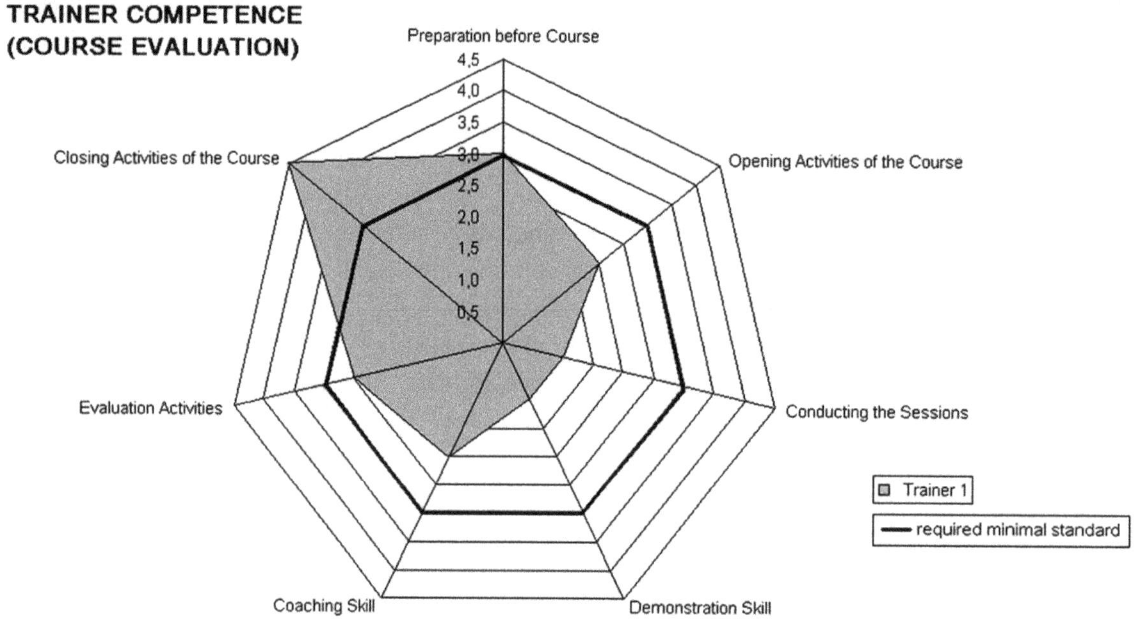

typically achieved greater efficiency reducing the costs per training. Such centers of excellence also provided "benchmarks" and "best practices" for use in quality improvement efforts of other facilities. The effectiveness of the cascade form of training and effective M&E is captured in achieved outcomes demonstrated by the steep infant mortality rate reduction in Turkey between years 1997, 2004 and 2010. It is certain that other factors apart from this project played their role in the graphed results (Figure 3). The described Strengthening Sexual and Reproductive Health In-Service Training Capacity project was one of the important factors responsible for this striking outcome.

Project Related Observations and Remarks

The success of the Turkish policy addressing national sexual and reproductive health issues was, to the authors understanding, achieved using a continuous dialogue with all affected stakeholders over time. The countrywide policy was well planned in advance and perfectly coordinated by responsible officials on the level of the MoH. International project partners drafted a list of potential opportunities how to arrive at the desired outcomes. These options, based on the existing Plan - Do - Study - Act (PDSA) predefined framework, were revised and customized in order to respect the logic and structure of the Turkish healthcare environment and the existing local healthcare professional's customs, habits and way of working. Close PDSA loops monitored and evaluated and then based on the findings readjusted the process to produce the best possible outcomes with the available financial, structural and human resources. Produced training materials, the training episodes, the organization of the training cascade itself and the monitoring, evaluation and benchmarking process were kept as simple and transparent as possible and brought to everyday life by the continuous face-to-face interaction of people involved in the process. The ownership of the process by all involved and continuous strengthening of people relations

Figure 3. Infant mortality rate reduction in Turkey between years 1997, 2004 and 2010
Source: Health for All Database WHO 2007/2013

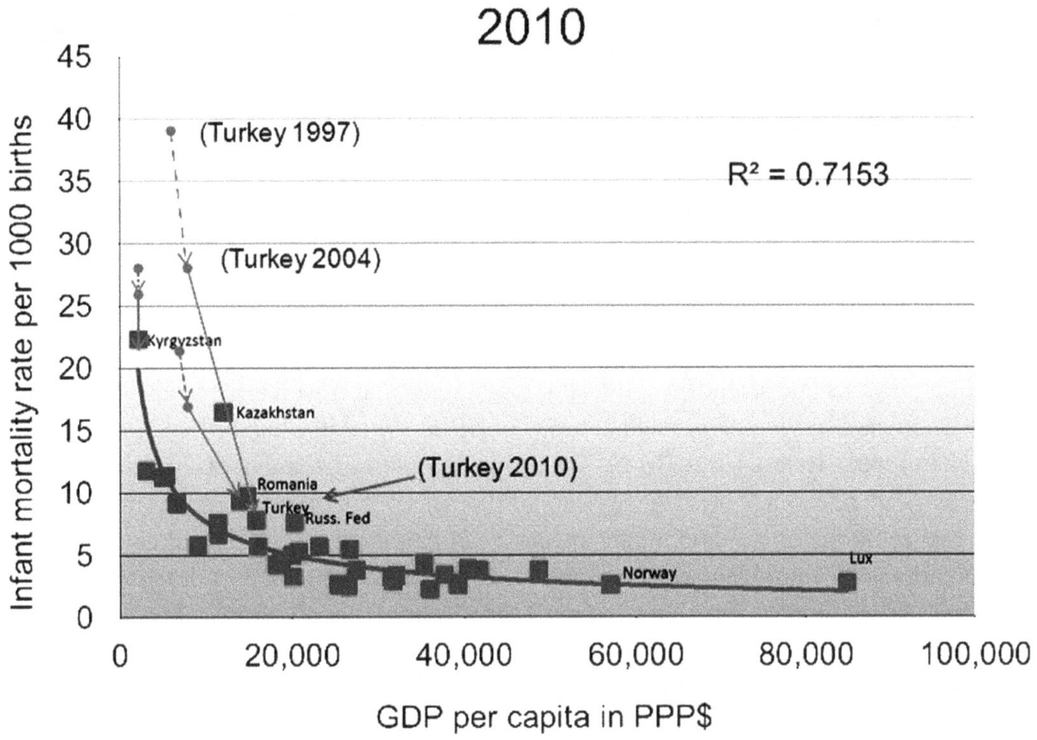

(meetings, shared photo-stories, issued certificates, continuous interaction with public media) formed the backbone of successful implementation of this project into a policy with tangible outcomes for the Turkish population.

CASE PROJECT 4: EUROPEAN REFERENCE NETWORKS (ERN) AND ERN ASSESSMENT MANUAL

Key concepts: momentum impact, harmonization, network, healthcare providers, patients, Member States, European Union, rights, European Reference Networks

Project Objectives

Health systems in the European Union seek to provide high-quality, cost-effective care. This is particularly difficult in the case of conditions requiring a concentration of resources or expertise, and even more so with rare or low-prevalence complex diseases or conditions. EU healthcare policy has furthered cooperation between EU countries, including networking. Some networks benefit from the EU's public health and research programs, especially in the areas of rare diseases, pediatric and neurological complex diseases. Such cooperation was based mainly on bilateral agreements or joint projects in specific fields. Moreover, healthcare access varies widely across the EU. More efficient and coordinated sharing of resources and expertise was thus needed, and can be achieved if the best specialists from across Europe could join their efforts to tackle complex or rare medical conditions that require highly specialized healthcare and a concentration of knowledge and resources. This is the purpose and role of the European Reference Networks which in the year 2016 is becoming a reality.

Project Description

It is difficult to look upon the creation of European reference networks from the perspective of traditional projects. It is better seen as an orchestrated effort. Development in the area how different stakeholders can collaborate, often using electronic platforms, puts us today in a situation which requests less traditional approaches. The ERNs are a good example of perfectly interlinked steps on micro, meso and macro levels of needs, opportunities and barriers assessment, mapping and harmonization of existing environments, legal frameworks and scientific and technology inputs that if well done leads to the provision of high-quality healthcare services. Expected benefits of ERNs stated in Chapter IV Cooperation between MS Article 12 European Reference Networks Framework are: - Improvement of high-quality specialized care, for patients with rare or low prevalence complex diseases or conditions, - Improvement of European cooperation and economy of scale on highly specialized healthcare, - Pooling of knowledge on certain diseases or treatments, - Improvement of diagnosis and treatment capacities where expertise is rare by developing and sharing clinical guidelines and patient pathways, - Facilitation of Helping Member States enhance the provision of highly specialized care, - Maximizing the speed and scale of incorporating innovation in medical science and health technologies, - Serving as focal points for medical training and research. Though the scope and complexity of the issue was unprecedented, by stepwise progression all the stated objectives were reached resulting in the Commission Delegated Decision of 10 March 2014 setting out criteria and conditions that European Reference Networks and healthcare providers wishing to join a European Reference Network must fulfill (Text with EEA relevance) (2014/286/EU). By this official document the European Commission declared that *Having regard to the Treaty on the Functioning of the European Union, Having regard to Directive 2011/24/EU of the European Parliament and of the Council of 9 March 2011 on the application of patients' rights in cross-border healthcare (1), and in particular point (a) of Article 12(4) thereof, Whereas: (1)Article 12 of Directive 2011/24/EU provides that the Commission is to support the Member States in the development of European Reference Networks ('Networks') between healthcare providers and centres of expertise in the Member States, in particular in the area of rare diseases (2). At the operational level, the Commission had to adopt a list of specific criteria and conditions to be fulfilled by European Reference Networks and healthcare providers wishing to join and become a Member of a Network* (Commission, 2014). It was necessary to: - Engage, attract, identify the right Networks and healthcare providers, - Establish a Network model with useful platforms and tools, - Foster commitment by Member States and ensure sustainability of established Networks, - Avoid fragmentation and/or duplication of efforts, - Develop and use standardized tools (clinical guidelines, registries, patient pathways, interoperable IT systems), - Devise an effective Network model & useful platforms and tools, and to also put in place assessment elements: - Assessment Manual and tool box, - Independent Assessment Bodies with solid background in assessment/certification of Healthcare providers, - Perform the assessment of Networks proposals (Competitive Call: deadline for proposals 23 November 2015), - Produce application forms, - Provide operational criteria (Guidance & Tools for applicants and assessment bodies) and - Assure close cooperation between Board of MS and Commission. Further reading on these issues is available at http://ec.europa.eu/health/ern/policy/index_en.htm.

Project Related Observations

As early as 2005 the DG SANCO Health Systems Working Party identified possible developments and needs (Health System Working Party Draft Work Programme February 2005). In this year also the ERN Rare Diseases was started. Among other objectives stated at this stage was providing information for decision-making in the area of health and health care services for use in the countries of EU. This would include issues as work on the Systems of Health Accounts, on how to compare hospital data or how to compare the utilization and costs of farmaceuticals in the EU, etc. The subjects would also include topics like comparing technology dissemination and utilization. Moreover, of course, cross-border issues (of both care and personnel) and issues of healthcare quality (comparing systems, guidelines, standards across Europe, etc.). An important aspect was also learning from each other, exchanging best practices (area of quality control and implementation of quality processes) and the potential of being able to benchmark our health systems, etc. would have to be focused upon. The basic concept was seen as sharing spare capacity and trans-national care. Cooperation between healthcare systems may bring benefits in some situations, such as in border regions or where there are limitations due to capacity constraints. "Cross-border care" is a general term which covers both cooperation in border regions and more generally care received in another Member State, without any implication of proximity. Cooperation between systems faces potential difficulties linked to different legal frameworks, liability issues, planning constraints of different systems, and reimbursement mechanisms, which should be addressed. Acquiring healthcare in the other Member States may have effects both in the country of provision and in the country of the beneficiary. Mapping of these areas led to following recommendations: - To invite the Commission to facilitate information sharing at European level on possible available healthcare, existing supply of care, entitlements and procedures, costs, prices, adverse incidents, patient records, nomenclature of conditions, treatments and products, and continuity and quality of care across the Union, as part of the overall framework for information discussed in the section on information below. The action could include support to networking and developing databases: - To evaluate existing cross-border health projects, in particular, Euregio projects, and to develop networking between projects in order to share best practice, - To invite the Commission to explore whether it is possible to draw up a clear and transparent framework for healthcare purchasing which competent bodies in the Member States could use when entering into agreements with each other, and to make any appropriate proposals, - To encourage ongoing work by the Commission, Council and Parliament to ensure clear, simple and transparent recognition procedures incorporating a high degree of automatic recognition as with the current sectoral rules in order to facilitate and develop mobility of health professionals. All this had to be done, since European centres of reference could provide healthcare services for conditions requiring a particular concentration of resources or expertise in order to provide high quality and cost-effective care, especially for rare diseases. Centres of reference could also contribute to medical training and research, information dissemination and evaluation. Any system of European centres of reference should be flexible, objective and transparent, with clear criteria, scientific and professional involvement, should ensure that centres are distributed across the enlarged European Union, and should leave choices open about the use of any centre of reference to the authorities responsible for the care concerned. The last step was the recommendation: - To invite the Commission, in collaboration with the Member and acceding States, to carry out a mapping exercise relating to centres of reference taking into account the principles set out above, and to explore how to foster networking and cooperation on these issues, including the organization, designation, and development of centres. After the mapping of European HC environment and after the creation of the legal framework for cross-border HC activities steps were initiated to facilitate the creation of ERNs and address the need for continuous management and quality evaluation of ERNs. During the Steering Committee of the ERN Assessment Manual and Toolbox Brussels in April 2015 following was proposed: - To base criteria and evaluation on feedback of those, who are being served by ERNs (patients, families and patient networks and referring medical professionals), - To produce the Assessment Manual and Toolbox to assure preferably basic admittance criteria for individual ERN members at the starting phase and only subsequently address the issue of periodic re-assessment that should include the participation of professionals from members of ERNs. It was also recommended to produce: - Checklist for self-assessment of the applicants, - Assessment manual and technical toolbox for Networks and healthcare providers, - Assessment manual and technical toolbox for Independent Assessment Bodies and to, - Assure that criteria and measures required are sufficiently generic (because of the wide diversity of approaches to management of rare diseases) and appropriate (the goal is to support the conception and creation of ERNs). The stated requirements were based on the Commission demand-objectives voiced in the Delegated Decision. The Board of Member States was acknowledged as the formal body in charge of the approval and termination of Networks and memberships as provided in the Commission Implementing Decision. The Board is constituted of representatives of the 28 EU Members States and the EEA countries. After necessary consultations and adjustment the European Reference Networks Implementation process, timeline, and milestones were presented by Enrique Terol from DG SANTE Directorate D European Commission during 2nd Conference on European Reference Networks „From planning to implementation" (8-9 October 2015, Lisbon). Networks criteria and capacities were defined as: - Knowledge and expertise to diagnose, follow up and manage patients, - Evidence of good outcomes, - Multi-disciplinary approach, - Capacity to produce good practice guidelines and to implement outcome measures and quality control, - Capability of performing research, teaching and training, - Capacity to collaborate with other centers of expertise and networks. How are thinks going? More than 50 interested groups or pilot networks are identified. Dynamic interaction of stakeholders with MS and Commission is taking place. Preparatory work of Network proposals is ongoing. Interaction among professionals of the same thematic diseases groups is in process. The active implication of EU patients and professional/scientific societies is seen. Strong support of the Commission advisory groups (in particular the RD expert group) exists (Terol, E., 2015).

The following steps were necessary for the successful establishment of European reference networks in the third quarter of 2016: - 2002 Free movement of patients, 2004 conceptual work and interaction between scientific bodies and Board of Member States initiated, - 2005 High Level Group on Health Services and Medical Care Centres of Reference report, - 2006 RD Task Force Working Group on centres of reference Public Health Programme First pilot networks projects, - 2011 Directive application of patients' rights in cross-border healthcare Article 12 ERN, - 2013 Eucerd Recommendations European Reference Networks (Rd Erns), - 2014 Commission Decisions on ERN, 2014 entry into force of legal acts, 2014 to 2015 the creation of the assessments manual and toolbox, 2015 to 2016 selection of independent assessment bodies for ERN assessment, early 2016 the official call for networks, second quarter of 2016th assessments of proposals. Though this looks simple to achieve, this in collaboration inputs and consensus of all Member States sets a starting point for dynamic improvement of HC services for European citizens. The Commission is aware, that Telemedicine and other IT solutions and tools are the cornerstone of the ERNs as stated in the material "European Reference Networks How digital solutions fit in?". The material calls for the urgent need of a ERN IT platform and also implies, that healthcare or expertise across borders implies necessarily: - Cross-border secure exchange of patient clinical information and data, - Communication in real time among healthcare providers and patients, - Broadband communication, - Integration of transnational research, - Telemedicine (transmission of images and other, T-radiology, dermatology, ophthalmology, electrophysiology, pathology etc.), - Interoperable and semantically compatible ICT systems (harmonized terminology, language translation), - Establishment and maintenance of shared databases and registries, - Knowledge and interactive support tools (Shared clinical guidelines, patient pathways, decision tools and algorithms, etc.), - Common reporting and notification systems, - Integrated Information and management system (activity, performance, common balanced scoreboard etc..), - Remote training and simulations solutions (Piha et al., 2015).

CONCLUSION

In today's dynamically developing environment system change strategies need to consider the rapid increase in turn-over time of breakthroughs influencing the applicability of historical lessons and experience. In previous centuries, we were limited in our ability to resolve health and healthcare issues because of the small volume of facts at our disposition, of course with limitations due to this situation. With the appearance of the Information society, we are confronted by an opposite situation. Healthcare professionals are unable to resolve these issues because of the overwhelming amount of facts and a large volume of data without appropriate context, since the data is not typically directly produced by the professional himself but rather is mediated via various digital systems and platforms. To use a parable, in previous centuries the professional was expected, after a brief interaction with the patient, to uncover where the patient's "life story" became corrupt and what to do in order to turn the situation into at least a relative "happy end". This is similar to seeing a 1-minute episode from a 2-hour movie and trying to guess what the film is about, what went wrong and how to fix the existing situation. As a result of digitalization and communication technologies development, we are now in a different position. Sooner or later a healthcare professional will have at his disposition (in some sort of a digital format) virtually the whole "life film" of a patient (or a cohort of patients). Wearable devices, smart devices, digital cameras, and other recording devices can capture, store and share anything from the rate of acceleration of an individual to what and when he ate (if he is an owner of a smart refrigerator). With genetic data, we have even data from the time when the "life film" was conceived. The future healthcare and HC systems will shift from retro-activity into pro-activity. To be of real help, the HC professional will have to be capable of generating an image of not what is wrong (in the traditional medicine the so-called diagnosis hypothesis) but what may become wrong if preventive measures are not taken. This is the driving force behind the shift towards proactive, predictive, preventive, personalized healthcare. Given the continuous heath and healthcare data supply, the future healthcare professionals will not have enough time to process the data stream manually. Researchers and technicians will have to produce such e-health platforms and system that will be capable (using methods of machine learning) to "crunch on demand" the available dataset (in the case of an individual patient the data-set of his "life story") and produce a life-film "trailer" informative enough to the healthcare professional and the patient himself to allow appropriate diagnostic, preventive and therapeutic interventions necessary. This does NOT to any degree implicate, that traditional healthcare professional skills (sometimes referred to as the art of medicine) will become obsolete. Since health and healthcare process is based on a human-human system interaction, there will always be a place for the skilled healthcare professional to produce a hypothesis of diagnosis based on data that is difficult to digitize (emotional, body language, olfactory, etc.). From the authors point of view, the introduction of e-health platforms and processes should be planned and done to aid the HC professional to come up with quicker and more accurate preventive and curative measures (care pathways) and at the same time with the help of e-health platforms provide the HC professional with the environment, where wrong, inaccurate or not enough personalized hypotheses could be rejected as quickly as possible. We will not successfully cope with challenges by designing electronic platforms as initial and standalone projects. We will not be successful unless we understand the environment where these platforms perform. We will not improve HC systems function if we use wrong policies and we will not have the chance of introducing right policies if we cannot explain our standpoints to policy makers. Implemented strategies depend on unexpected turning points. One good example demonstrating this is the recent report of the Emergency Care Research Institute Top 10 Patient Safety Concerns for Healthcare Organizations 2014 (ECRI Institute, 2014). Based on 300,000 reports, data integrity failures with IT systems (Electronic Medical Reports) represent the biggest risk to patient safety, only followed by patient handovers, errors in reporting patient findings, mislabeled laboratory samples, and other less frequent causes. The reasons for this rather unexpected finding are stated in the paper. Despite this, EMRs are still proposed to policymakers as a way of improving health systems functionality. We know the "what" but we are not so good in the "how." Given the unpredictability of the impacts of introduced systemic changes, my suggestion to healthcare professionals in the position, when they must interact with policy makers, is to get across the message, that even the best designed and implemented systemic change introduced into the complex existing health systems may produce unexpected results. A possible safeguard mechanism is to propose gradual step-wise system change and readjust as quickly as possible strategies based on feedback from the influenced system. Without trusted assurance that monitoring systems will be in place and will allow corrections, no change / disturbance should be allowed. We must also engage stakeholders to do things from „scratch" and limit the space for what the author of this article calls the „instant" effect. The vain belief (a by-product of the information/disinformation society) that all we need to do is to find a stored „document" and use it to solve the issues that need to be addressed. This approach works well if someone is doing a "repeat work" like spare part replacement in a device. Such approach fails in healthcare since no situation we encounter is a repeat! We always (on the level of individual patient care or the meso and macro level of populations) have to imagine the hypothesis of what is mal-functioning and if our hypothesis cannot be rejected by available scientific experiments (often in medicine stored in digital repositories such as the Cochrane Collaboration) we can start thinking about actions to take. In this sense, the designed and subsequently used platforms must enable all involved stakeholders a more sophisticated level of collaboration and cooperation in order to have the involved stakeholders interact with the HC system they would like to see improved. If it was known to Marcus Aurelius (Marcus Aurelius Antonius Augustus, lived 121-180) that „Everything we hear is an opinion not the fact. Everything we see is a perspective, not the truth" we should be cautious to make decisions and actions based on observation or mediated information unless we have had the chance and time to explore the context. Expected short-term development likely to impact the overall environment in which healthcare providers and other stakeholders operate was published in 2006: - Piecemeal, incremental approaches to healthcare change, sometimes with more results and unintended consequences. - A struggle to seek a viable balance in public and private health care spending. - An increasing portion of health related financial responsibility transfers to individual citizens. - The emergence of new and nontraditional local and global competitors and collaborators in care delivery to meet changing stakeholder needs. – The proliferation of health promotion and care delivery models and capabilities (Adams et al., 2006). Many of these are a result of Electronic

Healthcare. Electronic Healthcare (eHealth, sometimes e-health and e-Health) is a term dating back to the last century - at least 1999. (Della Mea, V., 2001) Usage of the term varies. The definition of the term continuously changes. To some, this term is synonymous with health informatics with a broad definition covering electronic/digital processes in health; others use it in the sense of healthcare practice using the Internet. (Eysenbach et al., 2001). It can also include health applications and links on mobile phones, referred to as m-health or mHealth. It uses information and communication technologies (ICT), which affect the health and health care and incorporates some services and systems to support preventive care, diagnosis, medical management. Since the beginning, eHealth has been perceived as an important tool for the improvement of healthcare quality improvement. Projects addressing HC policies aiming at the improvement of structure, functionality, effectivity and efficiency of complex systems can not even be initiated not alone become manageable and functional in our society without the inclusion of electronic healthcare. The „what" we know is always limited by the level of our literacy to interpret available facts correctly, but we are generally even worse off on the level of knowing "how". Most would agree that the valuable part of a company, or individual, lies in this "know how" area. This may well be the under-performing part of the health care systems. If there is a challenge (e.i. improvement of the level of know how to positively influence the behavior of the healthcare environment), there must be solutions. If our way of thinking created most of these challenges (sometimes politically incorrectly referred to as problems), then the same way of thinking, doing and attitudes have a low potential to solve the issues. Healthcare still has too many of the characteristics associated with the old-fashioned, individual, craft-based system which no longer sits well with what we know works better in the 21st century: teamwork, safety and improvement science, executed on an industrial scale (KPMG, 2013).

I would hesitate today to embark on any healthcare related strategy project without having partners aware of the following principles:

Principle 1: A living healthcare system is a self-generating network of communications. The aliveness of such system resides in its informal networks or communities of practice. Bringing life into human organizations means empowering their communities of practice.

Principle 2: You can never manage (direct) a healthcare system; you can only disturb it. A living network chooses which disturbances to notice and how to respond. The message will get through to people in the community of practice when it is meaningful to them. It becomes meaningful if they understand the context, in order to do so, they must become a part of the system and interact with it. Josef Ratzinger (Pope Benedict XVI) brilliantly shows, that only by the process of interaction (not by pure observation or even mediated observation) we may arrive at understanding (Ratzinger, J., 1968).

Principle 3: The creativity and adaptability of a living system express itself through the spontaneous emergence of a novelty at critical points of instability. This sets apart a living system from a mechanical system. Even in mechanics (physics) since Werner Karl Heisenberg we are aware of our limitations in computational predictability and the effect of the observer interacting with the observed. Unpredictability is a part of the blueprint of Nature. Every human organization contains both designed and emergent structures. The challenge is to find the right balance between the creativity of emergence and the stability of the design.

Principle 4: In addition to holding a clear vision, leadership and policy making involves facilitating the emergence of novelty by building and nurturing networks of communications; creating a learning culture in which questioning is encouraged, and innovation is rewarded; creating a climate of trust and mutual support; and recognizing viable novelty when it emerges, while allowing the freedom to make mistakes (Capra, F., 2009). These principles were discussed in Vienna in 2009 (Bourek et al., 2008).

Principle 5: Cultivating the habit of being progressive in seeking information, but being modest and conservative in applying it unless there was the opportunity for hands-on interaction with a system we try to change, and unless we are being a part of this system.

Principle 6: Awareness, that the Information Society also brings the provision of disinformation and necessity to work with "mediated" information. Unfortunately the old Czech proverb "lže jak když tiskne" (he lies like if he was printing) according to linguists does not appear in any other language. It is attributed to the times of Karel Havlíček Borovský (lived 1821-1856) and comments the level of honesty of the (then newspaper based) journalists - press. Today's level of ICT with social media where anyone can become a "journalist" multiplies this risk. The same observation and the use of the term "disinformation society" can be traced to an article by Robert F. Kennedy Jr. published in May 2005 in the Vanity Fair Magazine (Kennedy, R. F. Jr., 2005).

If we see the goals of health and health systems improvement as "cultivating the system in a way that lets ordinary people do extraordinary things instead of taking extraordinary people and getting very ordinary results from it", then the positive side of participating in projects aimed at improving health system quality and safety and interacting with policy makers on all hierarchical levels is the observed fact that every project always becomes a policy, but this policy is initially and predominantly limited to the confined community of practice that was at the conception and birth of such a project (the deviants). The policy (learned and accepted code of attitudes, conduct and possibly of behavior) will affect only the size of the population, which formed a part of the policy setting activity (project, training). From this point of view cascade projects stand a better chance of becoming an overall policy in a certain healthcare environment, and the author sees no waste of resources in "repeat projects", he actually deems these repeats beneficial as there is no other way how to increase the number of people "that have interacted with the system". During our projects we have noticed, that policy lifecycles are becoming shorter and shorter, and periodic adjustment needs to be performed due to the effect of continuously emerging singularities (unexpected and unforeseeable changes) resulting in unexpected system behavior. This happens in the area of opportunities as well as on the level of potential risks. In the authors hands the best method that works is to be as open as possible in introducing health system strategies to stakeholders and to do now (today, in the present) honestly, responsibly, with passion, using all available resources, information, knowledge, tools and aids in the current environment using his limited talent, physical capabilities, skills, intellect, intuition, emotions, feelings, beliefs, conscience, sub-consciousness, self-awareness and will (performing physically and mentally) all as best as he is capable and stay patient in waiting for the result. If such attitude is in harmony with your collaborators and people you interact with, results come.

ACKNOWLEDGMENT

The author would like to express his gratitude to Miloš Suchý, MD, who is his closest collaborator and idea driver in all projects related to performance measurement since 1993.

REFERENCES

Adams, J., Edgar, L., & Mounib, A. P. (2006). *Healthcare 2015: Win-win or lose-lose?* IBM Institute for Business Value. Retrieved May 10, 2009, from http://www.ibm.com/healthcare/hc2015

Bourek, A. (2002). The era of information in the Czech Republic: How healthcare is managing data sets and mind-sets. In Accountability through measurement: A global healthcare imperative. American Society of Quality (ASQ Quality Press).

Bourek, A. (2011). General principles and logic of quality management in health and healthcare. In E-Health Systems Quality and Reliability: Models and Standards. Hershey, PA: IGI Global Publishing. doi:10.4018/978-1-61692-843-8.ch001

Bourek, A. (2014). Introducing Healthcare System Change Strategies to Policy Makers in the Open Society and Digital Environment: What Works Now, But May Not Work in the Near Future. *International Journal of Reliable and Quality E-Healthcare*, *1*(2), 36–59. doi:10.4018/ijrqeh.2014040103

Bourek, A., Tůma, P., & Bourková, A. (2008). *Indicators as signals for assuring living and healthy health care organizations.* Paper presented at the WHO Vienna Public Healthcare Conference Performance Assessment in Healthcare Delivery PATH II, Vienna, Austria.

Capra, F. (2009). *Management.* Retrieved May 4, 2009, from http://www.fritjofcapra.net/management.html

Commission. (2014). *Commission delegated decision of 10 March 2014 setting out criteria and conditions that European Reference Networks and healthcare providers wishing to join a European Reference Network must fulfil.* Retrieved June 15, 2016 from: http://ec.europa.eu/health/ern/docs/ern_delegated-decision_20140310_en.pdf

Della Mea, V. (2001). What is e-Health (2): The death of telemedicine? *Journal of Medical Internet Research*, *3*(2), e22. doi:10.2196/jmir.3.2.e22 PMID:11720964

Donabedian, A. (1980). Explorations in Quality Assessment and Monitoring: Vol. 1. *The Definition of Quality and Approaches to its Assessment.* Ann Arbor, MI: Health Admin Press.

Dörner, D. (1975). Wie Menschen eine Welt verbessern wollten. *Bild der Wissenschaft*, *12*, 48–53.

ECRI Institute. (2014). *TOP 10 Patient Safety Concerns for Healthcare Organizations 2014.* Retrieved June 19, 2014 from https://www.ecri.org/PatientSafetyTop10

Eysenbach, G., & Diepgen, T. L. (2001). The role of e-health and consumer health informatics for evidence-based patient choice in the 21st century. *Clinics in Dermatology*, *19*(1), 11–17. doi:10.1016/S0738-081X(00)00202-9 PMID:11369478

Funke, J. (1991). Solving complex problems: Human identification and control of complex systems. In R. J. Sternberg & P. A. Frensch (Eds.), *Complex problem solving: Principles and mechanisms* (pp. 185–222). Hillsdale, NJ: Lawrence Erlbaum Associates.

Gray, J. A. M. (1996). *Evidence-based Healthcare.* Edinburgh, UK: Churchill Livingstone.

Haycock-Stuart, E. A., & Neil, M. (2005). Evaluation study of a resource for developing education, audit and teamwork in primary care. *Primary Health Care Research and Development*, *6*(3), 251–268. doi:10.1191/1463423605pc249oa

Iezzoni, L. I. (1996). Assessing quality using administrative data. *Annals of Internal Medicine*, *127*(8), 666–674. doi:10.7326/0003-4819-127-8_Part_2-199710151-00048 PMID:9382378

Institute of Medicine. (2001). *Crossing the Quality Chasm: A New Health System for the 21st Century*. Washington, DC: National Academy Press; doi:10.17226/10027

Johnston, G., Crombie, I. K., Davies, H. T. O., Alder, E. M., & Millard, A. (2000). Reviewing audit: Barriers and facilitating factors for effective clinical audit. *Quality in Health Care*, *9*(1), 23–36. doi:10.1136/qhc.9.1.23 PMID:10848367

Kennedy, R. F. Jr. (2005). *"The Disinformation Society," Crimes Against Nature*. New York: Harper Perennial.

Kiefe, C. I., Allison, J. J., Williams, O. D., Person, S. D., Weaver, M. T., & Weissman, N. W. (2001). Improving quality improvement using achievable benchmarks for physician feedback. A randomized controlled trial. *Journal of the American Medical Association*, *285*(22), 2871–2879. doi:10.1001/jama.285.22.2871 PMID:11401608

Kohn, L. T., Corrigan, J. M., & Donaldson, M. S. (Eds.). (1999). *To Err Is Human: Building a Safer Health System*. Washington, DC: National Academy Press. doi:10.17226/9728

KPMG. (2013). *KPMG Health Governace study*. Retrieved June 6, 2016 from https://www.kpmg.com/CN/en/IssuesAndInsights/ArticlesPublications/Documents/Global-perspectives-on-clinical-governance-o-201310.pdf

Lawrence, M., & Packwood, T. (1996). Adapting total quality management for general practice: Evaluation of a programme. *Quality in Health Care*, *5*(3), 151–158. doi:10.1136/qshc.5.3.151 PMID:10161529

Marshall, M. N., Shekelle, P. G., McGlynn, E. A., Campbell, S., Brook, R. H., & Roland, M. O. (2003). Can health care quality indicators be transferred between countries? *Quality & Safety in Health Care*, *12*(1), 8–12. doi:10.1136/qhc.12.1.8 PMID:12571338

Milne, R., & Clarke, A. (1990). Can readmission rates be used as an outcome indicator? *BMJ (Clinical Research Ed.)*, *301*(6761), 1139–1140. doi:10.1136/bmj.301.6761.1139 PMID:2252926

Piha, T., & Terol, E. (2015). *European Reference Networks. How digital solutions fit in?* Retrieved June 16, 2016 from http://www.expandproject.eu/wp-content/uploads/2015/09/Tapani-Piha-Enrique-Terol.pdf

Powell, A. E., Davies, H. T. O., & Thomson, R. G. (2003). Using routine comparative data to assess the quality of health care: Understanding and avoiding common pitfalls. *Quality & Safety in Health Care*, *12*(2), 122–128. doi:10.1136/qhc.12.2.122 PMID:12679509

Ratzinger, J. (1968). *Einführung in das Christentum. Vorlesungen über das Apostolische Glaubensbekenntnis*. München: Kösel–Verlag.

Suchý, M., Bourek, A., Klika, P., Dušek, L., Ryska, M., Bělina, F., & Kožený, P. (2011). Joint development of clinical practice guidelines and quality indicators as a tool for quality of care improvement. In P. A. Bath, T. Mettler, D. A. Raptis, & B. A. Sen (Eds.). *Proceedings of the 15th international Symposium on Health Information Management Rersearch - ISHIMR 2011*. Zurich: University of Zurich, University of St. Gallen and University of Sheffield.

Terol, E. (2015). *European Reference Networks Implementation process: timeline and milestones.* Retrieved June 16, 2016 from http://ec.europa.eu/health/ern/docs/ev_20151008_co011_en.pdf

The Economist. (2010). *Viktor Chernomyrdin, a Russian prime minister, died on November 3rd, aged 72.* Retrieved June 16, 2016, from http://www.economist.com/node/17414237

Thompson, J. W., Pinidiya, S. D., Ryan, K. W., McKinley, E. D., Alston, S., Bost, J. E., & Simpson, P. et al. (2003). Health plan quality-of-care information is undermined by voluntary reporting. *American Journal of Preventive Medicine*, *24*(1), 62–70. doi:10.1016/S0749-3797(02)00569-X PMID:12554025

Weingart, S. N., Iezzoni, L. I., Davis, R. B., Palmer, R. H., Cahalane, M., Hamel, M. B., & Banks, N. J. et al. (2000). Use of administrative data to find substandard care: Validation of the complications screening program. *Medical Care*, *38*(8), 796–806. doi:10.1097/00005650-200008000-00004 PMID:10929992

West, E. (2001). Management matters: The link between hospital organisation and quality of patient care. *Quality in Health Care*, *10*(1), 40–48. doi:10.1136/qhc.10.1.40 PMID:11239143

WHO. (2004). *World report on knowledge for better health: strengthening health systems. 1. Health systems plans 2. Health services research - utilization 3. Delivery of health care 4. Knowledge 5. Health policy 6. World health.* Geneva: World Health Organization. Retrieved June 14, 2016 from http://www.who.int/rpc/meetings/en/world_report_on_knowledge_for_better_health2.pdf

KEY TERMS AND DEFINITIONS

Difficult Problem: A problem (issue) with elements of complexity, dynamics, intransparency and polytely.

Electronic Health: In a broad sense the term covers electronic/digital processes in health. It can also include health applications on mobile devices, referred to as m-health or mHealth. It relates to the use of information and communication technologies (ICT), which affect the health and health care and incorporates some services and systems to support preventive care, diagnosis and medical management.

Participative Healthcare: The involvement of all stakeholders of the healthcare process in sharing information, opinion, decision-making and responsibility.

Personalized Healthcare: Type of care based on acknowledging that each person is an individual and that each individual responds differently to treatment modalities. It requires a move from the traditional one-size-fits-all paradigm.

Policy: A practical activity aimed at changing a certain situation. The noun "policy" can be interpreted as a course or principle of action adopted or proposed by the government, party, business, or individual. It is a verbalized intent, is implemented by means of procedures or protocols and helps with making decisions.

Predictive Healthcare: The use of the process of reviewing historical patient data, analyzing the results and predicting the optimal choice of treatment or behavior modality.

Proactive Healthcare: The commitment of all stakeholders of the healthcare process, where all parties take an active role in managing the patient's health to keep the patient healthy, acting in advance to deal with an expected difficulty.

Compilation of References

Abramowicz, W., Hofman, R., Suryn, W., & Zyskowski, D. (2008). SQuaRE based web services quality model. *Proceedings of the International MultiConference of Engineers and Computer Scientists, 2008*, 827–835.

Adams, J., Edgar, L., & Mounib, A. P. (2006). *Healthcare 2015: Win-win or lose-lose?* IBM Institute for Business Value. Retrieved May 10, 2009, from http://www.ibm.com/healthcare/hc2015

Adams, R., & Bischof, L. (1994). Seeded region growing. *IEEE Transaction on Pattern Analysis and Machine Learning, 16*(6), 641–647. doi:10.1109/34.295913

Adriaensens, S., Beyers, W., & Struyf, E. (2015). Impact of stuttering severity on adolescents' domain-specific and general self-esteem through cognitive and emotional mediating processes. *Journal of Communication Disorders, 58*, 43–57. doi:10.1016/j.jcomdis.2015.10.003 PMID:26484722

Aff, H. (2016, April1). (Millwood). Patients' and Consumers'. *Use of Evidence., 35*(4), 564–565. doi:10.1377/hlthaff.2016.0171

Akhtar, S. (2008). 2G-5G Networks: Evolution of Technologies, Standards, and Deployment. In Encyclopedia of Multimedia Technology and Networking (2nd ed.). Idea Group Publisher.

Allen, T. J. (1977). *Managing the Flow of Technology*. Cambridge, MA: MIT Press.

American College Health Association. (2007). National College Health Assessment Spring 2006 Reference Group data report. *Journal of Health., 55*, 195–206. PMID:17319325

American College of Physicians. (2008). *E-health and its impact on Medical Practice. Position paper*. Author.

American Health Information Management Association. (2013). *Analysis of Modifications to the HIPAA Privacy, Security, Enforcement, and Breach Notification Rules under the Health Information Technology for Economic and Clinical Health Act and the Genetic Information Nondiscrimination Act; Other Modifications to the HIPAA Rules*. Retrieved August 16, 2014, from http://library.ahima.org/PdfView?oid=106127

American Society of Human Genetics Social Issues Subcommittee on Familial Disclosure. (1998). ASHG STATEMENT Professional Disclosure of Familial Genetic Information. *American Journal of Human Genetics, 62*(2), 474–483. doi:10.1086/301707 PMID:9537923

Anastasiou, A., Giokas, K., Koutsouris, D. (2015). Monitoring of compliance on an individual treatment through mobile innovations. *EMBC*, 7320-7323.

Ancelle, J. A. G. (2015). Assistive Technologies at the Edge of Language and Speech Science for Children with Communication Disorders: VocalIDTM, Free SpeechTM, and SmartPalateTM. In N. R. Silton (Ed.), *Recent Advances in Assistive Technologies to Support Children with Developmental Disorders* (pp. 255–277). Hershey, PA: IGI Global. doi:10.4018/978-1-4666-8395-2.ch012

Anderson, K. J. (2001). Internet use among college students: An exploratory study. *Journal of American College Health, 50*(1), 21–26. doi:10.1080/07448480109595707 PMID:11534747

Anderson, P., & Blackwood, A. (2004). *Mobile and PDA technologies and their future use in education. JISC TechWatch.* Bristol: JISC.

Anonymous. (2007). *Healthcare's most expensive piece of paper.* DialogMEDICAL. Retrieved May 10, 2013, from http://www.dialogmedical.com/wp- content/uploads/2010/04/ROI%20White%20Paper%2005-07.pdf

Ansari, H., Bakhtiar, M., Ghanadzade, M., Packman, A., & Seifpanahi, S. (2010). Investigation of the reliability of the SSI-3 for preschool Persian-speaking children who stutter. *Journal of Fluency Disorders, 35*(2), 87–91. doi:10.1016/j.jfludis.2010.02.003 PMID:20609330

Antonino, P. O., Schneider, D., Hofmann, C., & Nakagawa, E. Y. (2011). Evaluation of AAL platforms according to architecture-based quality attributes. In *Ambient Intelligence* (pp. 264–274). Springer Berlin Heidelberg. doi:10.1007/978-3-642-25167-2_36

Anya, O., Tawfik, H., Nagar, A., & Amin, S. (2009). E-workbench: A Case for Collaborative Decision Support in E-health. Paper presented at the 11th International Conference on Computer Modelling and Simulation.

Apostol, T. M. (1988). *Calculus.* Barcelona: Reverté.

Appelbaum, P. S., & Thomas, G. (1995). The MacArthur Treatment Competence Study. I: Mental illness and competence to consent to treatment. *Law and Human Behavior, 19*(2), 105–126. doi:10.1007/BF01499321 PMID:11660290

Apple Inc. (2011). *iPhone Facetime.* Retrieved from http://www.apple.com/iphone/features/facetime.html

Arbyn, M., Herbert, A., Schenck, U., Nieminen, P., Jordan, J., McGoogan, E., & Martin-Hirsch, P. et al. (2007). European guidelines for quality assurance in cervical cancer screening: Recommendations for collecting samples for conventional and liquid-based cytology. *Cytopathology, 18*(3), 133–139. doi:10.1111/j.1365-2303.2007.00464.x PMID:17573762

Arkin, E. B. (1999). Cancer risk communication-what we know. *Journal of the National Cancer Institute. Monographs, 1999*(25), 182–185. doi:10.1093/oxfordjournals.jncimonographs.a024200 PMID:10854479

Arnett, J. J. (2000). Emerging adulthood: A theory of development from the late teens through the twenties. *The American Psychologist, 55*(5), 469–480. doi:10.1037/0003-066X.55.5.469 PMID:10842426

Assembling Reconfigurable Endoluminal Surgical System. (2014). CORDIS. Retrieved June 8, 2016, from http://cordis.europa.eu/publication/rcn/10899_en.html

Athanasiadi, E., Pouliakis, A., Bilirakis, E., Fragoulakis, V., Bilirakis, C., & Karakitsos, P. (2014). Quality Indicators for Cervical Cancer Screening Programs: The Role of Computerized Systems.[IJRQEH]. *International Journal of Reliable and Quality E-Healthcare, 3*(4), 19–37. doi:10.4018/ijrqeh.2014100102

Atzori, L., Iera, A., & Morabito, G. (2010). The Internet of Things: A survey. *Computer Networks, 54*(15), 2787–2805. doi:10.1016/j.comnet.2010.05.010

Austin, C. J., & Boxerman, S. B. (1998). *Information systems for health services administration* (5th ed.). Chicago, IL: Health Administration Press.

Australian Bureau of Statistics (ABS). (2011). *Households using the Internet.* Retrieved September 12, 2012, from: http://www.abs.gov.au/ausstats/abs@.nsf/mf/8146.0

Australian Institute for Primary Care. (2008). *System reform and development for chronic disease management.* Australian Institute for Primary Care. Retrieved October 21, 2009, from: http://www.health.gov.au/internet/nhhrc/publishing.nsf/Content/038-aipclatrobe/$FILE/038%20Australian%20Institute%20for%20Primary%20Care,%20La%20Trobe%20University%20Attachment%20B.pdf

Australian Institute of Health and Welfare. (2011). *Authoritative information and statistics to promote better health and wellbeing.* Retrieved September 12, 2012, from: http://www.aihw.gov.au/cancer-control-health-priority-area/

Auyang, E. D., Santos, B. F., Enter, D. H., Hungness, E. S., & Soper, N. J. (2011). Natural orifice translumenal endoscopic surgery (NOTES®): A technical review. *Surgical Endoscopy*, *25*(10), 3135–3148. doi:10.1007/s00464-011-1718-x PMID:21553172

Avendaño, C., Mata, A., Villanueva, A. M., Martínez, V. S., & Sarmiento, C. A. (2010). Laptop expositions affect motility and induce DNA fragmentation in human spermatozoa in vitro by a non-thermal effect: A preliminary report. *Journal of Fertility and Sterility*, *94*(4), 73. doi:10.1016/j.fertnstert.2010.07.284

Ayuso, C., Millán, J. M., Mancheño, M., & Dal-Ré, R. (2013). Informed consent for whole-genome sequencing studies in the clinical setting. Proposed recommendations on essential content and process. *European Journal of Human Genetics*, *21*(10), 1054–1059. doi:10.1038/ejhg.2012.297 PMID:23321621

Bae, J., Cho, H., Song, K., Lee, H., & Yoo, H. J. (2012). The signal transmission mechanism on the surface of human body for body channel communication. *IEEE Transactions on Microwave Theory and Techniques*, *60*(3), 582–593. doi:10.1109/TMTT.2011.2178857

Ballard, C., Gauthier, S., Corbett, A., Brayne, C., Aarsland, D., & Jones, E. (2011). Alzheimer's disease. *Lancet*, *377*(9770), 1019–1031. doi:10.1016/S0140-6736(10)61349-9 PMID:21371747

Bardaro, S. J., & Swanström, L. (2006). Development of advanced endoscopes for natural orifice transluminal endoscopic surgery (NOTES). *Minimally Invasive Therapy & Allied Technologies*, *15*(6), 378–383. doi:10.1080/13645700601038069 PMID:17190663

Barker, E. T., & Galambos, N. L. (2007). Body dissatisfaction, living away from parents, and poor social adjustment predict binge eating symptoms in young women making the transition to University. *Journal of Youth and Adolescence*, *36*(7), 904–911. doi:10.1007/s10964-006-9134-6

Barnes, T. D., Wozniak, D. F., Gutierrez, J., Han, T. U., Drayna, D., & Holy, T. E. (2016). A Mutation Associated with Stuttering Alters Mouse Pup Ultrasonic Vocalizations. *Current Biology*, *26*(8), 1009–1018. doi:10.1016/j.cub.2016.02.068 PMID:27151663

Baron, R. J., Fabens, E. L., Schiffman, M., & Wolf, E. (2005). Electronic health records: Just around the corner? Or over the cliff? *Annals of Internal Medicine*, *143*(3), 222–226. doi:10.7326/0003-4819-143-3-200508020-00008 PMID:16061920

Basu, P., Banerjee, D., Mittal, S., Dutta, S., Ghosh, I., Chowdhury, N., & Ratnam, S. et al. (2016). Sensitivity of APTIMA HPV E6/E7 mRNA test in comparison with hybrid capture 2 HPV DNA test for detection of high risk oncogenic human papillomavirus in 396 biopsy confirmed cervical cancers. *Journal of Medical Virology*, *88*(7), 1271–1278. doi:10.1002/jmv.24453 PMID:26693677

Beauchamp, T. L., & Childress, J. F. (1989). *Principles of Biomedical Ethics* (3rd ed.). New York: Oxford University Press.

Beer, D. (2013). *Popular Culture and New Media: The Politics of Circulation.* Houndmills, UK: Palgrave Macmillan. doi:10.1057/9781137270061

Behkamal, B., Kahani, M., & Akbari, M. K. (2009). Customizing ISO 9126 quality model for evaluation of B2B applications. *Journal of Information and Software Technology*, *51*(3), 599–609. doi:10.1016/j.infsof.2008.08.001

Belmont, J., & McGuire, A. L. (2009). The futility of genomic counseling: Essential role of electronic health records. *Genome Medicine*, *1*(5), 1. doi:10.1186/gm48 PMID:19439060

Bender, L. J., Yue, K. R. Y., To, J. M., Deacken, L., & Jadad, R. A. (2013). A lot of action, but not in the right direction: Systematic review and content analysis of smartphone applications for the prevention, detection, and management of cancer. *Journal of Medical Internet Research*, *15*(12), e287. doi:10.2196/jmir.2661 PMID:24366061

Benedetti, F. (2011). *The Patient's Brain: The neuroscience behind the doctor-patient relationship*. Oxford, UK: Oxford University Press.

Berg, M., & Mol, A. (Eds.). (1998). *Difference in Medicine; Unravelling Practices, Techniques, and Bodies*. Durham, NC: Duke University Press.

Bergmann, J., Bott, O. J., Pretschner, D. P., & Haux, R. (2007). An econsent-based shared EHR system architecture for integrated healthcare networks. *International Journal of Medical Informatics*, *76*(2-3), 130–136. doi:10.1016/j.ijmedinf.2006.07.013 PMID:16971171

Bernhardt, J., & Hubley, J. (2001). Health education and the Internet: The beginning of a revolution. *Health Education Research*, *16*(5), 643–645. doi:10.1093/her/16.6.643

Berwick, D. M. (1998). *Examining Errors in Health Care: Developing a Prevention, Education, and Research Agenda*. Paper presented at the American Hospital Association and Centennial Regional Leadership Forum, Cleveland, OH.

Betrán, A. P., Ye, J., Moller, A. B., Zhang, J., Gülmezoglu, A. M., & Torloni, M. R. (2016). The Increasing Trend in Caesarean Section Rates: Global, Regional and National Estimates: 1990-2014. *PLoS ONE*, *11*(2), e0148343. doi:10.1371/journal.pone.0148343 PMID:26849801

Bhatti, R., & Grandison, T. (2007). *Towards improved privacy policy coverage in healthcare using policy refinement*. Berlin: Springer. doi:10.1007/978-3-540-75248-6_11

Binkowska-Bury, M., & Januszewicz, P. (2010). Sense of coherence and health-related behaviour among University students--a questionnaire survey. *Journal of Public Health*, *18*(3), 145–150. PMID:21033609

Bird, T. (2001). Alzheimer's disease and other primary dementias. In D. Kasper, S. Hauser, D. Longo, & J. Jameson (Edits.), Harrison's Principles of Internal Medicine (pp. 2391-2399). McGraw-Hill.

Black, A., Car, J., Pagliari, C., Anandan, C., Cresswell, K., Bokun, T., & Sheikh, A. et al. (2011). The Impact of eHealth on the Quality and Safety of Health Care: A Systematic Overview. *PLoS Medicine*, *8*(1), e1000387. doi:10.1371/journal.pmed.1000387 PMID:21267058

Blake, A., & Isard, M. (1998). *Active contours: The application of techniques from graphics vision, control theory and statistics to visual tracking of shapes in motion*. London: Springer-Verlag. doi:10.1007/978-1-4471-1555-7

Blench, M. (2008). Global public health intelligence network (GPHIN). In *Proceedings of the conference of the American machine translation association (AMTA)*. Waikiki, HI: AMTA.

Blennow, K. (2005). *Amesterdão: European College of Neuropsychopharmacology*. ECNP.

Blennow, K., & Zetterberg, H. (2010). Is it time for biomarker-based diagnostic criteria for prodromal Azheimer's Disease? *Alzheimer's Research & Therapy*, *2*(2), 8. doi:10.1186/alzrt31 PMID:20441609

Boehm, B. W., Brown, J. R., & Kaspar, H. (1978). *Characteristics of software quality*. North Holland.

Boersma, P., & Weenink, D. (2009). *Praat Manual: doing phonetics by computer. 5.1.17.* [Computer program]. Available at: http://www.fon.hum.uva.nl/praat/download_win.html

Bogue, R. (2011). Robots in healthcare. *Industrial Robot: An International Journal, 38*(3), 218–223. doi:10.1108/01439911111122699

Bombardieri, M., & Fontana, F. A. (2008, September). A specialisation of the SQuaRE quality model for the evaluation of the software evolution and maintenance activity. In *Automated Software Engineering-Workshops, 2008. ASE Workshops 2008. 23rd IEEE/ACM International Conference on* (pp. 110-113). IEEE. doi:10.1109/ASEW.2008.4686328

Bonabeau, E., Dorigo, M., & Theraulaz, G. (1999). *Swarm intelligence: from natural to artificial systems (No. 1).* Oxford University Press.

Boonstra, H., & Nash, E. (2000). Minors and the right to consent to health care. *The Guttmacher Report on Public Policy, 3*(4), 4–8. PMID:12134879

Borzekowski, D. (2001). Adolescent cyber-surfing for health information: A new resource that crosses barriers. *Archives of Pediatrics & Adolescent Medicine, 155*(7), 813–817. doi:10.1001/archpedi.155.7.813 PMID:11434849

Bouillon, P., Flores, G., Starlander, M., Chatzichrisafis, N., Santaholma, M., Tsourakis, N., & Hockey, B. A. et al. (2007). A Bidirectional Grammar-Based Medical Speech Translator.*Workshop on Grammar-Based Approaches to Spoken Language Processing* (pp. 41–48). doi:10.3115/1626333.1626341

Bountris, P., Haritou, M., Pouliakis, A., Margari, N., Kyrgiou, M., Spathis, A., & Koutsouris, D. D. et al. (2014). An intelligent clinical decision support system for patient-specific predictions to improve cervical intraepithelial neoplasia detection. *Biomed Res Int, 341483.* doi:10.1155/2014/341483 PMID:24812614

Bourek, A. (2002). The era of information in the Czech Republic: How healthcare is managing data sets and mind-sets. In Accountability through measurement: A global healthcare imperative. American Society of Quality (ASQ Quality Press).

Bourek, A. (2011). General principles and logic of quality management in health and healthcare. In E-Health Systems Quality and Reliability: Models and Standards. Hershey, PA: IGI Global Publishing. doi:10.4018/978-1-61692-843-8.ch001

Bourek, A., Tůma, P., & Bourková, A. (2008). *Indicators as signals for assuring living and healthy health care organizations.* Paper presented at the WHO Vienna Public Healthcare Conference Performance Assessment in Healthcare Delivery PATH II, Vienna, Austria.

Bourek, A. (2014). Introducing Healthcare System Change Strategies to Policy Makers in the Open Society and Digital Environment: What Works Now, But May Not Work in the Near Future. *International Journal of Reliable and Quality E-Healthcare, 1*(2), 36–59. doi:10.4018/ijrqeh.2014040103

Bourgeois, F. C., Taylor, P. L., Emans, S. J., Nigrin, D. J., & Mandl, K. D. (2008). Whose personal control? Creating private, personally controlled health records for pediatric and adolescent patients. *Journal of the American Medical Informatics Association, 15*(6), 737–743.

Boyd, D. M., & Ellison, N. B. (2007). Social network sites: Definition, history, and scholarship. *Journal of Computer-Mediated Communication, 13*(1), 210–230. doi:10.1111/j.1083-6101.2007.00393.x

Boyer, C., & Geissbuhler, A. (2006). Health and the Internet for all. *International Journal of Medical Informatics, 75*(1), 1–3. doi:10.1016/j.ijmedinf.2005.07.039 PMID:16325462

Brachfeld, J. (2002). "Defensive Medicine" and malpractice suits. *Archives of Internal Medicine, 162*(22), 2631. doi:10.1001/archinte.162.22.2631 PMID:12456244

Brodie, M., Flournoy, E., Altman, D., Blendon, R. J., Benson, J. M., & Rosenbaum, M. D. (2000). Health information, the Internet, and the digital divide. *Health Affairs*, *19*(6), 255–265. doi:10.1377/hlthaff.19.6.255 PMID:11192412

Buchanan, A. (2004). Mental capacity, legal competence and consent to treatment. *Journal of the Royal Society of Medicine*, *97*(9), 415–420.

Buijink, A. W. G., Visser, B. J., & Marshall, L. (2013). Medical apps for smartphones: Lack of evidence undermines quality and safety. *Evidence-Based Medicine*, *18*(3), 90–92. doi:10.1136/eb-2012-100885 PMID:22923708

Bulian, D. R., Runkel, N., Burghardt, J., Lamade, W., Butters, M., Utech, M., & Lehmann, K. S. et al. (2014). Natural Orifice Transluminal Endoscopic Surgery (NOTES) for colon resections—analysis of the first 139 patients of the German NOTES Registry (GNR). *International Journal of Colorectal Disease*, *29*(7), 853–861. doi:10.1007/s00384-014-1883-1 PMID:24798629

Buzek, J., & Gyori, E. (2011). Directive 2011/24/EU of the European parliament and of the council. Official Journal of the European Union, 45-65.

Cain, J., Brent, I., & Fox, P. (2009). Web 2.0 and pharmacy education. *American Journal of Pharmaceutical Education*, *73*(7), 1–11. doi:10.5688/aj7307120 PMID:19960079

Calzolari, N., McNaught, J., Palmer, M., & Zampolli, A. (2002). International Standards for Language Engineering. Final Report.

Capra, F. (2009). *Management.* Retrieved May 4, 2009, from http://www.fritjofcapra.net/management.html

Care Continuum Alliance. (2012). *Advancing the Population Health Improvement Model.* Retrieved from http://www.fiercehealthit.com/story/hennepin-health-project-looks-build-countywide-ehr-program-national-implica/2012-01-10

Carroll, J. D., & Messenger, J. C. (2008). Medical simulation: The new tool for training and skill assessment. *Perspectives in Biology and Medicine*, *51*(1), 47–60. doi:10.1353/pbm.2008.0003 PMID:18192765

Carta, R., Sfakiotakis, M., Pateromichelakis, N., Thoné, J., Tsakiris, D. P., & Puers, R. (2011). A multi-coil inductive powering system for an endoscopic capsule with vibratory actuation. *Sensors and Actuators. A, Physical*, *172*(1), 253–258. doi:10.1016/j.sna.2011.03.036

Carvalho, D., & Biswas, D. (2013). Health care social media: Expectations of users in a developing country. *Med 2.0*, *9*(2), e4. doi: 10.2196/med20.2720

Caughey, G. E., Kalisch Ellett, L. M., & Wong, T. Y. (2014). Development of evidence-based Australian medication-related indicators of potentially preventable hospitalisations: A modified RAND appropriateness method. *BMJ Open*, *4*(4), e004625. doi:10.1136/bmjopen-2013-004625 PMID:24776711

Caughlin, J. P., & Sharabis, L. L. (2013). A Communicative Interdependence Perspective of Close Relationships: The Connections Between Mediated and Unmediated Interactions Matter. *Journal of Communication*, *63*, 873–893.

Cavalcanti, A., Shirinzadeh, B., & Kretly, L. C. (2008). Medical nanorobotics for diabetes control. *Nanomedicine; Nanotechnology, Biology, and Medicine*, *4*(2), 127–138. doi:10.1016/j.nano.2008.03.001 PMID:18455965

Chalana, V., & Kim, Y. (1997). A methodology for evaluation of boundary detection algorithms on medical images. *IEEE Transactions on Medical Imaging*, *16*(5), 642–652. doi:10.1109/42.640755 PMID:9368120

Chang, D., Thyer, I., Hayne, D., & Katz, D. (2014). Using mobile technology to overcome language barriers in medicine. *Annals of the Royal College of Surgeons of England*, *96*(6), e23–e15. doi:10.1308/003588414X13946184903685 PMID:25198966

Charles, C., Whelan, T., & Gafni, A. (1999). What do we mean by partnership in making decisions about treatment? *British Medical Journal*, *319*(7212), 780–782. doi:10.1136/bmj.319.7212.780 PMID:10488014

Charles, S., Nicole, E., & Cliff, L. (2008). Social capital, self-esteem, and use of online social network sites: A longitudinal analysis. *Journal of Applied Developmental Psychology*, *29*(200), 434–445.

Chaudhry, B., Jerome, W., Shinyi, W., Maglione, M., Mojica, W., & Roth, E. et al.. (2006). Systematic Review: Impact of Health Information Technology on Quality, Efficiency, and Costs of Medical Care. *Annals of Internal Medicine*, *144*(10), E12–W18. doi:10.7326/0003-4819-144-10-200605160-00125 PMID:16702590

Chen, C. H. (1988). *Signal processing handbook*. Marcel Dekker Incorporated.

Chetney, R. (2003). The Cardiac Connection Program. *Home Healthcare Nurse*, *21*(10), 680–686. doi:10.1097/00004045-200310000-00007 PMID:14557707

Cheung, K., Yip, K., Townsend, J., & Scotch, M. (2008). HCLS 2.0/3.0: Health care and life sciences data mashup using Web 2.0/3.0. *Journal of Biomedical Informatics*, *41*(5), 694–705. doi:10.1016/j.jbi.2008.04.001 PMID:18487092

Chlamtac, I., Conti, M., & Liu, J. J.-N. (2003). Mobile ad hoc networking: Imperatives and challenges. *Ad Hoc Networks*, *1*(1), 13–64. doi:10.1016/S1570-8705(03)00013-1

Clayton, E. W., Steinberg, K. K., Khoury, M. J., Thomson, E., Andrews, L., Kahn, M. J. E., & Weiss, J. O. et al. (1995). Informed consent for genetic research on stored tissue samples. *Journal of the American Medical Association*, *274*(22), 1786–1792. doi:10.1001/jama.1995.03530220052033 PMID:7500511

Cocosila, M., & Archer, N. (2010). Adoption of mobile ICT for health promotion: An empirical investigation. *Electronic Markets*, *20*(3-4), 241–250. doi:10.1007/s12525-010-0042-y

Cohen, E., Riesenfeld, R. F., & Elber, G. (2010). *Geometric modeling with splines: An introduction*. A.K. Peters Ltd.

Coiera, E., & Clark, R. (2004, March/April). e-Consent: The design and Implementation of consumer consent mechanisms in an electronic environment. *Journal of the American Informatics Association*, *11*(2). PMID:14662803

Commission. (2014). *Commission delegated decision of 10 March 2014 setting out criteria and conditions that European Reference Networks and healthcare providers wishing to join a European Reference Network must fulfil*. Retrieved June 15, 2016 from: http://ec.europa.eu/health/ern/docs/ern_delegateddecision_20140310_en.pdf

Compbell, D. (June, 2004). Case and Commentary – Listen to the family. *Morbidity & Mortality Rounds on the Web. AHRQ*. Retrieved August 8, 2013, from http://webmm.ahrq.gov/case.aspx?caseID=62

Conture, E. (1990). *Stuttering*. Englewood Cliffs, NJ: Prentice-Hall.

Coquillard, G., Palao, B., & Patterson, B. K. (2011). Quantification of intracellular HPV E6/E7 mRNA expression increases the specificity and positive predictive value of cervical cancer screening compared to HPV DNA. *Gynecologic Oncology*, *120*(1), 89–93. doi:10.1016/j.ygyno.2010.09.013 PMID:20950847

Cordero, F., Botta, M., & Calogero, R. A. (2007). Microarray data analysis and mining approaches. *Briefings in Functional Genomics & Proteomics*, *6*(4), 265–281. doi:10.1093/bfgp/elm034 PMID:18216026

Cormode, G., & Krishnamurthy, B. (2008). Key differences between Web 1.0 and Web 2.0. *First Monday*, *13*(6). doi:10.5210/fm.v13i6.2125

Costello, J. M., & Ingham, R. J. (1984). Assessment strategies for stuttering. In R. Curlee & W. H. Perkins (Eds.), *Nature and treatment of stuttering: New directions* (pp. 303–333). San Diego, CA: College-Hill Press.

Cote, M. A., Syryn, W., Martin, A. R., & Laport, Y. C. (2004). Evolving a Corporate Software Quality Assessment Exercise: A Migration Path to ISO/IEC-9126. *Software Quality Professional*, *6*(3), 1–17.

Coughlin, J. F., Pope, J. E., & Leedle, B. R. Jr. (2006). Old Age, New Technology, and Future Innovations in Disease Management and Home Health Care. *Home Health Care Management & Practice*, *18*(3), 196–207. doi:10.1177/1084822305281955

Courtenay, W. (2000). Construction of masculinity and their influence on men's well-being: A theory of gender and health. *Social Science & Medicine*, *50*(10), 1385–1401. doi:10.1016/S0277-9536(99)00390-1 PMID:10741575

Courtot, M., Mungall, C., Brinkman, R. R., & Ruttenberg, A. (2011). Building the OBO foundry - One policy at a time. In *CEUR Workshop Proceedings* (Vol. 833, pp. 377–380).

Cramton, C. (2001). The Mutual Knowledge Problem and Its Consequences for Dispersed Collaborations. *Organization Science*, *12*(3), 346–371. doi:10.1287/orsc.12.3.346.10098

Cretin, S., Shortell, S. M., & Keeler, E. B. (2004). An Evaluation of Collaborative Interventions to Improve Chronic Illness Care. *Evaluation Review*, *28*(1), 28–51. doi:10.1177/0193841X03256298 PMID:14750290

Cummings, J. (2004). *La neuropsiquiatria de la enfermedad de Alzheimer y demencias relacionadas.* Altas Medical Publishing Ltd.

Cummins, J. (2010). *Few hospitals use social media effectively, says study.* Health Leaders Media. Retrieved from October 13, 2011, from http://www.healthleadersmedia.com/content/TEC-245418/Few-Hospitals-Use-Social-Media-Effectively-Says-Study.html

Curlee, R. F. (1981). Observer agreement on disfluency and stuttering. *Journal of Speech and Hearing Research*, *24*(4), 595–560. doi:10.1044/jshr.2404.595 PMID:7035743

Curtis, E. M., van der Velde, R., Moon, R. J., van den Bergh, J. P., Geusens, P., de Vries, F., & Harvey, N. C. et al. (2016). Epidemiology of Fractures in the United Kingdom 1988-2012: Variation with Age, Sex, Geography, Ethnicity and Socioeconomic Status. *Bone*, *9*(87), 19–26. doi:10.1016/j.bone.2016.03.006 PMID:26968752

Cusack, C. M., Knudson, A. D., Kronstadt, J. L., Singer, R. F., & Brown, A. L. (2010). *Practice-Based Population Health: Information Technology to Support Transformation to Proactive Primary Care.* Retrieved from https://pcmh.ahrq.gov/sites/default/files/attachments/Information%20Technology%20to%20Support%20Transformation%20to%20Proactive%20Primary%20Care.pdf

Cutler, D. M., Feldman, N. E., & Horwitz, J. R. (2005). U. S. Adoption of Computerized Physician Order Entry Systems. *Health Affairs*, *24*(6), 1654–1663. doi:10.1377/hlthaff.24.6.1654 PMID:16284040

Cylus, J., Richardson, E., Findlay, L., Longley, M., O'Neill, C., & Steel, D. (2015). United Kingdom: Health System review. *Health Syst Transit.*, *17*(5), 1–126. PMID:27049966

Dadkhah, M., Kumar, N., & Yoon, J. (2013). Design and simulation of a 3D actuation system for magnetic nano-particles delivery system. In *Intelligent Robotics and Applications* (pp. 177–187). Springer Berlin Heidelberg. doi:10.1007/978-3-642-40852-6_20

Dalal, A. K., Dykes, P. C., Collins, S., Lehmann, L. S., Ohashi, K., Rozenblum, R., & Bates, D. W. et al. (2016). A web-based, patient-centered toolkit to engage patients and caregivers in the acute care setting: A preliminary evaluation. *Journal of the American Medical Informatics Association*, *23*(1), 80–87. doi:10.1093/jamia/ocv093 PMID:26239859

Danforth, R.M., Pitt, H.A., Flanagan, M.E., Brewster, B.D., Brand, E.W., & Frankel, R.M. (2014). Surgical inpatient satisfaction: What are the real drivers? *Surgery, 56*(2), 328-35.

Dang, J., Hedayati, A., Hampel, K., & Toklu, C. (2008). An ontological knowledge framework for adaptive medical workflow. *Journal of Biomedical Informatics*, *41*(5), 829–836. doi:10.1016/j.jbi.2008.05.012 PMID:18602872

Davis, D., O'Brien, M. A., Freemantle, N., Wolf, F. M., Mazmanian, P., & Taylor-Vaisey, A. (1999). Impact of formal continuing medical education: Do conferences, workshops, rounds, and other traditional continuing education activities change physician behavior or health care outcomes? *Journal of the American Medical Association*, *282*(9), 867–874. doi:10.1001/jama.282.9.867 PMID:10478694

Davis, R. L. (2005). Computerized Physician Order Entry Systems: The Coming of Age for Outpatient Medicine. *PLoS Medicine*, *2*(9), e290. doi:10.1371/journal.pmed.0020290 PMID:16173835

Del Carmen, M. G., & Joffe, S. (2005). Informed consent for medical treatment and research: A review. *The Oncologist*, *10*(8), 636–641. doi:10.1634/theoncologist.10-8-636 PMID:16177288

Della Mea, V. (2001). What is e-Health (2): The death of telemedicine? *Journal of Medical Internet Research*, *3*(2), e22. doi:10.2196/jmir.3.2.e22 PMID:11720964

Dennis, A. R., Fuller, R. M., & Valacich, J. S. (2008). Media, Tasks and Communication Processes: A Theory of Media Synchronicity. *Management Information Systems Quarterly*, *32*(3), 575–600.

Department of Health and Ageing. (2008). *Towards a National Primary Health Care Strategy: a discussion paper from the Australian Government*. Retrieved Feburary 6, 2009, from http://www.health.gov.au/primaryhealthstrategy

Directive, E. (1995). 95/46/EC of the European Parliament and of the Council of 24 October 1995 on the protection of individuals with regard to the processing of personal data and on the free movement of such data. *Official Journal of the EC, 23*(6).

Donabedian, A. (1976). *Benefits in medical care programs*. Cambridge, MA: Harvard University Press.

Donabedian, A. (1980). Explorations in Quality Assessment and Monitoring: Vol. 1. *The Definition of Quality and Approaches to its Assessment*. Ann Arbor, MI: Health Admin Press.

Donabedian, A. (2005, December). Evaluating the Quality of Medical Care.[A.B.]. *The Milbank Quarterly*, *83*(4), 691–729. RetrievedAugust302009. doi:10.1111/j.1468-0009.2005.00397.x PMID:16279964

Dörner, D. (1975). Wie Menschen eine Welt verbessern wollten. *Bild der Wissenschaft*, *12*, 48–53.

Downing, A., Rudge, G., Cheng, Y., Tu, Y.-K., Keen, J., & Gilthorpe, M. S. (2007). Do the uk government's new quality and outcomes framework (qof) scores adequately measure primary care performance? a cross-sectional survey of routine healthcare data. *BMC Health Services Research*, *7*(1), 166. doi:10.1186/1472-6963-7-166 PMID:17941984

Dromey, G. R. (1995). A model for software product quality. *Software Engineering. IEEE Transactions on*, *21*(2), 146–162.

Drösler, S. E., Klazinga, N. S., Romano, P. S., Tancredi, D. J., Gogorcena Aoiz, M. A., Hewitt, M. C., & Kelley, E. et al. (2009). Application of patient safety indicators internationally: A pilot study among seven countries. *International Journal for Quality in Health Care*, *21*(4), 272–278. doi:10.1093/intqhc/mzp018 PMID:19395469

Dunn, J. R., & Hayes, M. V. (1999). Toward a lexicon of population health. *Canadian Journal of Public Health*, *90*(Suppl 1), S7–S10. PMID:10686751

Duque-Ramos, A., Fernández-Breis, J. T., Stevens, R., & Aussenac-Gilles, N. (2011). OQuaRE: A SQuaRE-based approach for evaluating the quality of ontologies. *Journal of Research and Practice in Information Technology*, *43*(2), 159.

Durso, S. C. (2001). Technological advances for improving medication adherence in the elderly. *Annals of Long Term Care: Clinical Care and Aging*, *9*, 43–48.

Duvlis, S., Popovska-Jankovic, K., Arsova, Z. S., Memeti, S., Popeska, Z., & Plaseska-Karanfilska, D. (2015). HPV E6/E7 mRNA versus HPV DNA biomarker in cervical cancer screening of a group of Macedonian women. *Journal of Medical Virology*, *87*(9), 1578–1586. doi:10.1002/jmv.24199 PMID:25880030

EAGLES. (1999). *The EAGLES 7-step recipe EAGLES Evaluation Working*. ISSCO, UNIGE. Retrieved May 2016 from http://www.issco.unige.ch/en/research/projects/eagles/ewg99/7steps.html

Ebina, Y., Yaegashi, N., Katabuchi, H., Nagase, S., Udagawa, Y., Hachisuga, T., & Yoshikawa, H. et al. (2015). Japan Society of Gynecologic Oncology guidelines 2011 for the treatment of uterine cervical cancer. *International Journal of Clinical Oncology*, *20*(2), 240–248. doi:10.1007/s10147-015-0806-7 PMID:25800808

eBizMBA Rank. (2010). Retrieved March 13, 2010, from http://www.ebizmba.com/articles/health-websites

ECRI Institute. (2014). *TOP 10 Patient Safety Concerns for Healthcare Organizations 2014*. Retrieved June 19, 2014 from https://www.ecri.org/PatientSafetyTop10

Edwards, N., & McDowell, I. (1998). *Proposal for a Population Health PhD Program submitted to the Ontario Council of Graduate Studies*. Ottawa, Canada: University of Ottawa, Institute of Population Health.

Elenko, E., Underwood, L., & Zohar, D. (2015). Defining digital medicine. *Nature Biotechnology*, *33*(5), 456–461. doi:10.1038/nbt.3222 PMID:25965750

Ellison, N., Steinfield, C., & Lampe, C. (2007). The benefits of Facebook "friends:" Social capital and college students' use of online social network sites. *Journal of Computer-Mediated Communication, 12*, 1143–1168.

Elwyn, G., Quinlan, C., Mulley, A., Agoritsas, T., Vandvik, P. O., & Guyatt, G. (2015). Trustworthy Guidelines – Excellent; Customized Care Tools – Even Better. *BMC Medicine*, *1*(13), 199. doi:10.1186/s12916-015-0436-y PMID:26324120

eMobility. (2007). In D. Bourse & R. Tafazolli (Eds.), *Beyond 3G / 4G Radio Access Technologies (RATs) and Standards Roadmaps* (eMobility Technology Platform Whitepaper). Retrieved from http://www.ist-emobility.org/

Epp, J. (1986). *Achieving Health for All: A Framework for Health Promotion*. Ottawa, Canada: Minister of Supply and Services Canada.

Erden, F., Velipasalar, S., Alkar, A. Z., & Cetin, A. E. (2016). *Sensors in Assisted Living*. Retrieved May 30, 2016, from https://www.researchgate.net/profile/Fatih_Erden2/publication/297659778_Sensors_in_Assisted_Living_A_survey_of_signal_and_image_processing_methods/links/56e18f9508ae40dc0abf5111.pdf

Ernst & Young. (2012). Mobile technology poised to enable a new era in health care. *EYGM Limited.* Retrieved April 5, 2013, from http://www.ey.com/Publication/vwLUAssets/mHealth_Report_January_2013/$FILE/mHealth%20Report_Final.pdf

Escoffery, C., Miner, K., Adame, D., Butler, S., McCormick, L., & Mendell, E. (2005). Internet use for health information among college students. *Journal of American College Health*, *53*(4), 183–188. doi:10.3200/JACH.53.4.183-188 PMID:15663067

Estrella, P., Popescu-Belis, A., & King, M. (2010). The FEMTI guidelines for contextual MT evaluation: Principles and resources. *Evaluation of Translation Technology*, *8*, 43.

European Commission. Directorate-General for Health and Consumer Protection. (2008). *European guidelines for quality assurance in cervical cancer screening*. Retrieved from http://bookshop.europa.eu/en/european-guidelines-for-quality-assurance-in-cervical-cancer-screening-pbND7007117/

European Commission. Directorate-General for Health and Consumer Protection., & International Agency for Research on Cancer. (2008). European guidelines for quality assurance in cervical cancer screening. Office for Official Publications of the European Communities.

European Union. (2010). *ICT & Ageing-European study on users, markets and technologies.* European Commission. Retrieved from http://scholar.google.com/scholar?hl=en&btnG=Search&q=intitle:ICT+&+Ageing+European+Study+on+Users+,+Markets+and+Technologies+Final+Report#0\nhttp://scholar.google.com/scholar?hl=en&btnG=Search&q=intitle:ICT+&+Ageing-European+Study+on+Users,+Markets+and+T

Evans, D. C., Nichol, W. P., & Perlin, J. B. (2006). Effect of the implementation of an enterprise-wide Electronic Health Record on productivity in the Veterans Health Administration. *Health Economics, Policy, and Law*, *1*(2), 163. doi:10.1017/S1744133105001210 PMID:18634688

Evans, R. G., & Stoddart, G. L. (1990). Producing health, consuming health care. *Social Science & Medicine*, *31*(12), 1347–1363. doi:10.1016/0277-9536(90)90074-3 PMID:2126895

Eviatar, H., & Somorjai, R. L. (1996). A fast, simple active contour algorithm for biomedical images. *Pattern Recognition Letters*, *17*(9), 969–974. doi:10.1016/0167-8655(96)00054-2

Eysenbach, G., & Diepgen, T. L. (2001). The role of e-health and consumer health informatics for evidence-based patient choice in the 21st century. *Clinics in Dermatology*, *19*(1), 11–17. doi:10.1016/S0738-081X(00)00202-9 PMID:11369478

Fang, H., Wang, C., Li, S., Wang, K. W., & Xu, J. (2015). A comprehensive study on the locomotion characteristics of a metameric earthworm-like robot. *Multibody System Dynamics*, *35*(2), 153–177. doi:10.1007/s11044-014-9428-5

Faresi, A. L. A., Wijesekera, D., & Moidu, K. (2010). A comprehensive privacy-aware authorization framework founded on HIPAA privacy rules. In *Proceedings of the 1st ACM International Health Informatics Symposium.* ACM.

Fath-Allah, A., Cheikhi, L., Al-Qutaish, R. E., & Idri, A. (2014). A Comparative Analysis of E-Government Quality Models. *International Journal of Social, Behavioral, Educational, Economic Business and Industrial Engineering*, *8*(11), 3526–3530.

Federal/Provincial/Territorial Advisory Committee on Population Health. (1994). *Strategies for Population Health: Investing in the Health of Canadians*. Ottawa, Canada: Minister of Supply and Services Canada.

Feigenbaum, A. (1961). *Total Quality Control*. New York: McGraw-Hill.

Fell, J., Röschke, J., & Beckmann, P. (1995). Non-linear analysis of sleep eeg data in schizophrenia: Calculation of the principal lyapunov exponent. *Journal of Psychiatric Research*, *56*(3), 257–269. doi:10.1016/0165-1781(95)02562-B

Feng, Y., Li, W., Li, M., & Sun, L. (2007, December). Structure optimization of the endoscopic robot ciliary leg based on dimensional analysis. In *Robotics and Biomimetics, 2007. ROBIO 2007. IEEE International Conference on* (pp. 109-114). IEEE.

Ferenczy, A., & Franco, E. (2002). Persistent human papillomavirus infection and cervical neoplasia. *The Lancet Oncology*, *3*(1), 11–16. doi:10.1016/S1470-2045(01)00617-9 PMID:11905599

Ferri, C., Prince, M., Brayne, C., Brodaty, H., Fratiglioni, L., Ganguli, M., & Rimmer, E. et al. (2005). Global prevalence of dementia: A Delphi consensus study. *Lancet*, *366*(9503), 2112–2117. doi:10.1016/S0140-6736(05)67889-0 PMID:16360788

Fillmore, H., DuBard, C. A., Ritter, G. A., & Jackson, C. T. (2014). Health care savings with the patient-centered medical home: Community Care of North Carolina's experience. *Population Health Management*, *17*(3), 141–148. doi:10.1089/pop.2013.0055 PMID:24053757

Finkelstein, J., Eckersberger, E., Sadri, H., Taneja, S. S., Lepor, H., & Djavan, B. (2010). Open Versus Laparoscopic Versus Robot-Assisted Laparoscopic Prostatectomy: The European and US Experience. *Reviews in Urology, 12*(1), 35–43. PMID:20428292

Firth-Cozens, J. (2004). Organisational trust: The keystone to patient safety. *Quality & Safety in Health Care, 13*(1), 56–61. doi:10.1136/qshc.2003.007971 PMID:14757801

Fisher, C. B. (2002). Goodness-of-Fit Ethic for Informed Consent. *A. Fordham Urb. LJ, 30*, 159. PMID:15868667

Fox, S., & Jones, S. (2009). *The social life of health information*. Pew Internet and American Life Project. Retrieved March 13, 2010, from http://www.pewinternet.org/Reports/2009/8-The-Social-Life-of-Health-Information.aspx

Fox, J., Patkar, V., & Thomson, R. (2006). Decision support for health care: The proforma evidence base. *Informatics in Primary Care, 14*(1), 49–54. PMID:16848966

Fox, S., & Rainie, L. (2006). The Online Health Care Revolution: How the Web Helps American Take better Care of Themselves. *ElectronicHealthcare, 8*(5), 110–113.

Fox, S., Rainie, L., & Horrigan, J. (2000). The online health care revolution: How the web helps Americans take better care of themselves. *Pew Internet and American Life Project, 91*, 235–245.

Frampton, S., & Charmel, P. (2009). *Putting Patients First: Best Practices in Patient-Centered Care*. San Francisco: Jossey-Bass.

Frattasi, S., Fitzek, F., & Prasad, R. (2005). Cooperative Services for 4G. In *Proceedings of the 14th IST Mobile & Wireless Communications Summit*. European Association for Signal Processing (EURASIP).

Fuchs, N. E. E., Kaljurand, K., & Kuhn, T. (2008). *Discourse representation structures for ace 6.0*. Department of Informatics, University of Zurich. Retrieved from http://citeseerx.ist.psu.edu/viewdoc/download?doi=10.1.1.148.6989&rep=rep1&type=pdf

Fuchs, N. E., & Schneider, G. (2006). Attempto Controlled English Meets the Challenges of Knowledge Representation, Reasoning, Interoperability and User Interfaces. American Association for Artificial Intelligence.

Fulton, M. M., & Riley Allen, E. (2005). Polypharmacy in the elderly: A literature review. *Journal of the American Academy of Nurse Practitioners, 17*(4), 123–132. doi:10.1111/j.1041-2972.2005.0020.x PMID:15819637

Funke, J. (1991). Solving complex problems: Human identification and control of complex systems. In R. J. Sternberg & P. A. Frensch (Eds.), *Complex problem solving: Principles and mechanisms* (pp. 185–222). Hillsdale, NJ: Lawrence Erlbaum Associates.

Fu, X., Hogrefe, D., Narayanan, S., & Soltwisch, R. (2004). QoS and Security in 4G Networks. In *Proceedings of the 1st CIC/IEEE Global Mobile Congress (GMC 2004)* (pp. 117-122).

Gafni, R. (2009). Quality Metrics for PDA-based M-Learning Information Systems. *Interdisciplinary Journal of E-Learning and Learning Objects, 5*, 359–287.

Gagliardi, A. R., Brouwers, M. C., Palda, V. A., Lemieux-Charles, L., & Grimshaw, J. M. (2011). How can we improve guideline use? a conceptual framework of implementability. *Implementation Science; IS, 6*(1), 26. doi:10.1186/1748-5908-6-26 PMID:21426574

Gajanayake, R., Sahama, T., & Iannella, R. (2014). The role of perceived usefulness and attitude on electronic health record acceptance. *International Journal of E-Health and Medical Communications, 5*(4), 108–119. doi:10.4018/ijehmc.2014100107

Gani, A., Li, X., Yang, L., & Zakaria, O. (2008). Radio Frequency Combination for TCP/IP Suite Protocol Improvement in 4G Mobile Internet Networks. *International Journal of Communication*, *2*(1), 27–36.

Gans, D. N. (2016). Patient-centered care: A short-term investment for a long-term return. *MGMA Connexion*, *16*(2), 22–23. PMID:27049157

Garde, S., Knaup, P., Hovenga, E. J., & Heard, S. (2007). Towards Semantic Interoperability for Electronic Health Records--Domain Knowledge Governance for open EHR Archetypes. *Methods of Information in Medicine*, *46*(3), 332–343. PMID:17492120

Garzon, G., Gil, A., Alvaro, A., Rodrigo, R., Cerezo, M., & Dominguez, C. (2012). Relationship between process indicators measured using electronic records and intermediate health outcomes in patients with diabetes. *Revista de calidad asistencial: organo de la Sociedad Espanola de Calidad Asistencial, 28* (4), 207–216.

Gaston, C. M., & Mitchell, G. (2005). Information giving and decision-making in patients with advanced cancer: A systematic review. *Social Science & Medicine*, *61*(10), 2252–2264. doi:10.1016/j.socscimed.2005.04.015 PMID:15922501

Gawel, M., Szmidt-Salkowska, E., & Kowalski, J. (2009). The value of quantitative EEG in differential diagnosis of Alzheimer's disease subcortical vascular dementia. *Journal of the Neurological Sciences*, *283*(1-2), 127–133. doi:10.1016/j.jns.2009.02.332 PMID:19268969

Gehl, R. W. (2011). The archive and the processor: The internal logic of Web 2.0. *New Media & Society*, *13*(8), 1228–1244. doi:10.1177/1461444811401735

Geissler, H., Hasenbein, M., Kanatouri, S., & Wegener, R. (2014). E-Coaching: Conceptual and Empircal Findings of a Virtual Coaching Programme. *International Journal of Evidence Based Coaching and Mentoring*, *12*(2), 165–187.

Genetic Information Non-discrimination Act of 2008 (GINA). *Pub. L. 110-233*, 122 Stat. 883, codified as amended in scattered sections of 26, 29, and 42 U.S.C.

Ginsburg, L., Gilin, D., Tregunno, D., Norton, P. G., Flemons, W., & Fleming, M. (2009). Advancing measurement of patient safety culture. *Health Services Research*, *44*(1), 205–224. doi:10.1111/j.1475-6773.2008.00908.x PMID:18823446

Ginter, P. M., Swayne, L. E., & Duncan, W. J. (1998).Strategic management of health care organizations (3rd ed.). Malden, MA: Blackwell Publishers, Inc. Harper, P. (2005).Combining data mining tools with health care models for improved understanding of health processes and resourse utilization. Clinical and Investigative Medicine, 28(6), 338-341.

Glouberman, S., & Hayes, M. (1998). *Population Health, Sustainable Development and Policy Futures. A think piece for Health Canada*. Ottawa, Canada: Canadian Policy Research Networks.

Gonzales, R. C., & Woods, R. E. (1992). *Digital Image Processing*. Addison-Wisley.

González, G. G., Morales, D. R., Palomino, M. Á. R., Gómez, D. T., Barrera, V. H., & De Miguel, Á. G. (2012). Evaluación sobre historia clínica electrónica. asociación entre indicadores de proceso medidos sobre historia electrónica y resultados intermedios en salud, en pacientes con hipertensión. *Atencion Primaria*, *44*(12), 709–719. doi:10.1016/j.aprim.2012.06.004 PMID:22980946

Goodacre, S., Campbell, M., & Carter, A. (2013). What do hospital mortality rates tell us about quality of care? *Emergency Medicine Journal*, *2013*(Sep), 23. doi:10.1136/emermed-2013-203022 PMID:24064042

Gorini, S., Quirini, M., Menciassi, A., Pernorio, G., Stefanini, C., & Dario, P. (2006, February). A novel SMA-based actuator for a legged endoscopic capsule. In *Biomedical Robotics and Biomechatronics, 2006. BioRob 2006. The First IEEE/RAS-EMBS International Conference on* (pp. 443-449). IEEE. doi:10.1109/BIOROB.2006.1639128

Gostin, L. O., & Hodge, J. G. Jr. (1999). Genetic privacy and the law: An end to genetics exceptionalism. *Jurimetrics*, 21–58. PMID:12465649

Gostin, L. O., Turek-Brezina, J., Powers, M., Kozloff, R., Faden, R., & Steinauer, D. D. (1993). Privacy and security of personal information in a new health care system. *Journal of the American Medical Association*, *270*(20), 2487–2493. doi:10.1001/jama.1993.03510200093038 PMID:8192748

Gould, J. (2010). The role of regional collaboratives: The California Perinatal Quality Care Collaborative model. *Clinics in Perinatology*, *37*(1), 71–86. doi:10.1016/j.clp.2010.01.004 PMID:20363448

Governo, M., Riva, V., Fiorini, P., & Nugent, P. P. (2003). *MEDICATE Teleassistance System*. The 11th International Conference on Advance Robotics.

Grady, R. B. (1992). *Practical software metrics for project management and process improvement*. Prentice-Hall, Inc.

Grami, A., & Schell, B. H. (2004). Future Trends in Mobile Commerce: Service Offerings, Technological Advances and Security Challenges. In *Proceedings of the Second Annual Conference on Privacy, Security and Trust.*

Gray, J. A. M. (1996). *Evidence-based Healthcare*. Edinburgh, UK: Churchill Livingstone.

Greenhalgh, T., Procter, R., Wherton, J., Sugarhood, P., & Shaw, S. (2012). The organising vision for telehealth and telecare: Discourse analysis. *BMJ Open*, *2*(4), e001574. doi:10.1136/bmjopen-2012-001574 PMID:22815469

Griffith, T. L., Sawyer, J. E., & Neale, M. A. (2003). Virtualness and Knowledge in Teams: Managing the Love Triangle of Organizations, Individuals, and Information Technology. *Management Information Systems Quarterly*, *27*(2), 265–287.

Grimshaw, J., Eccles, M., Thomas, R., MacLennan, G., Ramsay, C., Fraser, C., & Vale, L. (2006). Toward evidence-based quality improvement. *Journal of General Internal Medicine*, *21*(S2), S14–S20. PMID:16637955

Grimson, J., Stephens, G., Jung, B., Grimson, W., Berry, D., & Pardon, S. (2001). Sharing health- care records over the internet. *IEEE Internet Computing*, *5*(3), 49–58. doi:10.1109/4236.935177

Grisso, T., & Appelbaum, P. S. (1998). *Assessing competence to consent to treatment: A guide for physicians and other health professionals*. Oxford University Press.

Grol, R. (2001). Improving the quality of medical care: Building bridges among professional pride, payor profit, and patient satisfaction. *Journal of the American Medical Association*, *286*(20), 2578–2585. doi:10.1001/jama.286.20.2578 PMID:11722272

Großkopf, S., Park, S. Y., & Kim, M. H. (1998). An improved Active Contour Model for Segmentation of Medical Images. *Proc.3rd Korea-Germany Joint Conference on Advanced Medical Image Processing.*

Gruber, T. R. (1993). A translation approach to portable ontology specifications. *Knowledge Acquisition*, *5*(2), 199–220. doi:10.1006/knac.1993.1008

Gruber, T. R. (1995). Toward principles for the design of ontologies used for knowledge sharing? *International Journal of Human-Computer Studies*, *43*(5), 907–928. doi:10.1006/ijhc.1995.1081

Gunter, T. D., & Terry, N. P. (2005). The emergence of national electronic health record architectures in the United States and Australia: Models, costs, and questions. *Journal of Medical Internet Research*, *7*(1), e3. doi:10.2196/jmir.7.1.e3 PMID:15829475

Gwyther, L. P. (2001). *Caring for People with Alzheimer's Disease: A Manual for Facility Staff.* Washington, DC: American Health Care Association.

Gymrek, M., McGuire, A. L., Golan, D., Halperin, E., & Erlich, Y. (2013). Identifying personal genomes by surname inference. *Science*, *339*(6117), 321–324. doi:10.1126/science.1229566 PMID:23329047

Hackworth, B. A., & Kunz, M. B. (2011). Healthcare and social media: Building relationship via social networks. Morehead State University. *Academy of Health Care Management Journal*, *7*(2), 34–45.

Haggerty, K., & Ericson, R. (2000). The surveillant assemblage. *The British Journal of Sociology*, *51*, 605–622. doi:10.1080/00071310020015280 PMID:11140886

Hall, D. E., Prochazka, A. V., & Fink, A. S. (2012). Informed consent for clinical treatment. *Canadian Medical Association Journal*, *184*(5), 533–540. doi:10.1503/cmaj.112120 PMID:22392947

Hallinan, D., & Friedewald, M. (2015). Open consent, biobanking and data protection law: can open consent be 'informed'under the forthcoming data protection regulation?. *Life Sciences, Society and Policy*, *11*(1), 1.

Hamilton, A., & Brady, R. (2012). Medical professional involvement in smartphone 'apps' in dermatology. *The British Journal of Dermatology*, *167*(1), 220–221. doi:10.1111/j.1365-2133.2012.10844.x PMID:22283748

Hamilton, N., & Bhatti, T. (1996). *Population Health Promotion: An Integrated Model of Population Health and Health Promotion*. Ottawa, Canada: Health Canada.

Haralick, R. M., & Shapiro, L. G. (1985). Image segmentation techniques. *Computer Vision Graphics and Image Processing*, *29*(1), 100–132. doi:10.1016/S0734-189X(85)90153-7

Haux, R. (2010). Medical informatics: Past, present, future. *International Journal of Medical Informatics*, *79*(9), 599–610. doi:10.1016/j.ijmedinf.2010.06.003 PMID:20615752

Haux, R., Howe, J., Marschollek, M., Plischke, M., & Wolf, K. (2008). Health-enabling technologies for pervasive health care: On services and ICT architecture paradigms. *Informatics for Health & Social Care*, *33*(2), 77–89. doi:10.1080/17538150802127140 PMID:18604752

Haycock-Stuart, E. A., & Neil, M. (2005). Evaluation study of a resource for developing education, audit and teamwork in primary care. *Primary Health Care Research and Development*, *6*(3), 251–268. doi:10.1191/1463423605pc249oa

Hayes, M., & Dunn, J. (1998). *Population Health in Canada: A Systematic Review*. Ottawa, Canada: Canadian Policy Research Networks.

Haykin, S. (1998). *Neural Networks*. Prentice Hall.

Haykin, S., & Veen, B. V. (2003). *Signals and Systems*. New York: John Wiley & Sons.

Head, A., & Eisenberg, M. (2011). How college students use the Web to conduct everyday life research. *First Monday*, *16*(4), 2. doi:10.5210/fm.v16i4.3484

Health Canada. (1996). *Towards a common Understanding: Clarifying the Core Concepts of Population Health - A Discussion*. Ottawa, Canada: Health Canada.

Health insurance portability and accountability act. U.S. department of health and human services. (2013). Retrieved February 20, 2014, from http://www.gpo.gov/fdsys/pkg/FR-2013-01-25/pdf/2013-01073.pdf

Heart, T., & Kalderon, E. (2013). Older adults: Are they ready to adopt health-related ICT? *International Journal of Medical Informatics*, *82*(11), e209–e231. doi:10.1016/j.ijmedinf.2011.03.002 PMID:21481631

Heath, M., & Appan, R. (2014). *Impact of information technology culture conflict on meaningful use of electronic health records system: A conceptual framework*. Academic Press.

He, L., & Zhao, C. (2008). 4G Technology Promote Mobile Learning for New Development. In *Proceedings of the 2008 International Symposium on Knowledge Acquisition and Modeling* (pp. 486-490). IEEE Computer Society. doi:10.1109/KAM.2008.151

Hendricks, C., Murdaugh, C., & Pender, N. (2006). The Adolescent Lifestyle Profile: Development and psychometric characteristics. *Journal of National Black Nurses' Association*, *17*(2), 1–5. PMID:17410753

Henry, M. R. (2003). The Bethesda System 2001: An update of new terminology for gynecologic cytology. *Clinics in Laboratory Medicine*, *23*(3), 585–603. doi:10.1016/S0272-2712(03)00053-2 PMID:14560530

Herold, R., & Beaver, K. (2004). *The practical guide to HIPAA privacy and security compliance*. CRC Press.

Herrero, R., Brinton, L. A., Reeves, W. C., Brenes, M. M., Tenorio, F., de Britton, R. C., & Rawls, W. E. et al. (1990). Sexual behavior, venereal diseases, hygiene practices, and invasive cervical cancer in a high-risk population. *Cancer*, *65*(2), 380–386. doi:10.1002/1097-0142(19900115)65:2<380::AID-CNCR2820650234>3.0.CO;2-9 PMID:2295062

Hewelt, M., & Kunde, A. (2014). *Integration of documentation task into medical treatment processes in the hospital*. Academic Press.

Hewitt, A., & Forte, A. (2006). *Crossing boundaries: Identity management and student/faculty relationships on the Facebook*. Poster presented at the ACM Special Interest Group on Computer-Supported Cooperative Work, Banff, Canada.

Hicks, L., O'Malley, A., Lieu, T., Keegan, T., McNeil, B., Guadagnoli, E., & Landon, B. (2010). Impact of health disparities collaboratives on racial/ethnic and insurance disparities in US community health centers. *Archives of Internal Medicine*, *170*(3), 279–286. doi:10.1001/archinternmed.2010.493 PMID:20142575

Higashino, T., Yamaguchi, H., Yasumoto, K., & Shimada, K. (2005). Toward Future Innovation of Mobile Communication Systems - Current Requirements for Research -. In *Proceedings of the 2nd International Conference on Mobile Computing and Ubiquitous Networking (ICMU 2005)*.

Higher Education. (2011). *Mental health issues among students to escalate*. Retrieved October 5, 2012, from http://www.theaustralian.com.au/higher-education/mental-health-issues-among-students-to-escalate/story-e6frgcjx-1226111953584

Hillestad, R., Bigelow, J., Bower, A., Girosi, F., Meili, R., Scoville, R., & Taylor, R. (2005). Can electronic medical record systems transform health care? Potential health benefits, savings, and costs. *Health Affairs*, *24*(5), 1103–1117. doi:10.1377/hlthaff.24.5.1103 PMID:16162551

Hillman, M. (2002). *Testimony before the Subcommittee on Health of the House Committee on Ways and Means, Hearing on Promoting Disease Management in Medicare*. Retrieved 10 June, 2015, from http://waysandmeans.house.gov/Legacy/health/107cong/4-16-02/4-16hill.htm

Hinds, P., & Bailey, D. (2003). Out of Sight, Out of Sync: Understanding Conflict in Distributed Teams. *Organization Science*, *14*(6), 615–632. doi:10.1287/orsc.14.6.615.24872

HIPAA Compliance Assistance. (2003). *Summary of the HIPAA privacy rule*. Office for Civil Rights. Retrieved February 20, 2014, from http://www.hhs.gov/ocr/privacy/hipaa/understanding/summary/privacysummary.pdf

Hirsch, F. (2007). *Le bégaiement Perturbation de l'organisation temporelle de la parole et conséquences spectrales*. (Ph.D dissertation). Marc Bloch Univ., Strasbourg.

Hitlin, P., & Rainie, L. (2005). Teens, technology, and school. *Pew Internet & American Life Project*, *93*, 124–201.

Hochman, N., & Schwartz, S. (2012). *Visualizing Instagram: Tracing Cultural Visual Rhythms AAAI Technical Report WS-12-03. Social Media Visualization.* Association for the Advancement of Artificial Intelligence. Retrieved June 11, 2012, from http://www.aaai.org/ocs/index.php/ICWSM/ICWSM12/paper/viewFile/4782/5091

Holder, A. R. (1987). Minors' rights to consent to medical care. *Journal of the American Medical Association, 257*(24), 3400–3402. doi:10.1001/jama.1987.03390240106033 PMID:3586272

Hong, J. W., & Leon-Garcia, A. (2005). Requirements for the Operations and Management of 4G Networks. In *Proceedings of the 19th International Telegraffic Congress* (pp. 981-990).

Horgan, A., & Sweeney, J. (2010). Young students' use of the Internet for mental health information and support. *ElectronicHealthcare, 17*(2), 117–123. PMID:20465756

Hovenga, E. J. (2010). *Health informatics: an overview* (Vol. 151). IOS Press.

Howe, R., & Spence, C. (2004). Population Health Management: Healthways PopWorks (Vol. 2). HCT Project. Retrieved from http://mthink.com/article/population-health-management-healthways-popworks/

Howell, P., & Au-Yeung, J. (2007). Phonetic complexity and stuttering in Spanish. *Clinical Linguistics & Phonetics, 21*(2), 111–127. doi:10.1080/02699200600709511 PMID:17364620

Howell, P., Au-Yeung, J., & Sackin, S. (2000). Internal Structure of Content Words Leading To Lifespan Differences in Phonological Difficulty in Stuttering. *Journal of Fluency Disorders, 25*(1), 1–20. doi:10.1016/S0094-730X(99)00025-X PMID:18259599

Howell, P., Au-Yeung, J., Yaruss, S., & Eldridge, K. (2006). Phonetic difficulty and stuttering in English. *Clinical Linguistics & Phonetics, 20*(9), 703–716. doi:10.1080/02699200500390990 PMID:17342878

Howell, P., Soukup-Ascencao, T., Davis, S., & Rusbridge, S. (2011). Comparison of alternative methods for obtaining severity scores of the speech of people who stutter. *Clinical Linguistics & Phonetics, 25*(5), 368–378. doi:10.3109/02699206.2010.538955 PMID:21434809

Hristova, L., & Hakama, M. (1997). Effect of screening for cancer in the Nordic countries on deaths, cost and quality of life up to the year 2017. *Acta Oncologica (Stockholm, Sweden), 36*(Suppl 9), 1–60. PMID:9143316

Huang, C.-Y., Yang, Y.-L., Tzeng, G.-H., Cheng, S.-T., & Lee, H.-Y. (2010). 4G Mobile phone consumer preference predictions by using the Rough Set Theory and flow graphs. In Proceedings of Technology Management for Global Economic Growth (PICMET'10) (pp. 1 - 10).

Huang, T. T., Harris, K. J., Lee, R. E., Nazir, N., Born, W., & Kaur, H. (2003). Assessing overweight, obesity, diet, and physical activity in college students. *Journal of American College Health, 52*(2), 83–86. doi:10.1080/07448480309595728 PMID:14765762

Hwang, J.-S., Consulta, R. R., & Yoon, H.-Y. (2007). 4G Mobile Networks–Technology Beyond 2.5G and 3G. In *Proceedings PTC'07.*

Hyppönen, H., Reponen, J., Lääveri, T., & Kaipio, J. (2014). User experiences with different regional health information exchange systems in Finland. *International Journal of Medical Informatics, 83*(1), 1–18. doi:10.1016/j.ijmedinf.2013.10.002 PMID:24200753

Iddan, G., Meron, G., Glukhovsky, A., & Swain, P. (2000). Wireless capsule endoscopy. *Nature, 405*(6785), 417. doi:10.1038/35013140 PMID:10839527

Iezzoni, L. I. (1996). Assessing quality using administrative data. *Annals of Internal Medicine*, *127*(8), 666–674. doi:10.7326/0003-4819-127-8_Part_2-199710151-00048 PMID:9382378

Institute of Medicine (U.S.). Committee for the Study of the Future of Public Health. (1988). The future of public health. Washington, DC: National Academy Press.

Institute of Medicine. (2001). *Crossing the Quality Chasm: A New Health System for the 21st Century*. Washington, DC: National Academy Press; doi:10.17226/10027

Institute of Medicine. (2001). *Crossing the Quality Chasm: A New Health System for the Twenty- first Century*. Washington, WA: National Academy Press.

Institute of Medicine. (2002). *The Future of the Public's Health in the 21st Century*. Washington, DC: National Academy Press.

Institute of Medicine. (2003). *Health Professions Education: A Bridge to Quality*. Washington, WA: National Academy Press.

Intuitive Surgical. (2002). *The da Vinci Surgical System*. Retrieved June 8, 2016, from http://www.intuitivesurgical.com/

Ioannidis, J. P. (2016). Evidence-Based Medicine Has Been Hijacked: A Report to David Sackett. *Journal of Clinical Epidemiology*, *73*, 82–86. doi:10.1016/j.jclinepi.2016.02.012 PMID:26934549

Iseki, F., & Baigalmaa, T. (1998). Extraction of 3D tree structure of blood vessels in lungs area from chest CT images. CARS 1998. Elsevier Science B.V.

Iseki, F., Kobatake, H., Omatsu, H., & Kakinuma, R. (1997). A new method to extract three dimensional tree structures of bronchus from chest CT images. *IEICE D-II*, J80-D-II, 10, 2841–2847. (in Japanese)

Ishikawa, K. (1976). *Guide to Quality Control*. Tokyo: Asian Productivity Organization.

ISO. (2003). *ISO 13485: Medical devices - Quality management systems - Requirements for regulatory purposes*. Geneva: International Organization for Standardization.

ISO. (2011). *ISO 25000: Systems and software engineering– Systems and software Quality Requirements and Evaluation (SQuaRE)–System and software quality models*. Geneva: International Organization for Standardization.

ISO. (2014). *ISO 25000: Systems and software engineering– Systems and software Quality Requirements and Evaluation (SQuaRE)–Guide to SQuaRE*. Geneva: International Organization for Standardization.

ISO/IEC. (1999). *ISO/IEC 14598-1: Information Technology, Software Product Evaluation*. Geneva: International Organization for Standardization.

ISO/IEC. (2001). *ISO/IEC, 9126: Software engineering–Product quality–Part 1: Quality model*. Geneva: International Organization for Standardization.

Istepanian, R., Laxminarayan, S., & Pattichis, C. (Eds.). (2006). *M-Health: Emerging Mobile Health Systems*. New York: Springer. doi:10.1007/b137697

Ivers, N. M., Grimshaw, J. M., Jamtvedt, G., Flottorp, S., O'Brien, M. A., French, S. D., & Odgaard-Jensen, J. et al. (2014). Growing literature, stagnant science? systematic review, meta-regression and cumulative analysis of audit and feedback interventions in health care. *Journal of General Internal Medicine*, *29*(11), 1534–1541. doi:10.1007/s11606-014-2913-y PMID:24965281

Ivers, N., Jamtvedt, G., Flottorp, S., Young, J. M., Odgaard-Jensen, J., French, S. D., & Oxman, A. D. et al. (2012). Audit and feedback: Effects on professional practice and healthcare outcomes. *The Cochrane Library*. PMID:22696318

Jackson, G., Powell, A., Ordin, D., Schlosser, J., Murawsky, J., Hersh, J., & Members, V. C. C. C. P. C. et al. (2010). Developing and sustaining quality improvement partnerships in the VA. *Journal of General Internal Medicine*, *25*(1), 38–43. doi:10.1007/s11606-009-1155-x PMID:20077150

Janevski, T. (2009). 5G Mobile Phone Concept. In *Proceedings of the 6th IEEE Consumer Communications and Networking Conference, 2009* (CCNC 2009). IEEE.

Jemal, A., Bray, F., Center, M. M., Ferlay, J., Ward, E., & Forman, D. (2011). Global cancer statistics. *CA: a Cancer Journal for Clinicians*, *61*(2), 69–90. doi:10.3322/caac.20107 PMID:21296855

Jeong, J. (2004). EEG dynamics in patients with Alzheimer's disease. *Clinical Neurophysiology*, *115*(7), 1490–1505. doi:10.1016/j.clinph.2004.01.001 PMID:15203050

Jha, V., Mclean, M., Gibbs, T. J., & Sandars, J. (2014). Medical professionalism across cultures: A challenge for medicine and medical education. *Medical Teacher*, *30*, 1–7. PMID:25073712

Jiao, Z., Wang, Z., Wang, G., Tian, H., Wu, H., & Wang, H. (2015). On the Granularity of Dialog Strategies: Insights from Large-scale Analyses of Two Commercial Travel Information Spoken Dialog Systems. In *AAAI 2015 Spring Symposium*.

Jimenez-Pernett, J., & Olry de Labry-Lima, A. (2010). Use of the internet as a source of health information by Spanish adolescents. *BMC Medical Informatics and Decision Making*, *10*(1), 6. doi:10.1186/1472-6947-10-6 PMID:20113486

Johansen, M., Pedersen, Å., & Ellingsen, G. (2015). The role of medical transcriptionists in producing high-quality documentation. *Studies in Health Technology and Informatics*, *218*, 114. PMID:26262537

Johnson, S. (2014). "Maternal devices", social media and the self-management of pregnancy, mothering and child health. *Societies*, *4*(2), 330–350. doi:10.3390/soc4020330

Johnson, W. (1963). *Diagnostic Methods in Speech Pathology*. New York: Herper & Row.

Johnson-Yale, S., Millermaier, S., & Seoane Perez, F. (2009). Everyday life, online: U.S. college students' use of the Internet. *First Monday*, *14*(10), 1.

Johnstone, P. A., Crenshaw, T., Cassels, D. G., & Fox, T. H. (2008). Automated data mining of a proprietary database system for physician quality improvement. *International Journal of Radiation Oncology, Biology, Physics*, *70*(5), 1537–1541. doi:10.1016/j.ijrobp.2007.08.056 PMID:18037576

Johnston, G., Crombie, I. K., Davies, H. T. O., Alder, E. M., & Millard, A. (2000). Reviewing audit: Barriers and facilitating factors for effective clinical audit. *Quality in Health Care*, *9*(1), 23–36. doi:10.1136/qhc.9.1.23 PMID:10848367

Jones, S., Johnson-Yale, C., Millermaier, S., & Seoane Perez, F. (2009). Everyday life, online: U.S. college students' use of the Internet. *First Monday*, *14*(10), 5. doi:10.5210/fm.v14i10.2649

Jonker, C., Launer, L., Hooijer, C., & Lindeboom, J. (1996). Memory complaints and memory impairment in older individuals. *Journal of the American Geriatrics Society*, *44*(1), 44–49. doi:10.1111/j.1532-5415.1996.tb05636.x PMID:8537589

Juste, F. S., Rondon, S., Sassi, F. C., Ritto, A. P., Colalto, C. A., & Andrade, C. R. (2012). Acoustic analyses of diadochokinesis in fluent and stuttering children. *Clinics (Sao Paulo)*, *67*(5), 409–414. doi:10.6061/clinics/2012(05)01 PMID:22666781

Kaiser, G. (1994). *A friendly guide to Wavelets*. Birkhäuser Verlag AG.

Kaljurand, K., & Fuchs, N. E. (2007). *Verbalizing OWL in Attempto Controlled English* (Vol. 258). OWLED.

Kalloo, A. N., Singh, V. K., Jagannath, S. B., Niiyama, H., Hill, S. L., Vaughn, C. A., & Kantsevoy, S. V. et al. (2004). Flexible transgastric peritoneoscopy: A novel approach to diagnostic and therapeutic interventions in the peritoneal cavity. *Gastrointestinal Endoscopy*, *60*(1), 114–117. doi:10.1016/S0016-5107(04)01309-4 PMID:15229442

Kamel Boulos, M. N., & Wheeler, S. (2007). The emerging Web 2.0 social software: An enabling suite of sociable technologies in health and health care education. *Health Information and Libraries Journal*, *24*(1), 2–23. doi:10.1111/j.1471-1842.2007.00701.x PMID:17331140

Karakitsos, P., Chrelias, C., Pouliakis, A., Koliopoulos, G., Spathis, A., Kyrgiou, M., & Paraskevaidis, E. et al. (2012). Identification of women for referral to colposcopy by neural networks: A preliminary study based on LBC and molecular biomarkers. *Journal of Biomedicine & Biotechnology*, *303192*. doi:10.1155/2012/303192 PMID:23093840

Karakitsos, P., Pouliakis, A., Meristoudis, C., Margari, N., Kassanos, D., Kyrgiou, M., & Paraskevaidis, E. et al. (2011). A preliminary study of the potential of tree classifiers in triage of high-grade squamous intraepithelial lesions. *Analytical and Quantitative Cytology and Histology*, *33*(3), 132–140. PMID:21980616

Karangelis, G. (2004). *3D simulation of external beam radiotherapy*. (Ph.D. thesis). University of Darmstadt, Darmstadt, Germany.

Karangelis, G., & Zimeras, S. (2002). An Accurate 3D Segmentation Method of the Spinal Canal Applied on CT Images. BVM 2002, Confedrence Proceedings, Bildverarbeitung für die Medizin 2002. Springer-Verlag.

Karangelis, G., and Zimeras, S. (2002). 3D segmentation method of the spinal cord applied on CT data. *Computer Graphics Topics, 14,* 28-29.

Kass, M., Witkin, A., & Terzopoulos, D. (1987). Snakes: Active contour models. *International Journal of Computer Vision*, *1*(4), 321–331. doi:10.1007/BF00133570

Kastania, A. N. (2010). Evaluation considerations for e-health systems. In A. Moumtzoglou & A. Kastania (Eds.), *E-Health Systems Quality and Reliability: Models and Standards*. Hershey, PA: IGI Global.

Kaye, J., Heeney, C., Hawkins, N., De Vries, J., & Boddington, P. (2009). Data sharing in genomics—re-shaping scientific practice. *Nature Reviews. Genetics*, *10*(5), 331–335. doi:10.1038/nrg2573 PMID:19308065

Kazakov, Y., Krötzsch, M. R., & Simančík, F. (2013). The Incredible ELK. *Journal of Automated Reasoning*, *53*(1), 1–61. doi:10.1007/s10817-013-9296-3

Kazandjian, V. A. (2014). Not Just Meaningful Data but Coordinated Data! Can Cloud Computing Promote Down-to-Earth E-Valuation of Disease and Healthcare? In Cloud Computing Applications for Quality Health Care Delivery. Hershey, PA: IGI Global. doi:10.4018/978-1-4666-6118-9.ch002

Kazandjian, V. A. (1996). The contribution of epidemiology to CQI: A commentary. *International Journal for Quality in Health Care*, *8*(4), 351–357. doi:10.1093/intqhc/8.4.351 PMID:8938496

Kazandjian, V. A. (1997). Genetic polymorphisms and breast cancer risk. *Journal of the American Medical Association*, *277*(7), 533. doi:10.1001/jama.1997.03540310031027 PMID:9032157

Kazandjian, V. A. (1999). Power to the people: Taking the assessment of physician performance outside the profession. *Canadian Medical Association Journal*, *161*(1), 44–45. PMID:10420865

Kazandjian, V. A. (2002). *Accountability through measurement: A global healthcare imperative*. Milwaukee, WI: ASQ Quality Press.

Kazandjian, V. A., Durance, P. W., & Schork, M. A. (1989). The extremal quotient in small-area variation analysis. *Health Services Research*, *124*(5), 665–684. PMID:2584039

Kazandjian, V. A., & Lied, T. R. (1999). *Healthcare Performance Measurement: Systems Design and Evaluation*. Milwaukee, WI: ASQ Quality Press.

Kazandjian, V. A., Wicker, K., Ogunbo, S., & Silverman, N. (2005). Understanding safer practices in health care: A prologue for the role of indicators. *Journal of Evaluation in Clinical Practice*, *11*(2), 161–170. doi:10.1111/j.1365-2753.2005.00516.x PMID:15813713

Kehoe, B., Kahn, G., Mahler, J., Kim, J. H., Lee, A., Nakagawa, K., . . . Goldberg, K. (2014, May). Autonomous multilateral debridement with the raven surgical robot. In *Robotics and Automation (ICRA), 2014 IEEE International Conference on* (pp. 1432-1439). IEEE. doi:10.1109/ICRA.2014.6907040

Kennedy, R. F. Jr. (2005). *"The Disinformation Society," Crimes Against Nature*. New York: Harper Perennial.

Kenneth, B. (2005). *Internet Enhances Patient Education*. U.S Publications. Retrieved from http:www.uspharmacist.com/oldformat.asp

Kerath, S. M., Klein, G., Kern, M., Shapira, I., Witthuhn, J., Norohna, N., & Taioli, E. et al. (2013). Beliefs and attitudes towards participating in genetic research–a population based cross-sectional study. *BMC Public Health*, *13*(1), 1. doi:10.1186/1471-2458-13-114 PMID:23388465

Khoury, M. J., & Dorman, J. S. (1998). The human genome epidemiology network. *American Journal of Epidemiology*, *148*(1), 1–3. doi:10.1093/aje/148.1.1 PMID:9663396

Kiefe, C. I., Allison, J. J., Williams, O. D., Person, S. D., Weaver, M. T., & Weissman, N. W. (2001). Improving quality improvement using achievable benchmarks for physician feedback. A randomized controlled trial. *Journal of the American Medical Association*, *285*(22), 2871–2879. doi:10.1001/jama.285.22.2871 PMID:11401608

Kilbridge, P. (2002). *Crossing the Chasm with Information Technology: Bridging the Quality Gap in Health Care*. CA: California HealthCare Foundation.

Kilo, C. M. (1998). A Framework for Collaborative Improvement: Lessons from the Institute for Healthcare Imrpovements Breakthrough Series. *Quality Management in Health Care*, *6*(4), 1–13. doi:10.1097/00019514-199806040-00001 PMID:10339040

Kim, B., Lee, S., Park, J. H., & Park, J. O. (2004, August). Inchworm-like microrobot for capsule endoscope. In *Robotics and Biomimetics, 2004. ROBIO 2004. IEEE International Conference on* (pp. 458-463). IEEE.

Kim, B., Lee, S., Park, J. H., & Park, J. O. (2005). Design and fabrication of a locomotive mechanism for capsule-type endoscopes using shape memory alloys (SMAs). *Mechatronics, IEEE/ASME Transactions on*, *10*(1), 77-86.

Kim, B., Park, S., & Park, J. O. (2009, July). Microrobots for a capsule endoscope. In *Advanced Intelligent Mechatronics, 2009. AIM 2009. IEEE/ASME International Conference on* (pp. 729-734). IEEE. doi:10.1109/AIM.2009.5229926

Kim, B., Park, S., Jee, C. Y., & Yoon, S. J. (2005, August). An earthworm-like locomotive mechanism for capsule endoscopes. In *Intelligent Robots and Systems, 2005. (IROS 2005). 2005 IEEE/RSJ International Conference on* (pp. 2997-3002). IEEE.

Kim, J., Gu, G. M., & Heo, P. (2016). Robotics for Healthcare. In Biomedical Engineering: Frontier Research and Converging Technologies (pp. 489-509). Springer International Publishing. doi:10.1007/978-3-319-21813-7_21

Kim, L., Tang, S. C., & Yoo, S. S. (2013, October). Prototype modular capsule robots for capsule endoscopies. In *Control, Automation and Systems (ICCAS), 2013 13th International Conference on* (pp. 350-354). IEEE. doi:10.1109/ICCAS.2013.6703922

Kindig, D. A. (2007). Understanding population health terminology. *The Milbank Quarterly, 85*(1), 139–161. doi:10.1111/j.1468-0009.2007.00479.x PMID:17319809

Kitchener, H., Canfell, K., Gilham, C., Sargent, A., Roberts, C., Desai, M., & Peto, J. (2014). The clinical effectiveness and cost-effectiveness of primary human papillomavirus cervical screening in England: Extended follow-up of the ARTISTIC randomised trial cohort through three screening rounds. *Health Technology Assessment, 18*(23), 1–196. doi:10.3310/hta18230 PMID:24762804

Knoppers, B. M. (2005). Consent revisited: Points to consider. *Health Law Review, 13*(2-3), 33–38. PMID:16459412

Kohn, L. T., Corrigan, J. M., & Donaldaon, M. S. (2000). *To err is human: building a safer health system.* Washington, DC: National Academy Press.

Kohn, L. T., Corrigan, J. M., & Donaldson, M. S. (Eds.). (1999). *To Err Is Human: Building a Safer Health System.* Washington, DC: National Academy Press. doi:10.17226/9728

Kohonen, T. (2001). *Self-Organizing Maps.* New York: Springer. doi:10.1007/978-3-642-56927-2

Komoto, S., Nishiwaki, Y., Okamura, T., Tanaka, H., & Takebayashi, T. (2014). Effect size and cost-effectiveness estimates of breast and cervical cancer screening reminders by population size through complete enumeration of Japanese local municipalities. *BMC Public Health, 14*(1), 43. doi:10.1186/1471-2458-14-43 PMID:24433346

Korp, P. (2006). Health on the Internet: Implications for health promotion. *Health Education Research, 21*(1), 78–86. doi:10.1093/her/cyh043 PMID:15994845

Kósa, G., Jakab, P., Hata, N., Jólesz, F., Neubach, Z., Shoham, M., . . . Székely, G. (2008, October). Flagellar swimming for medical micro robots: theory, experiments and application. In *Biomedical Robotics and Biomechatronics, 2008. BioRob 2008. 2nd IEEE RAS & EMBS International Conference on* (pp. 258-263). IEEE. doi:10.1109/BIOROB.2008.4762812

Kósa, G., Shoham, M., & Zaaroor, M. (2007). Propulsion method for swimming microrobots. *Robotics. IEEE Transactions on, 23*(1), 137–150.

Koshiol, J., Lindsay, L., Pimenta, J. M., Poole, C., Jenkins, D., & Smith, J. S. (2008). Persistent human papillomavirus infection and cervical neoplasia: A systematic review and meta-analysis. *American Journal of Epidemiology, 168*(2), 123–137. doi:10.1093/aje/kwn036 PMID:18483125

Kozar-Westman, M., Troutman-Jordan, M., & Nies, M. A. (2013). Successful aging among assisted living community older adults. *Journal ofNursing Scholarship, 45*(3), 238–46. http://doi.org/<ALIGNMENT.qj></ALIGNMENT>10.1111/jnu.12027

KPMG. (2013). *KPMG Health Governace study.* Retrieved June 6, 2016 from https://www.kpmg.com/CN/en/IssuesAndInsights/ArticlesPublications/Documents/Global-perspectives-on-clinical-governance-o-201310.pdf

Kraut, R., Galegher, J., & Egido, C. (1987). Relationships and Tasks in Scientific Research Collaboration. *Human-Computer Interaction, 3*(1), 31–58. doi:10.1207/s15327051hci0301_3

Kuperman, G. J., Bobb, A., Payne, T. H., Avery, A. J., Gandhi, T. K., Burns, G., & Bates, D. W. et al. (2007). Medication related clinical decision support in computerized provider order entry systems: A Review. *Journal of the American Medical Informatics Association, 14*(1), 29–40. doi:10.1197/jamia.M2170 PMID:17068355

Kyrgiou, M., Pouliakis, A., Panayiotides, J. G., Margari, N., Bountris, P., Valasoulis, G., & Paraskevaidis, E. et al. (2016). Personalised management of women with cervical abnormalities using a clinical decision support scoring system. *Gynecologic Oncology, 141*(1), 29–35. doi:10.1016/j.ygyno.2015.12.032 PMID:27016226

Ladhani, Z., Stevens, F. J., & Scherpbier, A. J. (2014). Does community health care require different competencies from physicians and nurses? *BMC Medical Education, 14*(1), 1. doi:10.1186/1472-6920-14-1 PMID:24387322

Lahiri, D. K., Farlow, M. R., Greig, N. H., & Sambamurti, K. (2002). Current drug targets for Alzheimer's disease treatment. *Drug Development Research, 56*(3), 267–281. doi:10.1002/ddr.10081

Lalonde, M. (1974). *A New Perspective on the Health of Canadians. A Working Document.* Ottawa, Canada: Minister of Supply and Services Canada.

Lampe, C., Ellison, N., & Steinfield, C. (2007). A familiar face(book): Profile elements as signals in an online social network.*Proceedings of the SIGCHI conference on human factors in computing systems* (pp. 435–444). New York: ACM. doi:10.1145/1240624.1240695

Landsberg, B., Plachta-Danielzik, S., Lange, D., Johannsen, M., Seiberl, J., & Müller, M. J. (2010). Clustering of lifestyle factors and association with overweight in adolescents of the Kiel Obesity Prevention Study. *Public Health Nutrition, 13*(10A), 1708–1715. doi:10.1017/S1368980010002260 PMID:20883570

Lash, S. (2007). Power after hegemony: Cultural studies in mutation? *Theory, Culture & Society, 24*(3), 55–78. doi:10.1177/0263276407075956

Laska, M. N., Pasch, K. E., Lust, K., Story, M., & Ehlinger, E. (2009). Latent Class Analysis of Lifestyle Characteristics and Health Risk Behaviors among College Youth. *Preventative Science, 5*, 12. PMID:19499339

Latour, B. (2005). *Reassembling the Social: An Introduction to Actor-Network-Theory.* Oxford, UK: Clarendon.

LaTour, K. M., & Eichenwald, S. (2006). *Health information management: Concepts, principles, and practice.* Ahima.

Law, A. V., Ray, M. D., Knapp, K. K., & Balesh, K. K. (2003). Unmet needs in medication use process: Perceptions of physician, pharmacists, and patients. *Journal of the American Pharmaceutical Association, 43*(3), 394–402. doi:10.1331/154434503321831111 PMID:12836790

Lawrence, M., & Packwood, T. (1996). Adapting total quality management for general practice: Evaluation of a programme. *Quality in Health Care, 5*(3), 151–158. doi:10.1136/qshc.5.3.151 PMID:10161529

Lehman, A. C., Rentschler, M. E., Farritor, S. M., & Oleynikov, D. (2007). The current state of miniature in vivo laparoscopic robotics. *Journal of Robotic Surgery, 1*(1), 45–49. doi:10.1007/s11701-007-0019-9 PMID:25484938

Lenaghan, S. C., Wang, Y., Xi, N., Fukuda, T., Tarn, T., Hamel, W. R., & Zhang, M. (2013). Grand challenges in bioengineered nanorobotics for cancer therapy. *Biomedical Engineering. IEEE Transactions on, 60*(3), 667–673.

Lesko, L. J. (2007). Personalized Medicine: Elusive Dream or Imminent Reality? *Clinical Pharmacology and Therapeutics, 81*(6), 807–816. doi:10.1038/sj.clpt.6100204 PMID:17505496

Li, W., Guo, W., Li, M., & Zhu, Y. (2006, June). A novel locomotion principle for endoscopic robot. In *Mechatronics and Automation,Proceedings of the 2006 IEEE International Conference on* (pp. 1658-1662). IEEE. doi:10.1109/ICMA.2006.257445

Liao, S. M. (2009). Is there a duty to share genetic information? *Journal of Medical Ethics, 35*(5), 306–309. doi:10.1136/jme.2008.027029 PMID:19407036

Lien, G. S., Liu, C. W., Jiang, J. A., Chuang, C. L., & Teng, M. T. (2012). Magnetic control system targeted for capsule endoscopic operations in the stomach—design, fabrication, and in vitro and ex vivo evaluations. *Biomedical Engineering. IEEE Transactions, 59*(7), 2068–2079.

Li, M., Yu, S., Zheng, Y., Ren, K., & Lou, W. (2013). Scalable and secure sharing of personal health records in cloud computing using attribute-based encryption. Parallel and Distributed Systems. *IEEE Transactions on Parallel and Distributed Systems, 24*(1), 131–143. doi:10.1109/TPDS.2012.97

Lin, P., Funk, T., Curwen, M., & Maucherat, R. (2016). *So You Want High Performance*. Retrieved March 28, 2016, from http://tomcat.apache.org/articles/performance.pdf

Lindenauer, P. K. (2008). Effects of quality improvement collaboratives. *British Medical Journal, 336*(7659), 1448–1449. doi:10.1136/bmj.a216 PMID:18577558

Lin, N. (1999). Building a network theory of social capital. *Connections, 22*, 28–51.

Li, R., Lu, B., & McDonald-Maier, K. D. (2015). Cognitive assisted living ambient system: A survey. *Digital Communications and Networks, 1*(4), 229–252. doi:10.1016/j.dcan.2015.10.003

Lisby, M., Nielsen, L. P., & Mainz, J. (2005). Errors in the medication process: Frequency, type, and potential clinical consequences. *International Journal for Quality in Health Care, 17*(1), 15–22. doi:10.1093/intqhc/mzi015 PMID:15668306

Liu, K., Hogan, W. R., & Crowley, R. S. (2011). Natural Language Processing methods and systems for biomedical ontology learning. *Journal of Biomedical Informatics, 44*(1), 163–179. doi:10.1016/j.jbi.2010.07.006 PMID:20647054

Liu, Y., Yu, H., & Yang, T. C. (2008). Analysis and Control of a Capsubot. *City, 10*, 2.

Loader, B. D., Hardey, M., & Keeble, L. (2008). Health informatics for older people: A review of ICT facilitated integrated care for older people. *International Journal of Social Welfare, 17*(1), 46–53. doi:10.1111/j.1468-2397.2007.00489.x

Locatelli, P., Restifo, N., Gastaldi, L., & Corso, M. (2012). Health Care Information Systems: Architectural Models and Governance. In C. Kalloniatis (Ed.), *Innovative Information Systems Modelling and Techniques* (pp. 71–96). Rijeka, Croatia: InTech. doi:10.5772/38212

Lowery, R., Galuska, D. A., Fulton, J. E., Wechsler, H., Kann, L., & Collins, J. L. (2000). Physical activity, food choice, and weight management goals and practices among U.S. college students. *American Journal of Preventive Medicine, 18*, 8–27. PMID:10736536

Lunshof, J. E., Chadwick, R., Vorhaus, D. B., & Church, G. M. (2008). From genetic privacy to open consent. *Nature Reviews. Genetics, 9*(5), 406–411. doi:10.1038/nrg2360 PMID:18379574

Lupton, D. (2012). M-health and health promotion: The digital cyborg and surveillance society. *Social Theory & Health, 10*(3), 229–244. doi:10.1057/sth.2012.6

Lupton, D. (2013). The digitally engaged patient: Self-monitoring and self-care in the digital health era. *Social Theory & Health, 11*(3), 256–270. doi:10.1057/sth.2013.10

Lupton, D. (2014). Health promotion in the digital era: A critical commentary. *Health Promotion International*. doi:10.1093/heapro/dau091

MacDonald, J., & Martin, R. (1973). Stuttering and disfluency as two reliable and unambiguous response classes. *Journal of Speech and Hearing Research, 17*(4), 691–699. doi:10.1044/jshr.1604.691 PMID:4783809

Macedo, M., & Isaías, P. (2011). A methodology to develop a clinical ontology for healthcare business. *Human Interface and the Management of Information. Interacting with Information*, 285–291.

Machado, J. C. (2002). Doença de Alzheimer. In E. V. Freitas, L. Py, A. L. Neri, F. A. Cançado, M. L. Gorzoni, & S. M. Rocha (Eds.), Tratado de Geriatria e Gerontologia (pp. 133-147). Rio de Janeiro: Guanabara Koogan.

Madden, M., & Zickuhr, K. (2011). *65% of online adults use social networking sites.* Washington, DC: Pew Internet and American Life Project, Pew Research Centre. Retrieved March 8, 2012, from http://www.pewinternet.org/~/media//Files/Reports/2011/PIP-SNS-Update-2011.pdf

Malhotra, A., & Majchrzak, A. (2014). Enhancing Performance of Geographically Distributed Teams Through Targeted Use of Information and Communication Technologies. *Human Relations*, *67*(4), 398–411. doi:10.1177/0018726713495284

Malik, A. I. (2005). The role of human papilloma virus (HPV) in the aetiology of cervical cancer. *JPMA. The Journal of the Pakistan Medical Association*, *55*(12), 553–558. PMID:16438278

Malik, J., Belongie, S., Leung, T., & Shi, J. (2001). Contour and texture analysis for image segmentation. *International Journal of Computer Vision*, *43*(1), 7–27. doi:10.1023/A:1011174803800

Malone, R. E. (2003). Distal nursing. *Social Science & Medicine*, *56*, 2317–2326.

Marcus, H., Nandi, D., Darzi, A., & Yang, G. Z. (2013). Surgical robotics through a keyhole: From today's translational barriers to tomorrow's "disappearing" robots. *Biomedical Engineering. IEEE Transactions on*, *60*(3), 674–681.

Marescaux, J., Dallemagne, B., Perretta, S., Wattiez, A., Mutter, D., & Coumaros, D. (2007). Surgery without scars: Report of transluminal cholecystectomy in a human being. *Archives of Surgery (Chicago, Ill.)*, *142*(9), 823–826. doi:10.1001/archsurg.142.9.823 PMID:17875836

Marshall, M. N., Shekelle, P. G., McGlynn, E. A., Campbell, S., Brook, R. H., & Roland, M. O. (2003). Can health care quality indicators be transferred between countries? *Quality & Safety in Health Care*, *12*(1), 8–12. doi:10.1136/qhc.12.1.8 PMID:12571338

Martin, R. R., Kuhl, P., & Haroldson, S. K. (1972). An experimental treatment with two preschool stuttering children. *Journal of Speech and Hearing Research*, *15*(4), 743–752. doi:10.1044/jshr.1504.743 PMID:4652394

Martin, R., & Haroldson, S. (1981). Stuttering identification: Standard definition and moment of stuttering. *Journal of Speech and Hearing Research*, *24*(1), 59–63. doi:10.1044/jshr.2401.59 PMID:7253630

Mascalzoni, D., Hicks, A., Pramstaller, P., & Wjst, M. (2008). Informed consent in the genomics era. *PLoS Medicine*, *5*(9), e192. doi:10.1371/journal.pmed.0050192 PMID:18798689

Massad, L. S. (2003). Guidelines for cervical cancer screening from the american cancer society: The Earth is moving. *Journal of Lower Genital Tract Disease*, *7*(2), 87–88. doi:10.1097/00128360-200304000-00002 PMID:17051050

Matos, E. E., Campos, F., Braga, R., & Palazzi, D. (2010). CelOWS: An ontology based framework for the provision of semantic web services related to biological models. *Journal of Biomedical Informatics*, *43*(1), 125–136. doi:10.1016/j.jbi.2009.08.008 PMID:19695346

Mattson, M. P. (2004). Pathways Towards and Away from Alzheimer's Disease. *Nature*, *430*(7000), 631–639. doi:10.1038/nature02621 PMID:15295589

Mavroidis, C., & Ferreira, A. (Eds.). (2013). *Nanorobotics: current approaches and techniques*. Springer Science & Business Media. doi:10.1007/978-1-4614-2119-1

McAulay, R., & Quatieri, T. (1986). Speech Analysis/Synthesis Based on a Sinusoidal Representation. *IEEE Transactions on Acoustics Speech, and Signal Processing, 34*(4).

McCall, J. A., Richards, P. K., & Walters, G. F. (1977). *Factors in software quality. Concept and definitions of software quality: final technical report*. Springfield: National Technical Information Service (NTIS), Report nr. RADC-TR-77-369 (I, II and III).

McCance, D. J. (1988). Human papillomavirus (HPV) infections in the aetiology of cervical cancer. *Cancer Surveys*, *7*(3), 499–506. PMID:2854000

McCarthy, D., Schoen, C., & Radley, D. (2014). State health system performance: A scorecard. *Journal of the American Medical Association*, *312*(2), 131–132. doi:10.1001/jama.2014.5374 PMID:24788783

McCartney, M. (2013). How do we know whether medical apps work? *BMJ (Clinical Research Ed.)*. doi:10.1136/bmj.f1811 PMID:23516158

McClean, M. D., & Tasko, S. M. (2004). Correlation of orofacial speeds with voice acoustic measures in the fluent speech of persons who stutter. *Experimental Brain Research*, *159*(3), 310–318. doi:10.1007/s00221-004-1952-8 PMID:15248043

McGlynn, E. A., & Asche, S. M. (1998). Developing a clinical performance measure. *American Journal of Preventive Medicine*, *14*(3), 14–21. doi:10.1016/S0749-3797(97)00032-9 PMID:9566932

McGrail, K., Ostry, A., & Thomas, V. (1998). *Determinants of Population Health: A Synthesis of the literature*. Paper prepared for the National Research and Development Program, Ottawa, Canada.

McGuire, A. L., & Beskow, L. M. (2010). Informed consent in genomics and genetic research. *Annual Review of Genomics and Human Genetics*, *11*(1), 361–381. doi:10.1146/annurev-genom-082509-141711 PMID:20477535

McKinney, M. (2013). Partway across the quality chasm: Providers improve performance, but good measurement still lacking. *Mod Healthc, 43*(22), 6-7.

Memon, M., Wagner, S., Pedersen, C., Beevi, F., & Hansen, F. (2014). Ambient Assisted Living Healthcare Frameworks, Platforms, Standards, and Quality Attributes. *Sensors (Basel, Switzerland)*, *14*(3), 4312–4341. doi:10.3390/s140304312 PMID:24599192

Menciassi, A., Valdastri, P., Quaglia, C., Buselli, E., & Dario, P. (2009, September). Wireless steering mechanism with magnetic actuation for an endoscopic capsule. In *Engineering in Medicine and Biology Society, 2009. EMBC 2009. Annual International Conference of the IEEE* (pp. 1204-1207). IEEE. doi:10.1109/IEMBS.2009.5332426

Mendes, D., Rodrigues, I. P., & Baeta, C. F. (2013). Enrichment/Population of customized CPR (Computer-based Patient Record) ontology from free-text reports for CSI (Computer Semantic Interoperability). *International Journal of E-Health and Medical Communications*. Retrieved from http://www.ejhi.net/ojs/index.php/ejhi/article/view/194

Mendes, D. J. M., Rodrigues, I. P., Baeta, C. F., & Solano-Rodriguez, C. (2015). Extended Clinical Discourse Representation Structure for Controlled Natural Language Clinical Decision Support Systems. *International Journal of Reliable and Quality E-Healthcare*, *4*(2), 1–11. doi:10.4018/IJRQEH.2015040101

Mercieca, C., Cassar, S., & Borg, A. A. (2014). Listening to patients: Improving the outpatient service. *International Journal of Health Care Quality Assurance*, *27*(1), 44–53. doi:10.1108/IJHCQA-03-2012-0033 PMID:24660517

Merker, J. (2014). *Establishing a clinical genomics program at an academic medical center*. Regional APC/PDAS Meeting, Kauuai.

Merlino, J. I., & Raman, A. (2013). Health care's service fanatics. *Harvard Business Review*, *91*(5), 108–116, 150. PMID:23898737

Mesulam, M. M. (2000). Aging Alzheimer Disease and Dementia. *Principies of Behavioural and Cognitive Neurology*, 439-522.

Meystre, S. M., Savova, G. K., Kipper-Schuler, K. C., & Hurdle, J. F. (2008). Extracting information from textual documents in the electronic health record: A review of recent research. *Yearbook of Medical Informatics*, 128–144. Retrieved from http://www.ncbi.nlm.nih.gov/pubmed/18660887 PMID:18660887

Milne, R., & Clarke, A. (1990). Can readmission rates be used as an outcome indicator? *BMJ (Clinical Research Ed.)*, *301*(6761), 1139–1140. doi:10.1136/bmj.301.6761.1139 PMID:2252926

MIM Software Inc. (2011). Retrieved from www.mimsoftware.com

Minkoff, H. (2012). Fear of litigation and cesarean section rates. *Seminars in Perinatology*, *36*(5), 390–394. doi:10.1053/j.semperi.2012.04.025 PMID:23009974

Misra, D. P., Guyer, B., & Allston, A. (2003). Integrated perinatal health framework. A multiple determinants model with a life span approach. *American Journal of Preventive Medicine*, *25*(1), 65–75. doi:10.1016/S0749-3797(03)00090-4 PMID:12818312

Mitra, A., Willyard, J., Platt, C., & Parson, M. (2005). Exploring Web usage and selection criteria among male and female students. *Journal of Computer-Mediated Communication*, *10*(3), 10.

MobiSante. (2011). Retrieved from http://mobisante.com/

Mölsä, P. M. (1986). Survival and cause of death in Alzheimer's disease and multi-infarct dementia. *Acta Neurologica Scandinavica*, *7*, 74–103. PMID:3776457

Monge, P., & Contractor, N. (2003). *Theories of Communication Networks*. New York, NY: Oxford Univ.

Monge, P., & Eisenberg, E. (1990). Communication Networks and New Media in Organizations. In J. Fulk & C. Steinfield (Eds.), *Organizations and Communication Technology* (pp. 143–172). Thousand Oaks, CA: Sage.

Monsonego, J., Hudgens, M. G., Zerat, L., Zerat, J. C., Syrjanen, K., & Smith, J. S. (2012). Risk assessment and clinical impact of liquid-based cytology, oncogenic human papillomavirus (HPV) DNA and mRNA testing in primary cervical cancer screening (the FASE study). *Gynecologic Oncology*, *125*(1), 175–180. doi:10.1016/j.ygyno.2012.01.002 PMID:22233689

Montfort, A.P.W.P. & Helm, M.H.J. (2006). Telemonitoring of Patients with Chronic Heart Failure. *Disease Management & Health Outcomes*, *14*(1), 33–35.

Mori, K., Hasegawa, J., Toriwaki, J., Anno, H., & Katada, K. (1995). Automated extraction and visualization of bronchus from 3D CT images of lung. *Proc. of 1st International Conference on Computer Vision, Virtual Reality and Robotics in Medicine (CVRMed'95)*. doi:10.1007/978-3-540-49197-2_71

Mosemghvdlishvili, L., & Jansz, J. (2012). Negotiability of technology and its limitations. *Information Communication and Society*, *16*(10), 1596–1618. doi:10.1080/1369118X.2012.735252

Moses, H., Matheson, D. H., Dorsey, E. R., George, B. P., Sadoff, D., & Yoshimura, S. (2013). The anatomy of health care in the United States. *Journal of the American Medical Association*, *310*(18), 1947–1963. doi:10.1001/jama.2013.281425 PMID:24219951

Moumtzoglou, A. (2010). E-health as the realm of Healthcare Quality: A mental image of the future. In A. Moumtzoglou & A. Kastania (Eds.), *E-Health Systems Quality and Reliability: Models and Standards*. Hershey, PA: IGI Global.

Moumtzoglou, A., & Pouliakis, A. (2015). Mapping Population Health Management Roadmap into Cervical Cancer Screening Programs. *International Journal of Reliable and Quality E-Healthcare*, *4*(3), 1–18. doi:10.4018/IJRQEH.2015070101

Mowafey, S., & Gardner, S. (2013). Towards ambient intelligence in assisted living: The creation of an Intelligent Home Care. *Science and Information Conference*. Retrieved from http://ieeexplore.ieee.org/xpls/abs_all.jsp?arnumber=6661717

Mulholland, W. F. (1998). Genetic privacy and discrimination: A survey of state legislation. *Jurimetrics*, *39*, 317. PMID:11762444

Mulligan, H. F., Anderson, T. J., Jones, R. D., Williams, M. J., & Donaldson, I. M. (2003). Tics and developmental stuttering. *Parkinsonism & Related Disorders*, *9*(5), 281–289. doi:10.1016/S1353-8020(03)00002-6 PMID:12781595

Murphy, D., Challacombe, B., Nedas, T., Elhage, O., Althoefer, K., Seneviratne, L., & Dasgupta, P. (2007). Equipment and technology in robotics (in Spanish; Castilian). *Archivos Espanoles de Urologia*, *60*(4), 349–355. PMID:17626526

Murray, E., Burns, J., See Tai, S., Lai, R., & Nazareth, I. (2005). Interactive Health Communication Applications for people with chronic disease. *Cochrane Database of Systematic Reviews*, *CD004274*(4). doi:10.1002/14651858.CD004274.pub4 PMID:16235356

Nadeem, E., Olin, S., Hill, L., Hoagwood, K., & Horwitz, S.Understanding the Components of Quality Improvement Collaboratives. (2013, June). A Systematic Literature Review. *The Milbank Quarterly*, *91*(2), 354–394. doi:10.1111/milq.12016 PMID:23758514

Nagel, R. N., & Rosenfield, A. (1972). Ordered search techniques in template matching. *Proceedings of the IEEE*, *60*(2), 242–244. doi:10.1109/PROC.1972.8611

Nagy, Z., Fluckiger, M., Oung, R., Kaliakatsos, I. K., Hawkes, E. W., Nelson, B. J., & Abbott, J. J. et al. (2009). Assembling reconfigurable endoluminal surgical systems: Opportunities and challenges. *International Journal of Biomechatronics and Biomedical Robotics*, *1*(1), 3–16. doi:10.1504/IJBBR.2009.030054

Nardi, B. (2005). Beyond Bandwidth: Dimensions of Connection in Interpersonal Communication. *Computer Supported Cooperative Work*, *14*(2), 91–130. doi:10.1007/s10606-004-8127-9

Nardi, B., & Whittaker, S. (2002). The Place of Face-to-Face Communication in Distributed Work. In P. Hinds & S. Kiesler (Eds.), *Distributed Work* (pp. 83–110). Cambridge, MA: MIT Press.

National Conference of State Legislatures. (2008). *Genetic privacy laws.* Congressional Research Service. Retrieved March 2008 from http://www.ncsl.org/research/health/genetic-privacy-laws.aspx

Natphopsuk, S., Settheetham-Ishida, W., Sinawat, S., Pientong, C., Yuenyao, P., & Ishida, T. (2012). Risk factors for cervical cancer in northeastern Thailand: Detailed analyses of sexual and smoking behavior. *Asian Pacific Journal of Cancer Prevention*, *13*(11), 5489–5495. doi:10.7314/APJCP.2012.13.11.5489 PMID:23317205

Nayar, R., & Wilbur, D. (2015). *The Bethesda system for reporting cervical cytology: definitions, criteria, and explanatory notes* (2nd ed.). New York: Springer. doi:10.1007/978-3-319-11074-5

Nembhard, I. M. (2009). Learning and Improving in Quality Improvement Collaboratives: Which Collaborative Features Do Participants Value Most? *Health Services Research, 44*(2), 358-378.

Németh, A. H., Kwasniewska, A. C., Lise, S., Schnekenberg, R. P., Becker, E. B., Bera, K. D., & Talbot, K. et al. (2013). Next generation sequencing for molecular diagnosis of neurological disorders using ataxias as a model. *Brain*, awt236. PMID:24030952

Nestor, P., Scheltens, P., & Hodges, J. (2004). Advances in the early detection of Alzheimer's disease. *Nature Medicine*, *10*, 34–41. PMID:15298007

Netter, F. H. (1997). Atlas of human anatomy. In NOVARTIS (2nd ed.). PLATE.

Newton, P. J., Davidson, P. M., Halcomb, E. J., Denniss, A. R., & Westgarth, F. (2006). A Introduction to the Collaborative Methodology and Its Potential Use for Management of Heart Failure. *The Journal of Cardiovascular Nursing*, *21*(3), 161–168. doi:10.1097/00005082-200605000-00002 PMID:16699354

Nicol, E. D., Mohanna, K., & Cowpe, J. (2014). Perspectives on clinical leadership: A qualitative study exploring the views of senior healthcare leaders in the UK. *Journal of the Royal Society of Medicine*, *107*(7), 277–286. doi:10.1177/0141076814527274 PMID:25013095

Nielsen's Internet & Technology Report. (2010). Retrieved March 13, 2011, from http://www.emerchant.com.au/blog/nielsen%E2%80%99s-2010-internet-technology-report/

Nijland, N., Seydel, E. R., van Gemert-Pijnen, J. E. W. C., Brandenburg, B., Kelders, S. M., & Will, M. (2009). *Evaluation of an Internet-Based Application for Supporting Self-Care of Patients with Diabetes Mellitus Type 2*. Paper presented at the International Conference on eHealth, Telemedicine, and Social Medicine. doi:10.1109/eTELEMED.2009.33

Niruthisard, S., & Trisukosol, D. (1991). Male sexual behavior as risk factor in cervical cancer. *Journal of the Medical Association of Thailand*, *74*(11), 507–512. PMID:1800607

Nishisaki, A., Keren, R., & Nadkarni, V. (2007). Does Simulation Improve Patient Safety?: Self-Efficacy, Competence, Operational Performance, and Patient Safety. *Anesthesiology Clinics*, *25*(2), 225–236. doi:10.1016/j.anclin.2007.03.009 PMID:17574187

Noonan, D. P., Vitiello, V., Shang, J., Payne, C. J., & Yang, G. Z. (2011, September). A modular, mechatronic joint design for a flexible access platform for MIS. In *Intelligent Robots and Systems (IROS), 2011 IEEE/RSJ International Conference on* (pp. 949-954). IEEE. doi:10.1109/IROS.2011.6094907

Norén, G. N., Bate, A., Hopstadius, J., Star, K., & Edwards, I. R. (2008). Temporal Pattern Discovery for Trends and Transient Effects: Its Application to Patient Records.*Proceedings of the Fourteenth International Conference on Knowledge Discovery and Data Mining SIGKDD 2008*, p. 963-971, Las Vegas NV. doi:10.1145/1401890.1402005

Norman, C., & Skinner, H. (2006). Ehealth Literacy: Essential skills for consumer health in a networked world. *Journal of Medical Internet Research*, *8*(2), 9. doi:10.2196/jmir.8.2.e9 PMID:16867972

Nöthlings, U., Ford, E., Kröger, J., & Boeing, H. (2010). Lifestyle factors and mortality among adults with diabetes: Findings from the European Prospective Investigation into Cancer and Nutrition–Potsdam study. *Journal of Diabetes*, *2*(2), 112–117. doi:10.1111/j.1753-0407.2010.00069.x PMID:20923493

Noy, N. F., & McGuinness, D. L. (2001). *Ontology development 101: A guide to creating your first ontology*. Retrieved February 20, 2014, from http://protege.stanford.edu/publications/ontology_development/ontology101.pdf

O'Daniel, J., Scott, J., Varga, E., Speights, V., & Gordon, E. (2012). Lecture iv: Genomic medicine: Communicating with the patient. *TRiG Curriculum: Lecture 4.*

O'Keefe, C. M., Greenfield, P., & Goodchild, A. (2005). A decentralized approach to electronic consent and health information access control. *Journal of Research and Practice in Information Technology*, *37*(2), 161–178.

O'Leary, C. (2010). Informed consent-principles and practice. *ASA Newsletter*, *74*(2), 20–21.

O'Reilly, T. (2007). What is Web 2.0: Design patterns and business models for the next generation of software. *Communications & Stratégies*, *65*(1), 17.

Office of National Statistics. (2009). *National Omnibus Survey*. Retrieved April 23, 2012, from http://www.statistics.gov.uk/default.asp

Ogbuji, C. (2011). A Framework Ontology for Computer-Based Patient Record Systems. In *Proceedings of the ICBO: International Conference on Biomedical Ontology* (pp. 217–223).

Oleynikov, D., Rentschler, M., Hadzialic, A., Dumpert, J., Platt, S. R., & Farritor, S. (2005). Miniature robots can assist in laparoscopic cholecystectomy. *Surgical Endoscopy And Other Interventional Techniques*, *19*(4), 473–476. doi:10.1007/s00464-004-8918-6 PMID:15742124

Olson, G., & Olson, J. (2000). Distance Matters. *Human-Computer Interaction*, *15*(2), 139–178. doi:10.1207/S15327051HCI1523_4

O'Neill, S., & Brady, R. R. W. (2012). Colorectal smartphone apps: Opportunities and risks. *Colorectal Disease*, *14*(9), e530–e534. doi:10.1111/j.1463-1318.2012.03088.x PMID:22646729

Onslow, M., Andrews, C., & Lincoln, M. (1994). A control/experimental trial of operant treatment for early stuttering. *Journal of Speech and Hearing Research*, *37*(6), 1244–1259. doi:10.1044/jshr.3706.1244 PMID:7877284

Onslow, M., Costa, L., & Rue, S. (1990). Direct early intervention with stuttering: Some preliminary data. *The Journal of Speech and Hearing Disorders*, *55*(3), 405–416. doi:10.1044/jshd.5503.405 PMID:2381182

Oracle corporation. (2016a). *MySQL 5.7 Reference Manual*. Retrieved from http://dev.mysql.com/doc/refman/5.7/en/ha-overview.html

Oracle corporation. (2016b). *MySQL web site*. Retrieved May 5, 2016, from http://www.mysql.com/

Orhan, M. (2014). Extending the Individual Level of Virtuality: Implications of Task Virtuality in Virtual and Traditonal Settings. *American Scientist*, *4*, 400–412.

Oudshoorn, N. (2009). Physical and digital proximity: Emerging ways of health care in face-to-face and telemonitoring of heart-failure patients. *Sociology of Health & Illness*, *31*(3), 390–405. doi:10.1111/j.1467-9566.2008.01141.x PMID:19144084

Ovretveit, J. (2002). How to run an effective improvement collaborative. *International Journal of Health Care Quality Assurance*, *15*(4/5), 192–196. doi:10.1108/09526860210437403

Ozdalga, E., Ozdalga, A., & Ahuja, N. (2012). The smartphone in medicine: A review of current and potential use among physicians and students. *Journal of Medical Internet Research*, *14*(5), e128. doi:10.2196/jmir.1994 PMID:23017375

Padayachee, I., Kotze, P., & van der Merwe, A. (2010). ISO 9126 external systems quality characteristics, sub-characteristics and domain specific criteria for evaluating e-Learning systems. In *SACLA 2010 Conference*.

Pal, N. R., & Pal, S. K. (1993). A review on image segmentation techniques. *Patt. Rec.*, *26*(9), 1277–1294. doi:10.1016/0031-3203(93)90135-J

Papanicolaou, G., & Traut, H. (1941). The diagnostic value of vaginal smears in carcinoma of the uterus. *American Journal of Obstetrics and Gynecology*, *42*, 193–206.

Parchman, M. L., & Burge, S. K. (2004). The patient-physician relationship, primary care attributes, and preventive services. *Family Medicine*, *36*(1), 22–27. PMID:14710325

Park, H., Park, S., Yoon, E., Kim, B., Park, J., & Park, S. (2007, April). Paddling based microrobot for capsule endoscopes. In *Robotics and Automation, 2007 IEEE International Conference on* (pp. 3377-3382). IEEE. doi:10.1109/ROBOT.2007.363994

Park, S., Park, H., Park, S., & Kim, B. (2006). A paddling based locomotive mechanism for capsule endoscopes. *Journal of Mechanical Science and Technology, 20*(7), 1012-1018.

Park, S., Bergs, R. A., Eberhart, R., Baker, L., Fernandez, R., & Cadeddu, J. A. (2007). Trocar-less instrumentation for laparoscopy: Magnetic positioning of intra-abdominal camera and retractor. *Annals of Surgery*, *245*(3), 379–384. doi:10.1097/01.sla.0000232518.01447.c7 PMID:17435544

Pate, C., & Turner-Ferrier, J. (2010).Expoloring linkages between Quality, E-health and Healthcare Education. In: Moumtzoglou A. and Kastania A. (eds) E-Health Systems Quality and Reliability: Models and Standards, IGI Global, Hershey, P.A.

Patil, S., & Davies, P. (2014). Use of Google Translate in medical communication: evaluation of accuracy. British Medical Journal,349.

Paul, H. A., Bargar, W. L., Mittlestadt, B., Musits, B., Taylor, R. H., Kazanzides, P., & Hosainpour, A. et al. (2012). PUMA-560 Robot Manipulator Position Computed Torque Control Methods Using MATLAB/SIMULINK and Their Integration into Graduate Nonlinear Control and MATLAB Courses. *International Journal of Robotics and Automation*, *3*(3), 167–191.

Pearson, M. (2001). The role of national guidelines in the prevention of healthcare-associated infections. *Japanese Pharmacology and Therapeutics, 29*(10), 667-679.

Perkins, W. H. (1990). What is stuttering? *The Journal of Speech and Hearing Disorders*, *55*(3), 370–382. doi:10.1044/jshd.5503.370 PMID:2199728

Perrucci, G. P., Fitzek, F. H. P., Zhang, Q., & Katz, M. D. (2009). Cooperative Mobile Web Browsing. *EURASIP Journal on Wireless Communications and Networking*, *2009*, 1–9. doi:10.1155/2009/543054

Petersen, A. (2007). 'Biobanks'" engagements": Engendering trust or engineering consent?'. *Genomics. Social Policy*, *3*(1), 1–13.

Peters, H., Hulstijn, W., & Van Lieshout, P. (2000). Recent Developments in Speech Motor Research into Stuttering. *Folia Phoniatrica et Logopaedica*, *52*(1-3), 103–119. doi:10.1159/000021518 PMID:10474010

Petronio, S. (2012). *Boundaries of privacy: Dialectics of disclosure*. Suny Press.

Petrova, A., Ma, Y., Tsatsaronis, G., Kissa, M., Distel, F., Baader, F., & Schroeder, M. (2015). Formalizing biomedical concepts from textual definitions. *Journal of Biomedical Semantics*, *6*(1), 22. doi:10.1186/s13326-015-0015-3 PMID:25949785

Pew Internet & American Life Project. (2009). *Usage over time*. Retrieved April 4, 2012, from http://pewInternet.org//trends/UsageOverTime_Jan_2009.xls

Pezard, L., Jech, R., & Ruzicka, E. (2001). Investigation of non-linear properties of multichannel eeg in the early stages of parkinson's disease. *Clinical Neurophysiology*, *112*(1), 38–45. doi:10.1016/S1388-2457(00)00512-5 PMID:11137659

Phelps, G., & Barach, P. (2014). Why has the safety and quality movement been slow to improve care? *International Journal of Clinical Practice*, *68*(8), 932–935. doi:10.1111/ijcp.12413 PMID:25074334

Piha, T., & Terol, E. (2015). *European Reference Networks. How digital solutions fit in?* Retrieved June 16, 2016 from http://www.expandproject.eu/wp-content/uploads/2015/09/Tapani-Piha-Enrique-Terol.pdf

Plant, R. L., & Younger, R. M. (2000). The interrelationship of subglottic air pressure, fundamental frequency, and vocal intensity during speech. *Journal of Voice*, *14*(2), 170–177. doi:10.1016/S0892-1997(00)80024-7 PMID:10875568

Pomares-Quimbaya, A., Amórtegui, M. P., González, R. A., Muñoz, O., Bohórquez, W. R., García, O. M., & Ascanio, M. M. (2015). A system for the semi-automatic evaluation of clinical practice guideline indicators. *International Journal of Reliable and Quality E-Healthcare*, *4*(1), 1–10.

Porth, C., & Matfin, G. (2009). *Pathophysiology: Concepts of altered health states*. Philadelphia, PA: Wolters Kluwer Health/ Lippencott Williams & Wilkins.

Pouliakis, A., & Karakitsos, P. (2012). *Advantages Of A Hierarchical Software Deployment Strategy For The Hellenic Cervical Cancer Prevention Screening Program.* Paper presented at the 37th European Congress of Cytology, Dubrovnik-Cavtat, Croatia.

Pouliakis, A., Karakitsou, E., Iliopoulou, D., Koutsouri, G., & Karakitsos, P. (2013). *Roaming Women In The Hellenic Population Based Cervical Cancer Screening Program. Secure Access Of Medical Records And High Flexibility.* Paper presented at the 18th International Congress of Cytology, Paris, France.

Pouliakis, A., Athanasiadi, E., Karakitsou, E., Archondakis, S., Mourtzikou, A., Stamouli, M., & Karakitsos, P. et al. (2014). ISO 15189:2012 Management Requirements for Cytopathology Laboratory Information Systems. *International Journal of Reliable and Quality E-Healthcare*, *3*(3), 37–57. doi:10.4018/ijrqeh.2014070103

Pouliakis, A., Iliopoulou, D., & Karakitsou, E. (2012). Design and Implementation Issues of an Information System Supporting Cervical Cancer Screening Programs. *Journal of Applied Medical Sciences*, *1*(1), 61–91.

Pouliakis, A., Karakitsou, E., Chrelias, C., Pappas, A., Panayiotides, I., Valasoulis, G., & Karakitsos, P. et al. (2014). The Application of Classification and Regression Trees for the Triage of Women for Referral to Colposcopy and the Estimation of Risk for Cervical Intraepithelial Neoplasia: A Study Based on 1625 Cases with Incomplete Data from Molecular Tests. *Biomed Res Int*, *2014*, 914740. PMID:26339651

Pouliakis, A., Margari, N., Spathis, A., Kottaridi, C., Stamouli, M., Mourtzikou, A., & Karakitsos, P. et al. (2014). ISO 15189:2012 Technical Requirements for Cytopathology Laboratory Information Systems. *International Journal of Reliable and Quality E-Healthcare*, *3*(3), 58–80. doi:10.4018/ijrqeh.2014070104

Powell, A. E., Davies, H. T. O., & Thomson, R. G. (2003). Using routine comparative data to assess the quality of health care: Understanding and avoiding common pitfalls. *Quality & Safety in Health Care*, *12*(2), 122–128. doi:10.1136/qhc.12.2.122 PMID:12679509

Prado-Velasco, M., & Fernández-Peruchena, C. (2011). An Advanced Concept of Altered Auditory Feedback as a Prosthesis-Therapy for Stuttering Founded on a Non-Speech Etiologic Paradigm. In J. Pereira (Ed.), *Handbook of Research on Personal Autonomy Technologies and Disability Informatics* (pp. 76–118). Hershey, PA: IGI Global. doi:10.4018/978-1-60566-206-0.ch006

Presidential Commission for the Study of Bioethical Issues. (2013). Retrieved March 23, 2015, from http://www.bioethics.gov/sites/default/files/Informed%20Consent%20Background%20090413.pdf

Price, J. H., Easton, A. N., Telljohann, S. K., & Wallace, P. B. (1996). Perceptions of cervical cancer and Pap smear screening behavior by women's sexual orientation. *Journal of Community Health*, *21*(2), 89–105. doi:10.1007/BF01682301 PMID:8728358

Prince, A. E., & Roche, M. I. (2014). Genetic information, non-discrimination, and privacy protections in genetic counseling practice. *Journal of Genetic Counseling*, *23*(6), 891–902. doi:10.1007/s10897-014-9743-2 PMID:25063358

Pronovost, P. J., & Kazandjian, V. A. (1999). A new learning environment: Combining clinical research with quality improvement. *Journal of Evaluation in Clinical Practice*, *5*(1), 33–40. doi:10.1046/j.1365-2753.1999.00160.x PMID:10468382

Pullman, A. W., Masters, R. C., Zalot, L. C., Carde, L. E., Saraiva, M. M., & Dam, Y. Y. et al. (2009). Effect of the transition from high school to University on anthropometric and lifestyle variables in males. *Applied Physiology, Nutrition, and Metabolism*, *34*(2), 162–171. doi:10.1139/H09-007 PMID:19370046

Punam, T. (2011). A Study of Image Segmentation and Edge Detection Techniques. *International Journal on Computer Science and Engineering*, *3*(2), 899–904.

Ramirez, A., Walther, J. B., Burgoon, J. K., & Sunnafrank, M. (2002). Information-Seeking Strategies, Uncertainty, and Computer-Mediated Communication: Toward a Conceptual Model. *Human Communication Research*, *28*(2), 213–228.

Rashidi, P., & Mihailidis, A. (2013). A Survey on Ambient-Assisted Living Tools for Older Adults. *IEEE Journal of Biomedical and Health Informatics*, *17*(3), 579–590. doi:10.1109/JBHI.2012.2234129 PMID:24592460

Rashwan, A., Ormandjieva, O., & Witte, R. (2013). Ontology-based classification of non-functional requirements in software specifications: A new corpus and SVM-based classifier. In *Computer Software and Applications Conference (COMPSAC), 2013 IEEE 37th Annual* (pp. 381-386). IEEE. doi:10.1109/COMPSAC.2013.64

Ratzinger, J. (1968). *Einführung in das Christentum. Vorlesungen über das Apostolische Glaubensbekenntnis*. München: Kösel–Verlag.

Rayner, M., Armando, A., Bouillon, P., Ebling, S., Gerlach, J., Halimi, S., & Tsourakis, N. et al. (2016). Helping domain experts build phrasal speech translation systems. *Lecture Notes in Computer Science*, *9577*, 41–52. doi:10.1007/978-3-319-33500-1_4

Rebello, K. J. (2004). Applications of MEMS in surgery. *Proceedings of the IEEE*, *92*(1), 43–55. doi:10.1109/JPROC.2003.820536

Reddy, P., Rankins, D., Timoshanko, A., & Dunbar, J. (2011). Life! in Australia: Translating prevention research into a large-scale intervention. *Br J Diabetes Vasc Dis*, *11*(4), 193–197. doi:10.1177/1474651411410724

Redman, R. W., & Lynn, M. R. (2004). Advancing patient-centred care through knowledge development. *Canadian Journal of Nursing Research*, *36*(3), 116–129. PMID:15551666

Reed, C., & Godden, A. (1997). An experimental treatment using verbal punishment with two preschool stutterers. *Journal of Fluency Disorders*, *2*(3), 225–233. doi:10.1016/0094-730X(77)90026-2

Rehm, H. L., Hynes, E., & Funke, B. H. (2016). The changing landscape of molecular diagnostic testing: Implications for Academic Medical Centers. *Journal of Personalized Medicine*, *6*(1), 8.

Reilly, E. D. (2003). *Milestones in computer science and information technology*. Greenwood Publishing Group.

Reiter, P. L., Katz, M. L., Ferketich, A. K., Ruffin, M. T., & Paskett, E. D. (2009). Measuring cervical cancer risk: Development and validation of the CARE Risky Sexual Behavior Index. *Cancer Causes & Control*, *20*(10), 1865–1871. doi:10.1007/s10552-009-9380-5 PMID:19543986

Rentschler, M. E., Dumpert, J., Platt, S. R., Iagnemma, K., Oleynikov, D., & Farritor, S. M. (2006). Modeling, analysis, and experimental study of in vivo wheeled robotic mobility. Mechanical Engineering Faculty Publications.

Rentschler, M. E., Dumpert, J., Platt, S. R., Ahmed, S. I., Farritor, S. M., & Oleynikov, D. (2006). Mobile in vivo camera robots provide sole visual feedback for abdominal exploration and cholecystectomy. *Surgical Endoscopy And Other Interventional Techniques*, *20*(1), 135–138. doi:10.1007/s00464-005-0205-7 PMID:16333551

Rentschler, M. E., Dumpert, J., Platt, S. R., Iagnemma, K., Oleynikov, D., & Farritor, S. M. (2007). An in vivo mobile robot for surgical vision and task assistance. *Journal of Medical Devices*, *1*(1), 23–29. doi:10.1115/1.2355686

Rentschler, M., Hadzialic, A., & Dumpert, J. (2004). In vivo robots for laparoscopic surgery. *Studies in Health Technology and Informatics*, *98*, 316–322. PMID:15544298

Riaño, D., Real, F., López-Vallverdú, J. A., Campana, F., Ercolani, S., Mecocci, P., & Caltagirone, C. (2012). An ontology-based personalization of health-care knowledge to support clinical decisions for chronically ill patients. *Journal of Biomedical Informatics*, *45*(3), 429–446. doi:10.1016/j.jbi.2011.12.008 PMID:22269224

Riley, G. (1972). A Stuttering Severity Instrument for Children and Adults. *The Journal of Speech and Hearing Disorders*, *37*(3), 314–322. doi:10.1044/jshd.3703.314 PMID:5057250

Riou, G., Favre, M., Jeannel, D., Bourhis, J., Le Doussal, V., & Orth, G. (1990). Association between poor prognosis in early-stage invasive cervical carcinomas and non-detection of HPV DNA. *Lancet*, *335*(8699), 1171–1174. doi:10.1016/0140-6736(90)92693-C PMID:1971033

Rioul, O., & Vetterli, M. (1992). Wavelets and Signal Processing. *IEEE Signal Processing Magazine*, *8*(4), 14–38. doi:10.1109/79.91217

Risk, A., & Dzenowagis, J. (2001). Review Of Internet Health Information Quality Initiatives. *Journal of Medical Internet Research*, *3*(4), 8. doi:10.2196/jmir.3.4.e28 PMID:11772543

Ritchie, M. D., Holzinger, E. R., Li, R., Pendergrass, S. A., & Kim, D. (2015). Methods of integrating data to uncover genotype-phenotype interactions. *Nature Reviews. Genetics*, *16*(2), 85–97. doi:10.1038/nrg3868 PMID:25582081

Riva-Posse, P., Busto-Marolt, L., Schteinschnaider, A., Martinez-Echenique, L., Cammarota, A., & Merello, M. (2008). Phenomenology of abnormal movements in stuttering. *Parkinsonism & Related Disorders*, *14*(5), 415–419. doi:10.1016/j.parkreldis.2007.11.006 PMID:18316236

Roach, J. C., Glusman, G., Smit, A. F., Huff, C. D., Hubley, R., Shannon, P. T., & Shendure, J. et al. (2010). Analysis of genetic inheritance in a family quartet by whole-genome sequencing. *Science*, *328*(5978), 636–639. doi:10.1126/science.1186802 PMID:20220176

Roberts, A., Gaizauskas, R., Hepple, M., Demetriou, G., Guo, Y., Roberts, I., & Setzer, A. (2009). Building a semantically annotated corpus of clinical texts. *Journal of Biomedical Informatics*, *42*(5), 950–966. doi:10.1016/j.jbi.2008.12.013 PMID:19535011

Rodenwaldt, J., Kopka, L., Roedel, R., Margas, A., & Grabbe, E. (1997). 3D Virtual Endoscopy of the Upper Airways: Optimization of the Scan Parameters in a Cadaver Phantom and Clinical Assessment. *Journal of Computer Assisted Tomography*, *21*(3), 405–411. doi:10.1097/00004728-199705000-00013 PMID:9135649

Rodrigues, P. M. (2011). *Diagnóstico da Doença de Alzheimer com base no Electroencefalograma.* (Master's thesis). Instituto Politécnico de Bragança, Bragança.

Rodrigues, P. M., & Teixeira, J. P. (2013). Alzheimer's Disease Recognition with Artificial Neural Networks. In R. Martinho, R. Rijo, M. Cruz-Cunha, & J. Varajão (Eds.), Information Systems and Technologies for Enhancing Health and Social Care (pp. 102-118). Hershey, PA: IGI Global.

Rodrigues, P. M., Freitas, D. R., & Teixeira, J. P. (2013). Detection of Alzheimer's Disease Electroencephalogram Temporal Events. *International Journal of Reliable and Quality E-Healthcare*, *2*(3), 44–61. doi:10.4018/ijrqeh.2013070104

Rodrigues, P., & Teixeira, J. (2010). Classification of Electroencephalogram Signals Using Artificial Neural Networks. *3rd International Conference on Biomedical Engineering and Informatics*. doi:10.1109/BMEI.2010.5639941

Rodrigues, P., & Teixeira, J. (2011). Artificial Neural Networks in the Discrimination of Alzheimer's disease. *Communications in Computer and Information Science*, *221*, 272–281. doi:10.1007/978-3-642-24352-3_29

Rogić Vidaković, M., Jerković, A., Jurić, T., Vujović, I., Šoda, J., Erceg, N., & Dogaš, Z. et al. (2016). Neurophysiologic markers of primary motor cortex for laryngeal muscles and premotor cortex in caudal opercular part of inferior frontal gyrus investigated in motor speech disorder: A navigated transcranial magnetic stimulation (TMS) study. *Cognitive Processing*, 1–14. PMID:27130564

Roncancio, C. (1997). Toward duration-based, constrained and dynamic event types. In *Active, real-time, and temporal database systems, second international workshop, proceedings* (pp. 176–193). doi:10.1007/3-540-49151-1_10

Rosen, A. K., Chen, Q., Borzecki, A. M., Shin, M., Itani, K. M., & Shwartz, M. (2014). Using Estimated True Safety Event Rates versus Flagged Safety Event Rates: Does It Change Hospital Profiling and Payment? *Health Services Research*, *49*(5), 1426–1445. doi:10.1111/1475-6773.12180 PMID:24779721

Rosse, C., & Mejino, J. L. Jr. (2003). A reference ontology for biomedical informatics: The Foundational Model of Anatomy. *Journal of Biomedical Informatics*, *36*(6), 478–500. doi:10.1016/j.jbi.2003.11.007 PMID:14759820

Rosser, B., & Eccleston, C. (2011). Smartphone applications for pain management. *Journal of Telemedicine and Telecare*, *17*(6), 308–312. doi:10.1258/jtt.2011.101102 PMID:21844177

Rothstein, M. A. (2014). Privacy and Confidentiality. Routledge Handbook of Medical Law and Ethics, 52.

Roussos, G., Marsh, A., & Maglavera, S. (2005). Enabling pervasive computing with smart phones. *IEEE Pervasive Computing / IEEE Computer Society [and] IEEE Communications Society*, *4*(2), 20–27. doi:10.1109/MPRV.2005.30

Ruan, C., & Yeo, S. S. (2009). Modeling of an Intelligent e-Consent System in a Healthcare Domain. *J. UCS*, *15*(12), 2429–2444.

Ruchlin, H. S., Dubbs, N. L., & Callahan, M. A. (2004). The role of leadership in instilling a culture of safety: Lessons from the literature. *Journal of Healthcare Management*, *49*(1), 47–58. PMID:14768428

Ruckenstein, M. (2014). Visualized and interacted life: Personal analytics and engagements with data doubles. *Societies*, *4*(1), 68–84. doi:10.3390/soc4010068

Russello, G., Dong, C., & Dulay, N. (2008). Consent-based workflows for healthcare management. In *Policies for Distributed Systems and Networks, POLICY. IEEE Workshop on* (pp. 153-161). doi:10.1109/POLICY.2008.22

Ryan, B. P., & Ryan, B. V. K. (1995). Programmed stuttering treatment for children: Comparison of two establishment programs through transfer, maintenance, and follow-up. *Journal of Speech and Hearing Research*, *38*(1), 61–75. doi:10.1044/jshr.3801.61 PMID:7731220

Saaty, T. L. (1994). How to make a decision: The Analytic Hierarchy Process. *Interfaces*, *24*(6), 19–43. doi:10.1287/inte.24.6.19

Sackett, D. L. (1997). Evidence-based medicine. *Seminars in Perinatology*, *21*(1), 3–5. doi:10.1016/S0146-0005(97)80013-4 PMID:9190027

Sackett, D. L., Rosenberg, W. M., Gray, J. A., Haynes, R. B., & Richardson, W. S. (1996). Evidence based medicine: What it is and what it isn't. *British Medical Journal, 312*(7023), 71–72.

Salgo v. Leland Stanford, Jr., Univ. Bd. of Trustees, 317 P. 2d 170, 181 (Cal. App. Ct. 1957).

Samwald, M., Fehre, K., de Bruin, J., & Adlassnig, K.-P. (2012). The arden syntax standard for clinical decision support: Experiences and directions. *Journal of Biomedical Informatics, 45*(4), 711 - 718. Retrieved from http://www.sciencedirect.com/science/article/pii/S1532046412000226

Sanchez, L. A., Le, M. Q., Rabenorosoa, K., Liu, C., Zemiti, N., Poignet, P., & Dario, P. (2013). A case study of safety in the design of surgical robots: The ARAKNES platform. In *Intelligent Autonomous Systems 12* (pp. 121–130). Springer Berlin Heidelberg. doi:10.1007/978-3-642-33932-5_12

Sanders, D. (2014). *A Landmark, 12-Point Review of Population Health Management Companies* (Executive Report). Retrieved from https://www.healthcatalyst.com/landmark-review-of-population-health-management-companies

Sanei, S., & Chambers, J. (2007). *EEG signal processing*. West Sussex, UK: Wiley-Interscience. doi:10.1002/9780470511923

Santhi, K. R., & Kumaran, G. S. (2006). Migration to 4 G: Mobile IP based Solutions. In *Proceedings of the Advanced International Conference on Telecommunications and International Conference on Internet and Web Applications and Services* (AICT/ICIW 2006). IEEE Computer Society.

Santo, A., Laizner, A. M., & Shohet, L. (2005). Exploring the value of audiotapes for health literacy: A systematic review. *Patient Education and Counseling, 58*(3), 235–243. doi:10.1016/j.pec.2004.07.001 PMID:16054796

Saranummi, N. (2005). PICNIC architecture. *Studies in Health Technology and Informatics, 115*, 37–60.

Saurin, J. C., Beneche, N., Chambon, C., & Pioche, M. (2016). Challenges and Future of Wireless Capsule Endoscopy. *Clinical Endoscopy, 49*(1), 26.

Sawyer, J., Chon, H., & Ambrose, N. (2009). Influences of Rate, Length, and Complexity on Speech Disfluency in a Single Speech Sample in Preschool Children Who Stutter. *Journal of Fluency Disorders, 33*(3), 220–240. doi:10.1016/j.jfludis.2008.06.003 PMID:18762063

Scheuner, M. T., de Vries, H., Kim, B., Meili, R. C., Olmstead, S. H., & Teleki, S. (2009). Are electronic health records ready for genomic medicine? *Genetics in Medicine, 11*(7), 510–517. doi:10.1097/GIM.0b013e3181a53331 PMID:19478682

Schiff, S. J., & Milton, J. G. (1993). Wavelet transforms for electroencephalographic spike and seizure detection.*Proceeding of the SPIE International Society for Optical Engineering.*

Schifrin, B. S., & Cohen, W. R. (2013). The effect of malpractice claims on the use of caesarean section. *Best Practice & Research. Clinical Obstetrics & Gynaecology, 27*(2), 269–283. doi:10.1016/j.bpobgyn.2012.10.004 PMID:23206669

Schlathoelter, T., Lorenz, C., Carlsen, I. C., Renisch, S., & Deschamps, T. (2002) Simultaneous segmentation and tree reconstruction of the airways for virtual bronchoscopy. *Proc. of SPIE on Medical Imaging 2002, 4684*, 103–113. doi:10.1117/12.467061

Schlecht, N. F., Kulaga, S., Robitaille, J., Ferreira, S., Santos, M., Miyamura, R. A., & Franco, E. L. et al. (2001). Persistent human papillomavirus infection as a predictor of cervical intraepithelial neoplasia. *Journal of the American Medical Association, 286*(24), 3106–3114. doi:10.1001/jama.286.24.3106 PMID:11754676

Schouten, L. M. T., Hulscher, M. E. J. L., van Everdingen, J. J. E., Huijsman, R., Niessen, L. W., & Grol, R. P. T. M. (2010). Short- and long-term effects of a quality improvement collaborative on diabetes management. *Implementation Science; IS, 5*(1), 94. doi:10.1186/1748-5908-5-94 PMID:21110898

Schouten, L. M. T., Hulscher, M. E., van Everdingen, J. J., Huijsman, R., & Grol, R. P. (2008). Evidence for the impact of quality improvement collaboratives: Systematic review. *BMJ (Clinical Research Ed.), 336*(7659), 1491–1494. doi:10.1136/bmj.39570.749884.BE PMID:18577559

Schulz, A. P., Seide, K., Queitsch, C., von Haugwitz, A., Meiners, J., Kienast, B., & Jürgens, C. (2007). Results of total hip replacement using the Robodoc surgical assistant system: Clinical outcome and evaluation of complications for 97 procedures. *International Journal of Medical Robotics and Computer Assisted Surgery*, *3*(4), 301–306. doi:10.1002/rcs.161 PMID:18000945

Secko, D. M., Preto, N., Niemeyer, S., & Burgess, M. M. (2009). Informed consent in biobank research: A deliberative approach to the debate. *Social Science & Medicine*, *68*(4), 781–789. doi:10.1016/j.socscimed.2008.11.020 PMID:19095337

Seeley, R., Stephens, T., & Tate, P. (2006). *Anatomy and Physiology (7th ed.).* Mcgraw-Hill.

Seeman, N. (2008). Web 2.0 and chronic illness: New horizons, new opportunities. *ElectronicHealthcare*, *6*(3), 104–110. PMID:18326388

Serban, R., ten Teije, A., van Harmelen, F., Marcos, M., & Polo-Conde, C. (2007). Extraction and use of linguistic patterns for modelling medical guidelines. *Artificial Intelligence in Medicine*, *39*(2), 137–149. doi:10.1016/j.artmed.2006.07.012 PMID:16963241

Sheppard, N. P., Safavi-Naini, R., & Jafari, M. (2009). A digital rights management model for healthcare. In Policies for Distributed Systems and Networks. *POLICY 2009.IEEE International Symposium* (pp. 106-109). doi:10.1109/POLICY.2009.8

Sherlock, E. (2009). *Disclosure of patient's genetic information without their consent- Is the "public interset" really a Sufficient Justification?* Genomics Law Report. retrieved March 2, 2015, from http://www.genomicslawreport.com/index.php/2009/11/10/disclosure-of-patients-genetic-information-without-their-consent-is-the-public-interest-really-a-sufficient-justification/

Shiffman, R. N., Karras, B. T., Agrawal, A., Chen, R., Marenco, L., & Nath, S. (2000). Gem: A proposal for a more comprehensive guideline document model using xml. *Journal of the American Medical Informatics Association*, *7*(5), 488–498. doi:10.1136/jamia.2000.0070488 PMID:10984468

Shim, J. P., & Shim, J. M. (2003). M-commerce Around the World: Mobile Services and Applications in Japan, Korea, Hong Kong, Finland, and the United States. *Decision Line*, *34*(5), 9–13.

Shimokawa, A., Yatomi, N., Anamizu, S., Torii, S., Isono, H., Sugai, Y., & Kohno, M. (2001). Influence of deteriorating ability of emotional comprehension on interpersonal behavior in Alzheimer-type dementia. *Brain and Cognition*, *47*(3), 423–433. doi:10.1006/brcg.2001.1318 PMID:11748898

Shortliffe, E. H., & Cimino, J. J. (2006). *Biomedical informatics.* Springer Science + Business Media, LLC.

Sicard, S., De Palma, N., & Hagimont, D. (2016). *J2EE Server Scalability through EJB Replication.* Retrieved April 30, 2016, from http://sardes.inrialpes.fr/papers/files/06-Sicard-SAC.pdf

Silva, S. (2009). *Classificação do grau de disfluência com e sem o uso de feedback acústico modificado em adolescentes e adultos gagos portugueses.* (Unpublished undergraduate dissertation). University Fernando Pessoa, Portugal.

Simalatsar, A., You, W., Gotta, V., Widmer, N., & De Micheli, G. (2014). Representation of medical guidelines with a computer interpretable model. *International Journal of Artificial Intelligence Tools*, *23*(03), 1460003. doi:10.1142/S0218213014600033

Simi, M., Valdastri, P., Quaglia, C., Menciassi, A., & Dario, P. (2010). Design, fabrication, and testing of a capsule with hybrid locomotion for gastrointestinal tract exploration. *Mechatronics. IEEE/ASME Transactions on Mechatronics*, *15*(2), 170–180. doi:10.1109/TMECH.2010.2041244

Singer, S. J., Falwell, A., Gaba, D. M., & Baker, L. C. (2008). Patient safety climate in US hospitals: Variation by management level. *Medical Care*, *46*(11), 1149–1156. doi:10.1097/MLR.0b013e31817925c1 PMID:18953225

Sittig, D. F., Ash, J. S., & Ledley, R. S. (2006). The story behind the development of the first whole-body computerized tomography scanner as told by Robert S. Ledley. *Journal of the American Medical Informatics Association*, *13*(5), 465–469. doi:10.1197/jamia.M2127 PMID:16799115

Sklar, D. P. (2016). Giving Voice to Patient-Centered Care. *Academic Medicine*, *91*(3), 285–287. doi:10.1097/ACM.0000000000001080 PMID:26907893

Smaling, J., & Holt, M. A. (2005, April). Integration and automation transform medication administration safety. *Health Care Management Technology*.

Smith, A. M., Heywood, W., Ryall, R., Shelley, J. M., Pitts, M. K., Richters, J., & Patrick, K. et al. (2011). Association between sexual behavior and cervical cancer screening. *Journal of Women's Health*, *20*(7), 1091–1096. doi:10.1089/jwh.2010.2585 PMID:21682554

Smith, B., Ashburner, M., Rosse, C., Bard, J., Bug, W., Ceusters, W., & Lewis, S. et al. (2007). The OBO Foundry: Coordinated evolution of ontologies to support biomedical data integration. *Nature Biotechnology*, *25*(11), 1251–1255. doi:10.1038/nbt1346 PMID:17989687

Smith, B., & Brochhausen, M. (2010). Putting Biomedical Ontologies to Work. *Methods of Information in Medicine*, *49*(2), 135–140. doi:10.3414/ME9302 PMID:20135080

Smith, J. S., Lindsay, L., Hoots, B., Keys, J., Franceschi, S., Winer, R., & Clifford, G. M. (2007). Human papillomavirus type distribution in invasive cervical cancer and high-grade cervical lesions: A meta-analysis update. *International Journal of Cancer*, *121*(3), 621–632. doi:10.1002/ijc.22527 PMID:17405118

Smith, R. A., Brooks, D., Cokkinides, V., Saslow, D., & Brawley, O. W. (2013). Cancer screening in the United States, 2013: A review of current American Cancer Society guidelines, current issues in cancer screening, and new guidance on cervical cancer screening and lung cancer screening. *CA: a Cancer Journal for Clinicians*, *63*(2), 88–105. doi:10.3322/caac.21174 PMID:23378235

Snyderman, R., & Williams, R. S. (2003). Prospective medicine: The next health care transformation. *Academic Medicine*, *78*(11), 1079–1084. doi:10.1097/00001888-200311000-00002 PMID:14604864

Soltani, S., & Mahnam, A. (2016). A practical efficient human computer interface based on saccadic eye movements for people with disabilities. *Computers in Biology and Medicine*, *70*, 163–173. doi:10.1016/j.compbiomed.2016.01.012 PMID:26848728

Sonka, M., Park, W., & Hoffman, E. A. (1996). Rule-based detection of intrathoracic airway trees. *IEEE Transactions on Medical Imaging*, *15*(3), 314–326. doi:10.1109/42.500140 PMID:18215912

Sosnowy, C. (2014). Practicing patienthood online: Social media, chronic illness, and lay expertise. *Societies*, *4*(2), 316–329. doi:10.3390/soc4020316

Spasic, I., Ananiadou, S., McNaught, J., & Kumar, A. (2005). Text mining and ontologies in biomedicine: Making sense of raw text. *Briefings in Bioinformatics*, *6*(3), 239–251. doi:10.1093/bib/6.3.239 PMID:16212772

Spathis, A., Kottaridi, C., Chranioti, A., Meristoudis, C., Chrelias, C., Panayiotides, I. G., & Karakitsos, P. et al. (2012). mRNA and DNA detection of human papillomaviruses in women of all ages attending two colposcopy clinics. *PLoS ONE*, *7*(11), e49205. doi:10.1371/journal.pone.0049205 PMID:23166611

Srirama, S. (2006). Publishing and Discovery of Mobile Web Services in Peer to Peer Networks. In *Proceedings of First International Workshop on Mobile Services and Personalized Environments (MSPE'06).*

Srirama, S. N., Jarke, M., Zhu, H., & Prinz, W. (2008). Scalable Mobile Web Service Discovery in Peer to Peer Networks. In *Proceedings of the 2008 Third International Conference on Internet and Web Applications and Services*, 2008 (pp. 668-674). IEEE Computer Society.

Srirama, S., Jarke, M., & Prinz, W. (2007). Mobile Web Service Discovery in Peer to Peer Networks. In *Proceedings of the 5th International Workshop on Ubiquitous Mobile Information and Collaboration Systems.*

Stadler, H. U., & Peter-Spörndli, U. (2007). The quest for machine translation quality at CLS Communication. *MT Summit XI*, 435-442.

Stallman, H. (2011). *Mental illness running high among uni students.* The World Today. Retrieved from http://www.abc.net.au/news/2010-11-23/mental-illness-running-high-among-uni-students/2348772

Stam, C. (2005). Nonlinear dynamical analysis of EEG and MEG: Review of an emerging field. *Clinical Neurophysiology*, *116*(10), 2266–2301. doi:10.1016/j.clinph.2005.06.011 PMID:16115797

Stansfield, S. (2005). Structuring information and incentives to improve health. *Bulletin of the World Health Organization*, *83*(8), 562–562. PMID:16184268

Stark, M., Pomati, S., D'Ambrosio, A., Giraudi, F., & Gidaro, S. (2015). A new telesurgical platform–preliminary clinical results. *Minimally Invasive Therapy & Allied Technologies*, *24*(1), 31–36. doi:10.3109/13645706.2014.1003945 PMID:25627435

Stefani, A., & Xenos, M. (2008). E-commerce system quality assessment using a model based on ISO 9126 and Belief Networks. *Software Quality Journal*, *16*(1), 107–129. doi:10.1007/s11219-007-9032-5

Steptoe, A., Wardle, J., Cui, W., Bellisle, F., Zotti, A. M., Baranyai, R., & Sanderman, R. (2002). Trends in smoking, diet, physical exercise and attitudes toward health in European University students from 13 countries. *Preventive Medicine*, *35*(2), 97–104. doi:10.1006/pmed.2002.1048 PMID:12200093

Stevens, D. J., Jackson, J. A., Howes, N., & Morgan, J. (2014). Obesity surgery smartphone apps: A review.[PubMed]. *Obesity Surgery*, *24*(1), 32–36. doi:10.1007/s11695-013-1010-3

Stewart, M., Brown, J. B., Weston, W. W., McWhinney, I. R., McWilliam, C. L., & Freeman, T. R. (2003). *Patient-centered Medicine: Transforming the Clinical Method.* Radcliffe Medical Press.

Strike, C., Goering, P., & Wasylenki, D. (2002). A population health framework for inner-city mental health. *Journal of Urban Health*, *79*(4), S13–S20. doi:10.1093/jurban/79.suppl_1.S13 PMID:12473695

Strouse, D. S. (2005). Informed consent to genetic research on banked human tissue. *Jurimetrics*, 135–152.

Struewingl, J. P., & Abeliovich, D. (1995). The carrier frequency of the BRCA1 185delAG mutation. *Nature Genetics*, 11.

Studdert, D. M., Mello, M. M., Levy, M. K., Gruen, R. L., Dunn, E. J., Orav, E. J., & Brennan, T. A. (2007). Geographic variation in informed consent law: Two standards for disclosure of treatment risks. *Journal of Empirical Legal Studies*, *4*(1), 103–124. doi:10.1111/j.1740-1461.2007.00083.x

Studer, R., Fensel, D., Decker, S., & Benjamins, V. R. (1999). Knowledge engineering: Survey and future directions. Lecture Notes in Computer Science, 1570, 1–23. http://doi.org/ doi:<ALIGNMENT.qj></ALIGNMENT>10.1007/10703016_1

Stutzman, F. (2006). *An evaluation of identity-sharing behavior in social network communities.Paper presented at the International Digital Media Arts.* Association and the Miami University Center for Interactive Media Studies CODE Conference, Oxford, OH.

Suarez-Coloma, J., Verdier, C., & Roncancio, C. (2014). Quality indices in medical alert systems. In *ICEIS 2014 - Proceedings of the 16th international conference on enterprise information systems,* (pp. 81–89). Retrieved from doi:10.5220/0004893900810089

Subversus Interactive. (2011). Retrieved from http://subvers.us/

Suchý, M., Bourek, A., Klika, P., Dušek, L., Ryska, M., Bělina, F., & Kožený, P. (2011). Joint development of clinical practice guidelines and quality indicators as a tool for quality of care improvement. In P. A. Bath, T. Mettler, D. A. Raptis, & B. A. Sen (Eds.). *Proceedings of the 15th international Symposium on Health Information Management Rersearch - ISHIMR 2011.* Zurich: University of Zurich, University of St. Gallen and University of Sheffield.

Summers, R., Feng, D., Holland, S., Sneller, M., & Shelhamer, J. (1996). Virtual Bronchoscopy: Segmentation Method for Real-Time Display. *Radiology*, *200*(3), 857–862. doi:10.1148/radiology.200.3.8756944 PMID:8756944

Suryn, W., & Laverdière, F. (2007). The Applicability Analysis of ISO/IEC 9126 Series of Standards in Telecom Sector: The Example of Softswitch Category of Software. *Software Quality Journal*, *15*(4), 417–448. doi:10.1007/s11219-007-9024-5

Swan, M. (2009). Emerging Patient-Driven Health Care Models: An Examination of Health Social Networks, Consumer Personalized Medicine and Quantified Self-Tracking. *International Journal of Environmental Research and Public Health*, *6*, 492–525.

Swanstrom, L. L., & Soper, N. J. (2013). *Mastery of endoscopic and laparoscopic surgery*. Lippincott Williams & Wilkins.

Tachikawa, K. (2003). A perspective on the evolution of mobile communications. *Communications Magazine, IEEE*, *41*(10), 66–73.

Teixeira, J. P. (2013). *Análise e Síntese da Fala - Modelação Paramétrica de Sinais Para Sistemas TTS*. Editorial Académica Espanhola.

Teixeira, J. P., Fernandes, M. G., & Costa, R. A. (2012). Measure and Comparison of Speech Pause Duration in Subjects with Disfluency Speech. *Procedia Technology*, *5*, 812–819. doi:10.1016/j.protcy.2012.09.090

Teixeira, J. P., Fernandes, M. G., & Costa, R. A. (2013). Pause Duration of Disfluent Speech. *International Journal of Reliable and Quality E-Healthcare*, *2*(3), 62–73. doi:10.4018/ijrqeh.2013070105

Teixeira, J. P., Freitas, D., Braga, D., Barros, M. J., & Latsch, V. (2001). *Phonetic Events from the Labeling the European Portuguese Database for Speech Synthesis, FEUP/IPB-DB*. Eurospecch.

Tennant, G. (2001). *Six Sigma, SPC and TQM in Manufacturing and Services*. Hampshire, UK: Gower Publishing, Ltd.

Terol, E. (2015). *European Reference Networks Implementation process: timeline and milestones*. Retrieved June 16, 2016 from http://ec.europa.eu/health/ern/docs/ev_20151008_co011_en.pdf

Terzopoulos, D., & Metaxas, D. (1987). Dynamic 3D models with local and global deformations: Deformable superquadrics. *IEEE Trans. Pattern Anal. Mach. Int.*, *13*(7), 703–714. doi:10.1109/34.85659

The Apache Software Foundation. (2016a). *The Apache Tomcat Connectors / mod_jk - ISAPI redirector - NSAPI redirector*. Retrieved May 9, 2016, from http://tomcat.apache.org/connectors-doc/index.html

The Apache Software Foundation. (2016b). *Apache Tomcat web site*. Retrieved May 8, 2016, from http://tomcat.apachc.org/

The Apache Software Foundation. (2016c). *Welcome to the Apache Web Services™ Project*. Retrieved 4th May, 2016, from https://ws.apache.org/

The Economist. (2010). *Viktor Chernomyrdin, a Russian prime minister, died on November 3rd, aged 72*. Retrieved June 16, 2016, from http://www.economist.com/node/17414237

Thompson, J. W., Pinidiya, S. D., Ryan, K. W., McKinley, E. D., Alston, S., Bost, J. E., & Simpson, P. et al. (2003). Health plan quality-of-care information is undermined by voluntary reporting. *American Journal of Preventive Medicine*, *24*(1), 62–70. doi:10.1016/S0749-3797(02)00569-X PMID:12554025

Titanic Medical. (2016). *The SPORT Surgical System*. Retrieved June 8, 2016, from http://www.titanmedicalinc.com/product/

Todd, H., Mirawwdeli, A., Costelloe, S, Cavenagh, P., Davis, S., & Howell, P. (2014). Scores on Riley's stuttering Severity Instrument Versions Three and Fur for samples os dofferent length and for different types of speech material. *Informa Healthcare, 28*(12), 912-926.

Tomita, L. Y., Longatto Filho, A., Costa, M. C., Andreoli, M. A., Villa, L. L., Franco, E. L., & Cardoso, M. A. (2010). Diet and serum micronutrients in relation to cervical neoplasia and cancer among low-income Brazilian women. *International Journal of Cancer*, *126*(3), 703–714. doi:10.1002/ijc.24793 PMID:19642096

Topol, E. (2012). *The Creative Destruction of Medicine*. New York, NY: Basic Books.

To, T., Williams, J. I., Wu, K., Theriault, M. E., & Goel, V. (2003). Comparison of methods to identify outliers observed in health services small area variation studies. *Statistical Methods in Medical Research*, *12*(6), 531–546. doi:10.1191/0962280203sm350oa PMID:14653355

Towards a National Primary Health Care Strategy: A discussion paper from the Australian Government. (2008). Department of Health and Ageing, Commonwealth of Australia. Retrieved October 6, 2011, from http://www.health.gov.au/primaryhealthstrategy

Toye, E., Sharp, R., Madhavapeddy, A., Scott, D., Upton, E., & Blackwell, A. (2007). Interacting with mobile services: An evaluation of camera-phones and visual tags. *Personal and Ubiquitous Computing*, *11*(2).

Transenterix. (2016). *The Telelap ALF-X Surgical Robotic System*. Retrieved June 8, 2016, from http://www.alf-x.com/en/

Tsai, P. H., Shih, C. S., & Yu, C. Y. (2008). *Smart Medication Dispenser Design, Architecture and Implementation* (Technical Report TR-IIS-08-010). Institute of Information Science, Academia Sinica.

Tsourakis, N., & Estrella, P. (2013). Evaluating the quality of mobile medical speech translators based on ISO/IEC 9126 series: Definition, weighted quality model and metrics. *International Journal of Reliable and Quality E-Healthcare*, *2*(2), 1–20. doi:10.4018/ijrqeh.2013040101

Tsui, Y. L., & Heng, P. A. (2000). Automated extraction of bronchus from 3D CT images of lung based on generic algorithm and 3D region growing. *Proc. of SPIE on Medical Imaging 2000*, *3979*, 906–916.

Uden-Kraan, C. F. (2009). Health-related Internet use by patients with somatic diseases: Frequency of use and characteristics of users. *Informatics for Health & Social Care*, *34*(1), 18–29. doi:10.1080/17538150902773272 PMID:19306196

Ullman-Cullere, M. H., & Mathew, J. P. (2011). Emerging landscape of genomics in the electronic health record for personalized medicine. *Human Mutation*, *32*(5), 512–516. doi:10.1002/humu.21456 PMID:21309042

Usher, W. (2009). Gold Coast general practitioners' understanding pertaining to reliability, interactive and usability components associated with health websites. *International Journal of Behaviour and Information Technology*, *28*(1), 39–44. doi:10.1080/01449290802187736

Usher, W. (2011). Types of social media (Web 2.0) usage by Australian Allied Health professionals' for early 21st century practice promotion and e-health care delivery. *Social Work in Health Care*, *50*(4), 305–329. doi:10.1080/00981389.2010.534317 PMID:21512953

Usher, W., Gudes, O., & Parekh, S. (2015). Exploring the use of technology pathways to access health information by Australian university students: A multi - dimensional approach. *Health Information Management Journal*, *4*, 1–12. PMID:26113541

Vallejo, M., Recas, J., del Valle, P. G., & Ayala, J. (2013). Accurate human tissue characterization for energy-efficient wireless on-body communications. *Sensors (Basel, Switzerland)*, *13*(6), 7546–7569. doi:10.3390/s130607546 PMID:23752565

Valls, A., Gibert, K., Sánchez, D., & Batet, M. (2010). Using ontologies for structuring organizational knowledge in Home Care assistance. *International Journal of Medical Informatics*, *79*(5), 370–387. doi:10.1016/j.ijmedinf.2010.01.012 PMID:20185360

Valtonen, E., Addams-Moring, R., Virtanen, T., Järvinen, A., & Moring, M. (2004). Emergency announcements to mobile user devices in geographically defined areas. In *Proceedings of the first International Workshop on Information Systems for Crisis Response and Management.*

Van der Ent, C. (2008). Quality assessment: Is the truth in the outcome*? The European Respiratory Journal*, *31*(1), 6–7. doi:10.1183/09031936.00141507 PMID:18166589

Van Lieshout, P., Hulstijn, W., & Peters, H. (2004). Searching for the weak link in the speech production chain of people who stutter: a motor skill approach. In B. Maassen, R. Kent, P. H. van Lieshout, & W. Hulstijn (Eds.), Speech motor control in normal and disordered speech. Oxford University Press.

Vanhoutte, S., Cosyns, M., van Mierlo, P., Batens, K., Corthals, P., De Letter, M., & Santens, P. et al. (2016). When will a stuttering moment occur? The determining role of speech motor preparation. *Neuropsychologia*, *86*, 93–102. doi:10.1016/j.neuropsychologia.2016.04.018 PMID:27106391

Vassilakos, P., Catarino, R., Frey Tirri, B., & Petignat, P. (2015). Cervical cancer screening in Switzerland: Time to rethink the guidelines. *Swiss Medical Weekly*, *145*, w14112. doi:10.4414/smw.2015.14112 PMID:25664576

Veacez, P. J. (2006). An individual based framework for a study on medical error. *International Journal for Quality in Health Care*, *18*(4), 314–319. doi:10.1093/intqhc/mzl011 PMID:16672255

Veillard, J., Gula, C., Huynh, T., & Klazinga, N. (2012). Measuring and reporting on quality of care and patient safety in Canada: Focusing on what matters. *Healthcare Papers*, *12*(1), 32–37, discussion 50–57. doi:10.12927/hcpap.2012.22863 PMID:22543328

VHA HANDBOOK 1004.05, Transmittal Sheet. (2005). *IMEDCONSENT™*. Retrieved August 17, 2013, from http://www.va.gov/vhapublications/ViewPublication.asp?pub_ID=1857

Vining, D., Shifrin, R., Haponik, E., Liu, K., & Choplin, R. (1994). Virtual Bronchoscopy (abstract). Radiology, 193, 261.

Virginia women's center - cancer family history questionnaire. (n.d.). Retrieved May 22, 2015, from https://www.virginiawomenscenter.com/assets/HEREDITARY_CANCER_RISK_ASSESSMENT_FORM.pdf

Visvanathan, A., Hamilton, A., & Brady, R. (2012). Smartphone apps in microbiology—Is better regulation required? *Clinical Microbiology and Infection*, *18*(7), E218–E220. doi:10.1111/j.1469-0691.2012.03892.x PMID:22563840

Viswanathan, V. (2001). *Load Balancing Web Applications*. Retrieved from http://onjava.com/pub/a/onjava/2001/09/26/load.html

Vitiello, V., Lee, S. L., Cundy, T. P., & Yang, G. Z. (2013). Emerging robotic platforms for minimally invasive surgery. *Biomedical Engineering. IEEE Reviews in*, *6*, 111–126.

Wachter, R.M. (2004). *The End of The Beginning: Patient Safety Five Years After 'To Err Is Human'*. Health Aff (Millwood).

Wallace, L. S., & Dhingra, L. K. (2014). A systematic review of smartphone applications for chronic pain available for download in the united states. *Journal of Opioid Management*, *10*, 63–68. doi:10.5055/jom.2014.0193 PMID:24604571

Wan, D. (1999). Magic Medicaine Cabinet: A situated portal for consumer healthcare. *Proceedings of First International Symposium on Handheld and Ubiquitous Computing (HUC '99)*. doi:10.1007/3-540-48157-5_44

Webster, A. J. (2002). Innovative health technologies and the social: Redefining health, medicine and the body. *Current Sociology*, *50*, 443–457.

Wegmüller, M. S. (2007). Intra-Body Communication for Biomedical Sensor Networks. *ETH*, (17323). http://doi.org/<ALIGNMENT.qj></ALIGNMENT>10.3929/ethz-a-005479240

Weingart, S. N., Iezzoni, L. I., Davis, R. B., Palmer, R. H., Cahalane, M., Hamel, M. B., & Banks, N. J. et al. (2000). Use of administrative data to find substandard care: Validation of the complications screening program. *Medical Care*, *38*(8), 796–806. doi:10.1097/00005650-200008000-00004 PMID:10929992

Wennberg, J. E., & Gittelsohn, A. (1973). Small area variations in health care delivery. *Science*, *182*(117), 1102–1108. doi:10.1126/science.182.4117.1102 PMID:4750608

Wentzensen, N., & Klug, S. J. (2008). Early detection of cervical carcinomas: Finding an overall approach. *Deutsches Ärzteblatt International*, *105*(37), 617–622. doi:10.3238/arztebl.2008.0617 PMID:19471627

Wentzensen, N., Schiffman, M., Palmer, T., & Arbyn, M. (2016). Triage of HPV positive women in cervical cancer screening. *Journal of Clinical Virology*, *76*(Suppl 1), S49–S55. doi:10.1016/j.jcv.2015.11.015 PMID:26643050

Wertheimer, A. I., & Santella, T. M. (2003). Medication compliance research. *Journal of Applied Research in Clinical and Experimental Therapeutics*, *3*(3), 254–261.

West, E. (2001). Management matters: The link between hospital organisation and quality of patient care. *Quality in Health Care*, *10*(1), 40–48. doi:10.1136/qhc.10.1.40 PMID:11239143

Wheatley, M. J. (1999). *Leadership and the new science: Discovering order in a chaotic world.* San Fransisco: Berrett-Koehler.

White, A. (2006). Men's Health in the 21st Century. *International Journal of Men's Health*, *5*(1), 1–17. doi:10.3149/jmh.0501.1

WHO. (1986). *Ottawa Charter for Health Population*. Retrieved from http://www.who.int/healthpromotion/conferences/previous/ottawa/en/

WHO. (2001). The International Classification of Functioning. *Disability and Health. World Health Organization*, *18*, 237. doi:10.1097/01.pep.0000245823.21888.71

WHO. (2004). *World report on knowledge for better health: strengthening health systems. 1. Health systems plans 2. Health services research - utilization 3. Delivery of health care 4. Knowledge 5. Health policy 6. World health.* Geneva: World Health Organization. Retrieved June 14, 2016 from http://www.who.int/rpc/meetings/en/world_report_on_knowledge_for_better_health2.pdf

Wickramasinghe, N., & Geisler, E. (Eds.). (2008). *Encyclopedia of Healthcare Information Systems*. Hershey, PA: Medical Information Science Reference. doi:10.4018/978-1-59904-889-5

Wieland, E. A., McAuley, J. D., Dilley, L. C., & Chang, S. E. (2015). Evidence for a rhythm perception deficit in children who stutter. *Brain and Language*, *144*, 26–34. doi:10.1016/j.bandl.2015.03.008 PMID:25880903

Williams, C., Lee, S., Fisher, R., & Dickerman, L. (1999). A comparison of statistical methods for prenatal screening for Down syndrome. *Applied Stochastic Models in Business and Industry*, *15*(2), 89–101. doi:10.1002/(SICI)1526-4025(199904/06)15:2<89::AID-ASMB366>3.0.CO;2-K

Wilson, J. (2006). 3G to Web 2.0? Can Mobile Telephony Become an Architecture of Participation? *The International Journal of Research into New Media Technologies*, *12*(2), 229–242.

Win, K., Song, H., Croll, P., & Cooper, J. (2002). Implementing patients consent in electronic health record systems. *Proceedings of CollECTeR*.

Wingate, M. (1964). A standard definition of stuttering. *The Journal of Speech and Hearing Disorders*, *29*(4), 484–489. doi:10.1044/jshd.2904.484 PMID:14257050

Win, K. T., & Fulcher, J. A. (2007). Consent mechanisms for electronic health record systems: A simple yet unresolved issue. *Journal of Medical Systems*, *31*(2), 91–96. doi:10.1007/s10916-006-9030-3 PMID:17489500

Win, K. T., Susilo, W., & Mu, Y. (2006). Personal health record systems and their security protection. *Journal of Medical Systems*, *30*(4), 309–315. doi:10.1007/s10916-006-9019-y PMID:16978011

Wirth, T., Parker, N., & Ylä-Herttuala, S. (2013). History of gene therapy. *Gene*, *525*(2), 162–169. doi:10.1016/j.gene.2013.03.137 PMID:23618815

Wofford, J., Smith, E., & Miller, D. (2005). The multimedia computer for office-based patient education: A systematic review. *Patient Education and Counseling*, *59*(2), 148–157. doi:10.1016/j.pec.2004.10.011 PMID:16257619

Wolf, J., Moreau, J., Akilov, O., Patton, T., English, J., Ho, J., & Ferris, L. (2013). Diagnostic inaccuracy of smartphone applications for melanoma detection. *JAMA Dermatology*, *149*, 422–426.

Wong, W., Liu, W., & Bennamoun, M. (2012). Ontology learning from text: A look back and into the future. *ACM Comput. Surv.*, *44*(4), 20:1–20:36. http://doi.org/<ALIGNMENT.qj></ALIGNMENT>10.1145/2333112.2333115

Wong, A. H., Gang, M., Szyld, D., & Mahoney, H. (2016). Making an "Attitude Adjustment": Using a Simulation-enhanced Interprofessional Education Strategy to Improve Teamwork and Communication. *Simulation in Healthcare*, *1*(2), 117–125. doi:10.1097/SIH.0000000000000133 PMID:27043097

Wong, C., Merchanta, R., & Morenoc, M. (2014). Using social media to engage adolescents and young adults with their health. *Health Care*, *31*(3), 56–58. PMID:25984444

Wood, G. (2004). Academic Original Sin: Plagiarism, the Internet, and Librarians. *Journal of Academic Librarianship*, *30*(3), 237–242. doi:10.1016/j.acalib.2004.02.011

Woo, S. H., Kim, T. W., Lee, J. H., Kim, P. U., Won, C. H., & Cho, J. H. (2009). Implemented edge shape of an electrical stimulus capsule. *International Journal of Medical Robotics and Computer Assisted Surgery*, *5*(1), 59–65. doi:10.1002/rcs.235 PMID:19170130

Woo, S. H., Kim, T. W., Mohy-Ud-Din, Z., Park, I. Y., & Cho, J. H. (2011). Small intestinal model for electrically propelled capsule endoscopy. *Biomedical Engineering Online*, *10*(1), 108. doi:10.1186/1475-925X-10-108 PMID:22177218

World Economic Forum. (2011). *Personal Data: The Emergence of a New Asset Class*. Geneva, Switzerland: World Economic Forum.

World Health Organisation (WHO). (2010). *The social determinants of health*. WHO. Retrieved November 2, 2012, from http://www.who.int/social_determinants/en/

Yairi, E. (1997). Disfluency characteristics of childhood stuttering. In R. F. Curlee & G. M. Siegel (Eds.), *Nature and treatment of stuttering: New directions* (2nd ed.; pp. 49–78). Boston: Allyn & Bacon.

Yaruss, J. (1999). Utterance length, syntactic complexity, and childhood stuttering. *Journal of Speech, Language, and Hearing Research: JSLHR*, *42*(2), 329–344. doi:10.1044/jslhr.4202.329 PMID:10229450

Yee, K. C., Miils, E., & Airey, C. (2008). Perfect match? Generation Y as change agents for information communication technology implementation in healthcare. *Studies in Health Technology and Informatics*, *136*, 496–501. PMID:18487780

Yeh, H. C., Hsiu, P. C. C., Shih, S., Tsai, P. H., & Liu, J. W. S. (2006). APAMAT: A Prescription Algebra for Medication Authoring Tool. *Proceedings of IEEE International Conference on Systems, Man and Cybernetics*. doi:10.1109/ICSMC.2006.384807

Yen, C. L. (2013). It is our destiny to die: The effects of mortality salience and culture-priming on fatalism and karma belief. *International Journal of Psychology*, *48*(5), 818–828. doi:10.1080/00207594.2012.678363 PMID:22551301

Yetisen, A. K., Martinez-Hurtado, J., da Cruz Vasconcellos, F., Simsekler, M. C. E., Akram, M. S., & Lowe, C. (2014). The regulation of mobile medical applications. *Lab on a Chip*, *14*(5), 833–840. doi:10.1039/c3lc51235e PMID:24425070

Ylisaukko-oja, A., Vildjiounatie, E., & Mantyjarvi, J. (2004). Five-Point Acceleration Sensing Wireless Body Area Network - Design and Practical Experiences.*Eighth International Symposium on Wearable Computers*. doi:10.1109/ISWC.2004.22

Yoo, H.-J., & Bae, J. (2013). Low energy wireless body area network systems. In *Wireless Symposium (IWS), 2013 IEEE International* (pp. 1–2). http://doi.org/ doi:10.1109/IEEE-IWS.2013.6616846

Yoo, I., Alafaireet, P., Marinov, M., Pena-Hernandez, K., Gopidi, R., Chang, J. F., & Hua, L. (2012). Data Mining in Healthcare and Biomedicine: A Survey of the Literature. *Journal of Medical Systems*, 1–18. PMID:21537851

Young, J., & Simon, W. (2005). iCon: Steve Jobs, the greatest second act in the history of business. *Studies in Health Technology and Informatics*, *23*, 45–50.

Young, M. A. (1975). Onset, prevalence, and recovery from stuttering. *The Journal of Speech and Hearing Disorders*, *40*(1), 49–58. doi:10.1044/jshd.4001.49 PMID:1123928

Young, T. K. (1998). *Population health: concepts and methods*. New York: Oxford University Press.

Yu, B., & Wijesekera, D. (2013). Building Dialysis Workflows into EMRs. *Procedia Technology*, *9*, 985-995.

Yu, B., Wijesekera, D., & Costa, P. (2014). An Ontology for Medical Treatment Consent. *The 9th International Conference on. Semantic Technologies for Intelligence, Defense, and Security - STIDS 2014.*

Yu, B., Wijesekera, D., & Costa, P. (2014). Consent-Based Workflow Control in EMRs. *HCIST- International Conference on Health and Social Care Information Systems and Technologies,* 72-79.

Yu, B., Wijesekera, D., Costa, P., & Hiremagalore, S. (2015). Genetic Counseling Using Workflow-based EMRs. *The 10th International Conference on. Semantic Technologies for Intelligence, Defense, and Security - STIDS2015.*

Yu, A. C. (2006). Methods in biomedical ontology. *Journal of Biomedical Informatics*, *39*(3), 252–266. doi:10.1016/j.jbi.2005.11.006 PMID:16387553

Zabulis, X., Sfakiotakis, M., & Tsakiris, D. P. (2008, August). Effects of vibratory actuation on endoscopic capsule vision. In *Engineering in Medicine and Biology Society, 2008. EMBS 2008. 30th Annual International Conference of the IEEE* (pp. 5901-5904). IEEE. doi:10.1109/IEMBS.2008.4650557

Zeltser, I. S., Bergs, R., Fernandez, R., Baker, L., Eberhart, R., & Cadeddu, J. A. (2007). Single trocar laparoscopic nephrectomy using magnetic anchoring and guidance system in the porcine model. *The Journal of Urology*, *178*(1), 288–291. doi:10.1016/j.juro.2007.03.001 PMID:17499803

Zhang, J., Chen, Y., Ashfaq, S., Bell, K., Calvitti, A., Farber, N. J., & Agha, Z. et al. (2016). Strategizing EHR use to achieve patient-centered care in exam rooms: A qualitative study on primary care providers. *Journal of the American Medical Informatics Association*, *23*(1), 137–143. doi:10.1093/jamia/ocv142 PMID:26568605

Ziegler, R. G., Jones, C. J., Brinton, L. A., Norman, S. A., Mallin, K., Levine, R. S., & Hoover, R. N. et al. (1991). Diet and the risk of in situ cervical cancer among white women in the United States. *Cancer Causes & Control*, *2*(1), 17–29. doi:10.1007/BF00052357 PMID:1873430

Zimeras, S. (2012). An efficient 3D segmentation method for spinal canal applied to CT volume sequence data. *International Journal of Reliable and Quality E-Healthcare*, *1*(1), 33–42.

Zimeras, S., Karangelis, G., & Firle, E. (2002). Object segmentation and shape reconstruction using computer-assisted segmentation tools. *Medical Imaging*.

Zinn, J. S., Shortell, S. M., & Scott, W. R. (2000). Organizational performance: Managing for success. In S. M. Shortell & A. D. Kaluzny (Eds.), *Health care management: Organization design and behavior* (4th ed., pp. 356–389). Albany, NY: Delmar.

Zouaq, A., & Nkambou, R. (2010). A Survey of Domain Ontology Engineering: Methods and Tools. *Advances in Intelligent Tutoring Systems*, 103–119. http://doi.org/<ALIGNMENT.qj></ALIGNMENT>10.1007/978-3-642-14363-2_6

Zygomalas, A., Giokas, K., & Koutsouris, D. (2012). Modular assembly micro-robots for natural orifice transluminal endoscopic surgery, the future of minimal invasive surgery. *International Journal of Reliable and Quality E-Healthcare*, *1*(4), 43–55. doi:10.4018/ijrqeh.2012100104

Zygomalas, A., Giokas, K., & Koutsouris, D. (2014). In Silico Investigation of a Surgical Interface for Remote Control of Modular Miniature Robots in Minimally Invasive Surgery. *Minimally Invasive Surgery*, *2014*, 307641. doi:10.1155/2014/307641 PMID:25295187

Zygomalas, A., Gkiokas, K., & Koutsouris, D. D. (2011). In silico development and simulation of a modular reconfigurable assembly micro-robot for use in natural orifice transluminal endoscopic surgery. *Hellenic Journal of Surgery*, *83*(4), 190–196. doi:10.1007/s13126-011-0037-y

Zygomalas, A., Kehagias, I., Giokas, K., & Koutsouris, D. (2015). Miniature surgical robots in the era of NOTES and LESS: Dream or reality? *Surgical Innovation*, *22*(1), 97–107. doi:10.1177/1553350614532549 PMID:24828382

About the Contributors

Anastasius Moumtzoglou is a Former Executive Board Member of the European Society for Quality in Health Care, President of the Hellenic Society for Quality & Safety in Health Care, holds B.A in Economics, MA in Health Services Management, MA in Macroeconomics, Ph.D. in Economics. He teaches the module of quality at the graduate and postgraduate level. He has also written three Greek books, which are the only ones in the Greek references. The first deals with "Marketing in Health Care", the following with "Quality in Health Care" and the third with "Quality and Patient Safety in Health Care." He has edited the books "E-Health Systems Quality and Reliability: Models and Standards", "E-health Technologies & Improving Patient Safety: Exploring Organizational Factors", "Cloud Computing Applications for Quality Health Care Delivery", "Laboratory Management Information Systems: Current Requirements and Future Perspectives", and " M-Health Innovations for Patient-Centered Care". He is the Editor-in-Chief of the "Advances in Healthcare Information Systems and Administration" book series and the International Journal of Reliable & Quality in Healthcare (IJRQEH). He has also served as the scientific coordinator of research programs in Greece and participated as a researcher in European research programs. In 2004, he was declared "Person of Quality," with respect to Greece.

***

Athanasios Anastasiou received his Bachelor degree in Electrical & Electronic Engineering from the University of Newcastle Upon Tyne, in 2005. In 2006, he received his M.Sc. degree in Digital Signal & Image Processing from the University of Central Lancashire. Likewise, in 2009 he obtained his second M.Sc. degree in Biomedical Engineering held by the University of Patras and the National Technical University of Athens (N.T.U.A.). Since 2011, he is a member of the Biomedical Engineering Laboratory of N.T.U.A., and a Ph.D. candidate in Biomedical Engineering (University of Patras and N.T.U.A.). His current research interests comprise Bioinformatics, Biosignal Processing, Digital Image Processing and technologies for assisted living. He is a Member of the Institute of Electrical and Electronics Engineers (IEEE) - EMBS Society and Computer Society, Member of the Institution of Engineering and Technology (IET) and a member of the Technical Chamber of Greece (TEE).

Greg Arling is Katherine Birck Professor of Nursing at Purdue University. He received his Ph.D. in Sociology from the University of Illinois and completed post-doctoral study in Health Systems Engineering at the University of Wisconsin. His research interests are in health care quality assessment, evaluation, and policy analysis. Much of his research has been with elderly populations in long-term care settings. He has helped develop comprehensive measures of care quality, assessed the accuracy and effectiveness of these measures, and applied them to quality improvement, public reporting and pay-for-performance. He also has studied transitions between care settings, such as hospital, nursing home, and community care. He has been a principal or co-investigator on projects supported by the Agency for Healthcare Research and Quality, Veterans Health Administration, National Institute on Aging, Centers for Medicare and Medicaid Services, and state Medicaid programs.

Priscilla Arling is an Associate Professor of Information Systems at Butler University in Indianapolis, Indiana. She earned her Ph.D. in Information and Decision Sciences from the Carlson School of Management at the University of Minnesota. Dr. Arling also earned an M.B.A. from the University of Missouri-Kansas City. Research interests include communication and quality in health care settings, social network analysis, knowledge work, electronic communication, and technology use in distributed work.

Ricardo Bohorquez is Full Professor of Cardiology at the Department of Internal Medicine, School of Medicine from Pontificia Universdiad Javeriana at Bogota Colombia. Dr. Bohorquez attended Javeriana University, Bogota, Colombia, where he received an M.D. degree in 1984. His subsequent career includes residency in Internal Medicine at San Ignacio´s Hospital, 1989 Clinical Cardiology fellowship at Nueva Granada University at Bogota Colombia, 1990. Fellow observer at University of Alabama in Birmingham, 1994. His research has focused on cardiovascular risk factor, myocardial infarction, clinical cardiology, cardiac images and on development and implementation of Clinical Practice Guidelines in the Colombian Health System.

Konstantinos Bougoulias was born on July 8th, 1982 in Karditsa, Greece where he grew up, went to school and lived until 2000. He then moved to Athens to study at the National Technical University of Athens, being accepted at the local School of Electronic Engineering. During his years with the NTUA he got interested in software engineering, specifically in the field of electronic applications for computerization of medical data, thus his thesis was concentrated on the subject of designing and developing electronic health and medical records. Besides his work with the NTUA on the subject he began researching the electronic record keeping needs of various Medicine specialties and has been dealing with medical software development.

Aleš Bourek, MD, PhD. (born 28.06.1957) Works as CEO of the University Center for Healthcare Quality. He explores computer linguistics for medical information management. For 28 years he mentors students of the Masaryk University and abroad in information and communication use (skills, attitudes, benefits, limitations, risks and technologies) for professional needs. He is an active gynecologist and the head of L'ART Center for Assisted Reproduction (www.ivf.cz). He worked for DG SANCO, Council of Europe, WHO, World Bank and EFQM and collaborates with people and institutions interested in quality and accountability improvement in healthcare and healthcare education. He is a member of editorial boards of several journals, Vice-President of the European Society for Quality in Healthcare (www.esqh.net), executive board member of CEESTAHC (www.ceestahc.org) and European Health Futures Forum (www.ehff.org). He enjoys philosophy, skiing, hiking, spending time with family and friends and hosting people when they come to Czech Republic.

Alvaro Bustamante MD is studying at the Pontificia Universidad Javeriana Internal Medicine, currently in third year of residency. Dr. Bustamante graduated from medicine at the University of Rosario in 2010. His research interests include infectious diseases, cardiovascular diseases and is part of research groups in these areas and the development and implementation of clinical practice guidelines.

Paulo C. G. Costa, Ph.D, is a GMU Associate Professor of Systems Engineering and Operations Research. His research interests comprise the areas of probabilistic ontologies, decision support systems, cyber security, and multi-sensor data fusion. He is the inventor of PR-OWL, a probabilistic extension to OWL, a key contributor to UnBBayes-MEBN, an open source implementation of MEBN/PR-OWL, and has worked as a W3C invited expert in the area of uncertainty reasoning. Prof. Costa's academic service includes participation in technical program in several academic conferences and journals, as well as members of review boards in NSF, National Academies of Engineering, and others. He also has been actively involved as PI, co-PI, or technical lead in research projects related to his areas of expertise. He is an IEEE senior member and an elected member of the Board of Directors of the International Society for Information Fusion.

Rita Alexandra Santos da Costa has a Master degree in Biomedical Technology from Polytechnic Institute of Bragança, Portugal. Has a bachelor degree in Mechanical Engineering from Polytechnic Institute of Bragança, Portugal. Professional in the department of logistics from Portuguese Institute of Oncology in Porto (Portugal) where has acquiring knowledge of the entire logistics process, using logistics tool "Kanban System", in order to perform tasks such as managing services availability inside the organization, to optimize use of the resources, and managing stocks (Mainly medicines and medical equipment). Author of several scientific papers in international journals and conferences indexed by ISI. In the year of 2013, was honoured with the award of Best Student of the year (Master - Biomedical Technology).

Vassileia Costarides has graduated from National Technical University of Athens, from the school of Mining and Metallurgical Engineering with a specialization in Materials Engineering. She proceeded her studies in Biomedical Engineering and has worked in the medical device industry for 6 years as a technical specialist in the field of Neurology and Neuromodulation. Since 2013 she has been participating in projects regarding public health, medical device nomenclature, health technology assessment and medical device technical specifications. Among her interests is also quality in health care and she is an ISO9001:2008 and ISO13485:2003 auditor. She is currently a PhD candidate in Biomedical Engineering in the National Technical University of Athens and a member of the Biomedical Engineering Lab and Applied Informatics in the AiM research team focusing on User Interfaces and User Experience. She is also a member of the Technical Chamber of Greece.

Julian Camilo Daza MSc. works as an Assistant Researcher at San Ignacio's Hospital at Bogotá Colombia. Julian is a Systems Engineer from Pontificia Universidad Javeriana graduated in 2013 and has a Magister in Systems Engineer and Computer Science from Pontificia Universidad Javeriana in 2016. Julian has worked in multidisciplinary projects like digital media industries, web or mobile applications and medical research. His research interests cover medical image processing techniques related to alzheimer disease detection, 3D reconstruction of cardiovascular structures and Clinical Practice Guidelines analysis from structured and unstructured texts.

Paula Estrella is currently Adjunct Professor and member of the Natural Language Processing (NLP) research group at the Faculty of Mathematics, Astronomy, Physics and Computer Science (FaMAF) at the National University of Córdoba (UNC), Argentina. She holds a Msc. in Computer Science by FaMAF-UNC and a PhD. in Multilingual Information Processing by the Faculty of Translation and Interpreting at the University of Geneva, Switzerland. As part of her doctoral thesis she started working on the evaluation of NLP systems, focusing on the application of ISO standards and on user-centered evaluation of machine translation systems.

Olga Milena Garcia Morales MD is physician and epidemiologist from the University of Rosario, she is also specialist in internal medicine and fellowship of pulmonology from the Pontificia Universidad Javeriana. Her clinical work focuses on the management of patients in hospital areas with chronic diseases. Her research interests include venous thromboembolic disease, chronic obstructive pulmonary disease and electronic health record data analysis. Her research results have been published in scientific journals and books. She is currently working for the Department of Internal Medicine at the San Ignacio hospital and she is professor ad-honorem at the Pontificia Universidad Javeriana.

Angel Alberto García Peña MD, MSc. attended Javeriana University at Bogota, Colombia, where he received a M.D. degree in 2003. His subsequent career included a certification in quality health services at Rosario University in Colombia, residency in internal medicine and fellowship in cardiology at San Ignacio's Hospital Colombia and Heart Failure and Cardiac Transplant at Clinic Hospital in Barcelona, Spain. He has a master's degree in Clinical Epidemiology at Javeriana University and a master's degree in Transesophageal Echocardiography at Menendez Pelayo University. He is an assistant professor and clinical physician at San Ignacio´s Hospital and Pontificia Universidad Javeriana. His research has focused on epidemiology, cardiac images, cardiovascular risk factors, diabetes, and on development and implementation of Clinical Practice Guidelines in the Colombian Health System.

Rafael A. Gonzalez is a Systems Engineer from Javeriana University (Bogotá) with an MSc in Computer Science and a PhD in Systems Engineering (cum laude, Aart Bosman Award) from Delft University of Technology (The Netherlands). He has been lecturer in the areas of knowledge management, systems thinking and software engineering, as well as acting as IT consultant for the public and private sectors. His research interests are focused on development of information systems with a design science approach, centered on the issues of coordination, complexity and the interplay between ICT and society in domains such as healthcare and crisis management. He is currently Associate Professor at the Systems Engineering Department at Pontificia Universidad Javeriana.

Maria Goreti Fernandes has a Master degree in Biomedical Technology from Polytechnic Institute of Bragança, Portugal. She is Ph.D. Student of Mechanical Engineering from Faculty of Engineering of University of Porto, Portugal. Researcher of INEGI, Associated Laboratory for Energy, Transports and Aeronautics. Her research interests include product development, experimental mechanics, biomechanics, computational methods and rehabilitation. She is author of several scientific papers in national and international journals and conferences indexed by ISI and Scopus and book chapters. In the year of 2013, she was honoured with the award of Eng.ª Cruz Azevedo to distinguish annually the best scientific and technical paper.

Kostas Giokas, Esq has been an IT consultant since 1994, working in multiple firms and projects in London UK. He received a BSc in Information Systems from the University of Westminster a BSc in Electrical and Computer Engineering, an MSc in Electrical and Computer Engineering from NTUA and an MBA from the UK Open University. He joined the Biomedical Engineering Laboratory of the National Technical University of Athens as a Systems' Architect while consulting on National and European deployment projects. He is currently a Senior Research Scientist having lead more than 50 proposals and running several EU funded research projects. His research interests include most fields in the Health ICT domain, in particular mHealth. Since 2014 he is the Applied Informatics in mHealth (AiM) research team leader. He has published 50 papers and 15 chapters and has been invited as a speaker in major conferences and Healthcare Technology events.

Dimitra Iliopoulou graduated from the School of Electrical and Electronic Engineering at NTUA and is a post doctorate associate of the Biomedical Engineering Laboratory. Her research involves disease modelling (mainly diabetes mellitus and cervical cancer) and bioinformatics focusing on self-adaptive treatment planning, large data manipulation and systems interoperability. She is a member of the IEEE and the Greek Society of Biomedical Technology. She has published 10 scientific papers. She has worked in IT and Telecoms in several companies (Multimedia A.E. – DOL, Bull ATS, Datamed, Omnis M.). She has been active in several research projects in regards to the application of IT in health.

Vahé Kazandjian is the previous Principal for ARALEZ HEALTH LLC, a Baltimore, Maryland-based global consulting company for healthcare performance improvement and accountability. He was the architect of the first multi-national hospital quality assessment project, the Maryland Quality Indicator Project (QIP) which he directed from 1990-2000. Twenty countries and more than 1800 hospitals participated in the QIP. He also served as the Senior Vice President of the Maryland Hospital Association from 1987 till 2010. Dr. Kazandjian is Professor, The Johns Hopkins University, Bloomberg School of Public Health; Associate Professor (Adjunct), The University of Maryland, School of Medicine; and Professor (Adjunct) The Uniformed Health Services University, School of Medicine, Maryland. Since 2002, he serves as Advisor to the World Health Organization (WHO) to assist in hospital and healthcare systems performance assessment project in European countries. Dr. Kazandjian is the author of four healthcare books on quality of care improvement, five books of travel stories and poetry, and author/co-author of more than 80 peer-reviewed articles and book chapters. His poetry and photography have been featured in anthologies and his photographic work is now in gallery exhibit in Prescott, Arizona.

Ioannis Kouris, received his Degree in Electrical & Computer Engineering in 2005 (Greece), his Master Degree in Biomedical Engineering in 2008 (Greece) and his Doctorate in 2012 (Greece). Since 2008 he is member of NTUA's Biomedical Engineering Laboratory and he also has experience in developing medical software in participation with international companies. His research is focusing on chronic disease management solutions (Diabetes, COPD, Parkinson's Disease, Alzheimer's Disease), Decision Support Systems, activity recognition, telemedical technologies, mHealth, software engineering and IoT. He also has experience in integrating wireless technologies in health applications, such as Electronic Health Record Management tools and physical activity recognition using wireless sensors and mobile devices. He is active in European Research projects in regards to the integration of new technologies in health as researcher and technical manager. He has published 10 papers in scientific journals and 7 conference papers.

Dimitris Koutsouris was born in Serres, Greece in 1955. He received Diploma in Electrical Engineering in 1978 (Greece), DEA in Biomechanics in 1979 (France), Doctorat in Genie Biologie Medicale (France), Doctorat d' Etat in Biomedical Engineering 1984 (France). Since 1986 he was research associate on the USC (Los Angeles), Renè Dèscartes (Paris) and Assoc. Professor at the Dept. of Electrical & Computers Engineering of NTU of Athens. He is currently Professor & head of the Biomedical Engineering Laboratory. He has published over 100 research articles & book chapters & more than 150 conference communications. He has been the former elected president of the Hellenic Society of Biomedical Technology, principal investigator in many European & National Research programs, especially in the field of Telematics in Healthcare.

Georgia Koutsouri has obtained her Engineering Diploma from the Electrical and Computer Engineering (ECE) department of the University of Patras, Greece, in 2010. She has a PhD from the Biomedical Engineering Laboratory at the National Technical University of Athens, Greece. Her research interests include the areas of machine learning, data mining, neural networks and image processing techniques. From 2011 to 2012 she has worked at Datamed Systems Integrator and Consulting Services S.A. as ERP, HIS and LIS consultant in the Business Development Department. She also has some publications, is member of IEEE, ELEVIT and Technical Chamber of Greece and has participated on the organization of conferences.

Manuel José Lopes Completed PhD in Nursing Science from the University of Porto in 2005. He is Professor Coordinator at the University of Évora. He has published 44 articles in specialized journals and 3 papers in conference proceedings, has 8 book chapters and 8 books published. Has 1 software and other 76 items of technical production. 11 mentored doctoral theses and co-mentored one, mentored 15 master's theses and co-mentored 1 in the areas of Health Sciences, Other Medical Sciences and Sociology. Between 2006 and 2012 participated in four research projects, and coordinated three of these. Currently coordinating 1 research project. Active in the areas of Medical Sciences with emphasis in Health Sciences and Medical Sciences. In their professional activities interacted with 124 employees in co-authorship of scientific papers. In his curriculum DeGóis the most frequent terms in the context of scientific, technological and artistic-cultural production are: Nursing, Health, Epistemology of Nursing Science, Caring for cancer patients, Help Relationship, Aging, Health policy, elderly, Violence on elderly and social representations.

Edward Miech, EdD is a health services researcher with special expertise in implementation science. He has a doctorate in education from Harvard University and has in-depth experience as an investigator in program evaluation, assessment, qualitative research and mixed methods. A research topic of particular interest to Dr. Miech is examining the impact of local context on how implementation processes unfold across different settings. Dr. Miech is a Research Scientist in the Health Services Research division of the Regenstrief Institute and holds appointments as an Assistant Professor in the Department of Emergency Medicine and the Department of Internal Medicine at the Indiana University School of Medicine.

Oscar Muñoz is an Assistant Professor at the Department of Internal Medicine, School of Medicine, Javeriana University at Bogotá Colombia. Currently is Chief of General Internal Medicine Unit at San Ignacio's Hospital at Bogotá Colombia. Dr. Muñoz attended National University of Colombia, where he received an M.D. degree in 1998. His subsequent career included residency in internal medicine at San

Ignacio´s Hospital, a Master degree in Clinical Epidemiology at Javeriana University and currently is PhD candidate in Clinical Epidemiology. His research has focused on cardiovascular risk factor, diabetes, and on development and implementation of Clinical Practice Guidelines in the Colombian Health System.

David José Murteira Mendes, born in Évora (Portugal) in the 4th of July of 1966, achieved his PhD in Computer Science in Universidade de Évora (Portugal) in December 2014. Previously he owns a MSc in Applied Artificial Intelligence also from the same University, a MBA from Universidad de Extremadura (Badajoz, Spain) a BSc in Computer Science from Universidade Nova de Lisboa (Portugal). He has developed a Software Engineer career from 1989 and developed mainly software for government organizations in particular for Hospitals intended both for management and clinical support. He has special interest in scuba diving being an active PADI instructor and underwater photographer. His main research interests are related to Healthcare providing knowledge modelling and reasoning. He is currently R+D Manager for Healthcare Computing at DECSIS.

Irene Pimenta Rodrigues is since November 2002 Associate Professor in the Department of Computer Science of the School of Science and Technology of the University of Évora, where she entered in 1995. She currently teaches courses from the BSc in Informatics engineering, Database and Artificial Intelligence, from the Master in Informatics engineering, Applied Artificial Intelligence and Systems for Natural Language Processing, and in the Phd degree she teaches Knowledge Representation and Reasoning in Natural Language processing. She got a B.Sc. in Informatics Engineering in 1987 and a PhD. in Computer Science in 1995 by the New University of Lisbon. Her main research interests are within the area of Artificial Intelligence, more specifically on Natural Language Processing, Knowledge Representation, Information Retrieval and Biomedical Ontologies. Currently she works on natural language question answer systems, on the development of natural language tools such as named entity recognition, sentiment analysis and on the Automatic Medical Ontology Enrichment.

Alexandra Pomares-Quimbaya Ph.D. is Associate Professor at the Pontificia Universidad Javeriana. Throughout her research work, she has been involved in the area of business intelligence and data integration. Currently, she is working in a Colombian initiative that aims to improve the quality of the medical information available to promote value based medicine. Alexandra also teaches courses on information systems and data mining and directs ISTAR, a research group in information systems.

Abraham Pouliakis is physicist, holds an M.Sc. in electronics and radio-communications, and a Ph.D. degree from the Medical School (University of Athens) related to the application of neural networks in cytopathology. Since 1993 has participated in numerous National, European and European Space Agency Research projects related to information and communication technology, artificial intelligence applied in medicine, collaborative systems, e-learning, e-health and GIS. Currently is senior researcher in the Department of Cytopathology, University of Athens, School of Medicine, as well as responsible for quality control and assurance. He has more than 60 publications in international peer reviewed scientific magazines, more than 120 presentations in international and Greek conferences and is co-author of seven books chapters. His research interests are related to information and communication technology, image/signal processing and artificial intelligence including their applications in the fields of industry and health.

Marios Prasinos holds a BSc degree in computer science (University of Crete, Greece, 2010) and an MSc degree in engineering—economic systems (National Technical University of Athens, University of Piraeus, Greece, 2013). During his postgraduate studies, Prasinos collaborated with the Biomedical Engineering Laboratory of the Electrical and Computer Engineering School of National Technical University of Athens, Athens, Greece. For his master thesis, he designed and implemented an interactive software system for improving health compliance that includes web and mobile interfaces. From 2014, Prasinos is pursuing a PhD in computer science from City University London, London, U.K. He is a member of the Center for Adaptive Systems and has received a bursary associated with the European Union project EMBalance. The aim of this research is to apply machine learning techniques and build an advanced model which will contribute to the prevention, diagnosis, and therapy of balance health problems. Prasinos's research interests include health databases, health informatics, data mining, machine learning, and decision-support systems. Beyond research, Prasinos has worked in the software industry as a consultant and software engineer for more than two years.

Pedro Miguel Rodrigues was born in Coimbra, Portugal, in 1988. He received his graduation and Master graduation in biomedical engineering, in 2009 and 2011, respectively, both from the Polytechnic Institute of Bragança, Portugal. Currently, He is currently working toward the Ph.D. degree with the Faculty of Engineering of the University of Porto (FEUP) at the Department of Electrical and Computer Engineering - FEUP. He is author of a several research articles and his research interest areas are related with signal processing and pattern recognition. Recently his research has been mainly focused in processing and discrimination of biomedical signals, especially electroencephalogram signals obtained from patients with neurological diseases.

Artur Romão is director of Innovation and Development at DECSIS, where he supervises the R&D activities and strategy of the company, with special focus on data analytics, IoT, and cognitive computing applied to social economy. Before joining DECSIS, Artur was COO at Cortex Europe (data analytics), CTO at Saphety (electronic transactions and B2B ecommerce), manager at the Trusted Services division of Novis (telco operator), and a teacher and researcher at University of Évora. Artur holds an MSc. in Computer Science from the New University of Lisbon.

Alejandro Sierra MSc. is a systems engineer and computer scientist specialized in Data Management, Business Intelligence and Natural Language Processing. He obtained the Systems Engineering degree from the Pontificia Universidad Javeriana in Bogotá, Colombia and a M.Sc. degree in Computer Science from Saarland University in Saarbrücken, Germany where he focused on Information Retrieval writing his master thesis with the Max Plank Institute for Informatics. Besides his academic background he has gained experience from working with the government, consulting companies, software companies and lately working on research with Hospital Universitario San Ignacio. His research is focused on combining NLP techniques, data integration techniques and machine learning in the process of identifying entities inside the notes contained in Electronic Health Records.

João Paulo Teixeira completed his graduation in Electrical and Computers Engineering in the Faculty of Engineering of the University of Porto (FEUP) in 1993. He completed his Master graduation also in FEUP in the area of speech modulation for TTS Systems, in 1996. He finished his PhD in the same Institution in 2004 where a prosody model for TTS systems in Portuguese language was developed. He is Professor since 1995 in the Polytechnic Institute of Bragança teaching in the areas of digital electronics, signal processing and rehabilitation engineering. . He is author of 2 books, eleven chapter books, 25 review articles and 50 conference papers, all with revision by his peers. His research interest areas are related with signal processing and signal modulation. Recently he had worked with Artificial Neural Networks, Speech signal processing, EEG signals for discrimination of Alzheimer disease, ECG signal events detection and prediction of time series.

Nikos Tsourakis is a Research Associate at the Department of Translation Technology, University of Geneva, Switzerland. His research interests concentrate on multimodal interaction, voice user interfaces, multilingual dialogue systems, distributed systems and evaluation. He has more than 40 peer reviewed publications in relevant areas. He has also served as an expert reviewer for the European Commission in the context of FP7. Before joining TIM/FTI he worked as a software engineer developing telephone-based speech recognition applications. He has extensive experience in designing, building and evaluating systems targeted to end-users, and also solving problems from the back-end until the front-end of an application. He holds a BSc and an MSc in Computer Engineering, and an MSc in Engineering Management from TU Crete. He also holds a PhD from the University of Geneva.

Wayne Usher has had 28 years of practical experience in education, spanning across primary, secondary and higher educational settings. He brings a breadth and depth of knowledge associated with traditional and contemporary practices which influences the teacher experience. Dr Usher's research interests include school and community health, physical education, modern classroom practices and curriculum development / implementation. His past and current research examines 21st century pedagogical approaches that engage the teacher and the student in the co-construction of meaning, value, and knowledge associated with primary, secondary and higher educational settings. His research gives specific attention to communication technologies and how they are creating a paradigm shift surrounding traditional barriers of power and information dissemination. Other areas of research include the internet, WWW and social media applications. Current research includes combining spatial technologies, quantitative and qualitative theories to better examine distribution patterns associated with health and technology usage.

Duminda Wijesekera is a professor in the Department of Computer Science at George Mason University, Fairfax, Virginia and a visiting research scientist at the National Institute of Standards and Technology (NIST). His current research addresses (1) Security and safety of cyber physical systems, which includes safety and security of trains, aircraft, ships and automobiles, creating secure cognitive radio networks that ensure mandated safety guarantees. (2) Electronic support for medical procedures, which includes formulating, validating and verification of safety of medical workflows, privacy and security medical data. (3) Digital forensics, which includes creating potential scenarios from evidence and creating frameworks for argumentations, error management of forensic data and add odds ratio between different scenarios that fit evidence. Dr. Wijesekera received a PhD in Computer Science from the University of Minnesota in 1997 and a PhD in Mathematical Logic from Cornell University in 1990.

Bo Yu is a Research Faculty in the Department of Computer Science at George Mason University (GMU), Fairfax, Virginia and a visiting researcher at the National Institute of Standards and Technology (NIST). Her current researches focus on privacy and security of healthcare domain and its applications, which include three main areas. The first is formulating and enforcing medical procedures into existing Electronic Health Record (EHR) systems to improve the medical safety. The second is requiring electronic consents, which comply with various law governed by federal, state and organization to ensure privacy and security protection of medical data. The third area is developing web and mobile medical applications, which adopt two technologies using in the first two areas to further advance EHR systems. She received a PhD in Information Technology and a Master in Information Security and Assurance from George Mason University, VA in 2007.

Stelios Zimeras holds a BSc. (Hons) on Statistics and Insurance Sciences from University of Piraeus (5fth in the rank) and Ph.D. on Statistics from the University of Leeds, U.K. He had received a full scholarship (fees and maintenance) during his research studies (1993-1997) from the University of Leeds. Since 2012, he is a full time staff member (Assistant Prof) on statistics and probabilities at the Department of Mathematics, Division of Statistics and Financial-Actuarial Mathematics, University of the Aegean, Samos, Greece. He had worked as post-doc at University of Leeds, Department of Electrical Engineering (funded by EPSRC), at IRISA/INRIA-VISTA PROJECT institute, France (funded by EUMETSAT-ESA) and at MedCom GmbH, Germany (funded by Marie-Curie grants). Finally 2011-2012 he had worked during his sabbatical in University of Piraeus, Department of Digital Systems, in computer virus modelling. In 2011 he has nominated the Best Paper for the 5th International Conference on Energy and Development - Environment - Biomedicine 2011 (EDEB '11) with title "Spatial Uncertainty", pp. 203-208, by S. Zimeras, Y. Matsinos. He has involved in national and international projects (FP7, ESPA, Marie-Curie). His published material and presentations are on a number of topics of Data Processing, Statistical Simulations, Image analysis, Medical Image analysis, Spatial Statistics, Telemedicine, and Statistical Modelling with applications in biology, ecology, and medicine, statistical epidemiology, and Bayesian statistics. He has been a member of a number of professional and scientific societies and associations; while he is a reviewer for a number of conferences. Finally his is review for International Journal of Reliable and Quality E-Healthcare (IJRQEH) and for International Journal of Systems Biology and Biomedical Technologies (IJSBBT). In 2016 his is the co-author of the book with title: mHealth Ecosystems and Social Networks in Healthcare, Lazakidou, A.A., Zimeras, S., Iliopoulou, D., Koutsouris, D.-D. (Eds.), Springer Verlag, 240 pages, ISBN 978-3-319-23341-3.

Apollon N. Zygomalas was born in 1978 in Greece. He received his Medical Degree (MD) with Honors from the school of Medicine & Surgery at the "Università Politecnica delle Marche", Ancona, Italy. He qualified in General Surgery at the University Hospital of Patras, Greece. He was fully trained in Hepatobiliary and Pancreatic surgery, Bariatric surgery, Colorectal, Upper GI, Endocrine, Breast, General surgery and Trauma. He received his MSc in Medical Informatics-Life Science Informatics from the University of Patras with Honors. He studied the use of miniature robots in Natural Orifice Transluminal Endoscopic Surgery (NOTES). The Hellenic Surgical Society awarded his MSc scientific work with the First Prize on the application of new technology to the practice of surgery. He is currently a PhD candidate at the University of Patras in Medical Informatics. His study on computer assisted liver tumor surgery was awarded with the First Prize during the 2014 congress of the Hellenic Surgical Society. He has been awarded a graduate studies scholarship from the "ERSU di Ancona" and a grant for PhD studies from the "Onassis Foundation". The research work includes scientific presentations at conferences and publications of articles in English and Greek scientific journals, as well as active participation in specialized postgraduate courses. His research interests include computer assisted surgery, laparoscopic and robotic surgery. He regularly takes part in conferences, seminars and postgraduate courses. He is currently working as a fully private General surgeon in collaboration with the "OLYMPION" General Clinic of Patras and with the Metropolitan Hospital and Doctor's Hospital in Athens.

Index

Q

R

S

T

U

V

W

Z

www.ingramcontent.com/pod-product-compliance
Lightning Source LLC
LaVergne TN
LVHW060411300926
849162LV00006B/1400